Ibero-American Bioethics

Philosophy and Medicine

VOLUME 106

For other titles published in this series, go to
www.springer.com/series/6414

Leo Pessini · Christian de Paul de Barchifontaine
Fernando Lolas Stepke
Editors

Ibero-American Bioethics

History and Perspectives

Translated by
Jennifer Bulcock
Adail Sobral
Maria Stela Gonçalves

Springer

Editors
Leo Pessini
Centro Universitário São Camilo
São Paulo
Brazil

Christian de Paul de Barchifontaine
Centro Universitário São Camilo
São Paulo
Brazil

Fernando Lolas Stepke
Pan American Health Organization
Santigo
Chile
lolasf@chi.ops-oms.org

Translated by
Jennifer Bulcock
Rice University
Houston
USA

Adail Sobral
Universidade Católica de Pelotas
Rio Grande do Sul
Brazil

Maria Stela Gonçalves
Translator – Adail Transervices Ltd.
São Paulo
Brazil

ISBN 978-1-4020-9349-4 e-ISBN 978-1-4020-9350-0
DOI 10.1007/978-1-4020-9350-0
Springer Dordrecht Heidelberg London New York

Library of Congress Control Number: 2009933100

Printed on acid-free paper

Springer is part of Springer Science+Business Media (www.springer.com)

Foreword

This book is the first in a series of planned volumes focused on preserving the character of the development of bioethics in particular cultural contexts. As the first of these volumes, Leo Pessini, Christian de Paul de Barchifontaine, and Fernando Lolas Stepke's work has succeeded well. It has brought together accounts by scholars who were crucial to the emergence of bioethics in the Ibero-American cultural domain. This trail-blazing work in the history of bioethics will be of enduring significance. I am deeply in their debt for having shouldered this far from easy task.

Bioethics is the product of very particular socio-historical developments. Most prominent among them have been (1) the secularization of the dominant culture of North America, Western Europe, and now Central and South America as well, (2) a deflation of the status and authority of physicians as moral authorities able to guide their own profession, and (3) the salience of a post-traditional animus that gives central place to persons as isolated atomic sources of moral authority. Bioethics initially took shape in North America as a post-Christian, post-professional, post-traditional social movement. This bioethics sought to establish a moral discourse for the public forum, a moral practice able to give practical guidance in hospitals and other institutions, and a body of undergirding and justifying theoretical reflections. The emergence of bioethics in the 1970s recapitulated the Enlightenment aspiration to articulate a universal, rational, moral vision that could supersede Western Christian moral understandings. The latter had already taken on the aspiration of supporting a universal, rationally justifiable moral vision, given its moral–theological commitments to natural law. At the very time traditional Christian belief, medical ethics, and traditional moral authorities were displaced from the public forum, medical advances and the increased costs and power of medicine called out for moral guidance. Bioethics was crafted to fill the cultural–moral vacuum.

This original bioethics of the early 1970s, made in America, was with missionary zeal exported globally. There was a naïve and doctrinaire assumption that all humans share a common morality (the conflicts of the culture wars to the contrary notwithstanding), and that all, if only properly enlightened, would embrace the bioethics that took shape at Georgetown University and the Hastings Center. A global consensus, supporting a global bioethics, was seen as inevitable. This has not turned out to be the case. In the ruins of the Enlightenment, Hegel recognized that the dominant morality of every society is socio-historically conditioned, despite Kantian aspirations to a universal rational morality. Also, it is far from clear that Hegel's claims, that a dialectic in world history will move all to embrace a common understanding of all being free, will in fact prevail. In any event, bioethics has turned out not to be one, but many, with disparate histories and different foundational understandings. In part, this has been due to the force of local culture. In part, this has been due to the contributions and influences of particular persons and particular local events. As a result, in order to appreciate the variegated character of the development of bioethics worldwide, one must with care look at how it took shape locally. It is a story shaped by different personalities set within different cultures.

This volume in presenting the development of bioethics in the Ibero-American cultural domain offers a rich perspective on the constitution of a particular bioethical discourse. It gives voice to those who gave it shape. The essays allow the reader access in English to the various perspectives on this history, indeed, to the various first-person histories of this history. The essays have an importance in terms of the arguments and accounts of the authors. The essays in addition possess the status of indispensable primary sources for any future account of this history. No history, including this history, is a final history. No account is ever from nowhere. These essays give the reader an entrée into the various somewheres of the particular contributors to the complex phenomena of Ibero-American bioethics. Even if this phenomenon may have no Aristotelian essential core, it is bound together by a complex of heuristic family resemblances, as well as points of divergence. In all of this, Leo Pessini and his co-editors are to be praised. They have done, if not the impossible, then at least the improbable. They have articulated a powerful mosaic of reflections concerning the regional development of bioethics. This work is thrice over important in its own right. It has preserved the voice of those who gave shape to the local emergence of bioethics. It has preserved a sense of the importance of local culture, events, and persons. It offers competing, critical perspectives on the history of Ibero-American bioethics. It should inspire others to do likewise for their own cultures. This volume will surely guide all future attempts to give an account of the local emergence of bioethics.

The task of providing accounts of the local emergence of bioethics is important not only because the voices of the founders will soon be silent. Dead men write no autobiographies. One all too quickly loses the first-person perspective on the local concerns that fashion bioethics within a particular culture. Such regional explorations of the development of bioethics are likely crucial now, in that there are indications that the complex phenomenon of bioethics may be entering a period of critical self-regard. It is not just that the original bioethics once made in America is no longer uncritically accepted. It is not just that different cultures seek different guiding middle-level principles. In addition, the aspirations to a global bioethics are increasingly being brought into question as the demands of moral pluralism are taken more seriously. The character of bioethics is likely to change. The histories that will be written in the future will likely have a quite different bioethics to address. This volume offers a rich contribution to the appreciation of the first phase in the development of bioethics.

Manaus, Brazil H. Tristram Engelhardt, Jr.
19 September 2008

Contents

Notes on Contributors

Authors

Francesc Abel, S.J., M.D., Ph.D., is the founder of the first European Institute of Bioethics, the *Instituto Borja de Bioética* (1975), and he is its current President. The Center is located in Sant Cugat Del Vallès (Barcelona, Spain) and since 2000 has been part of Ramon Llull University (Barcelona).

Márcio Fabri dos Anjos, Ph.D., is a researcher and professor of bioethics at Saint Camillus University Center (Centro Universitário São Camilo). He is a charter member of the Brazilian Society of Bioethics and former president of the Brazilian Society of Theology and Sciences of Religion. He has edited and authored many books, including: *Teología y nuevos paradigms* (*Theology and New Paradigms*, 1999), *Novas gerações e vida religiosa* (*New Generations and Religious Life*, 2004); and the chapter "Power and Vulnerability: A contribution of developing countries to the ethical debate on genetics," in *Genetics, Theology, Ethics: An Interdisciplinary Conversation*, ed. L. S. Cahill, 2005.

Alberto Arellano-Méndez, J.D., is a researcher at the Health and Law Studies Group at the Legal Research Institute (IIJ-UNAM). He was a lecturer at UNAM Law School.

Marta Ascurra, Ph.D., is a biochemist specializing in genetics. She is a researcher and professor at the Institute of Research in Health Sciences of Asunción (Paraguay), and a Member of the National Commission for the Development of Bioethics – Paraguay. She is a consultant for the Latin-American and Caribbean Bioethics Network – UNESCO.

Christian de Paul de Barchifontaine, M.A., is a research and professor of bioethics at Saint Camillus University Center (Centro Universitário São Camilo), is the author of several books, including *Bioética e início da vida: alguns desafios* [(*Bioethics and Beginning of Life: Some Challenges* – Idéias e Letras, São Paulo, 2004)]: he co-authored the first didactic work on bioethics in Brazil, *Problemas atuais de bioética* (*Current Problems of Bioethics* – Ed. Loyola, 8th ed., 2007), and he is co-editor of *Bioética, alguns desafios* (*Bioethics: Some Challenges*. Loyola, São Paulo, 3rd ed., 2004). He is President of the Saint Camillus University Center (Centro Universitário São Camilo, São Paulo).

Jorge Biscaia, M.D., is Director of the Center for Bioethical Studies of Coimbra (Portugal). He is the author and editor of several bioethical works, including: Archer, L.; Biscaia, J.; Osswald, W.; Renaud, M. (eds.) – *Novos desafios à bioética* (*New Challenges to Bioethics* – Porto Editora, Porto, 2001); (Ed.) *Bem da pessoa, bem comum* (*People's Good – Common Good* – Gráfica de Coimbra, Coimbra, 1998); *Perder para encontrar* (*Lose to Find Out* – Gráfica de Coimbra, Coimbra, 2004); *Ao encontro da ternura* (*Towards Tenderness* – Gráfica de Coimbra, Coimbra, 2005).

Jennifer A. Bulcock is a graduate student in the Department of Philosophy, Rice University, Houston, TX. She is also co-managing editor of the *Journal of Medicine and Philosophy* and *Christian Bioethics*.

Daniel Bustos-Montero, Ph.D., is a professor of bioethics. He is a member of the Centro de Desarrolo Estratégico y Información en Seguridad Social y Salud. Caja Costarricense de Seguro Social in Costa Rica.

Debora Diniz, Ph.D., works at the University of Brasília and is Director of the NGO Anis: Institute of Bioethics, Human Rights and Gender. She is the author of books, papers, and documentaries on bioethical subjects. She is a Charter Member of the Board of Directors of the *International Association of Bioethics* (*IAB*).

James F. Drane, Ph.D., is Director of the James F. Drane Bioethics Institute in Edinboro University (Pennsylvania, USA). He has had a consulting role in the Pan-American Health Organization, the Program of Bioethics, since its establishment in 1994. He is co-author of *More Humane Medicine: A Liberal Catholic Bioethics* (Edinboro University Press, Edinboro, PA, 2003).

Javier Luna Orozco Eduardo, M.D., is a physician and one of the pioneers of bioethics in Bolivia. He is president of Bolivia's National Committee of Bioethics and has organized many bioethics conferences in Latin America. He also founded the first journal of bioethics in Bolivia, *Revista Boliviana de Bioética*.

H. Tristram Engelhardt, Jr., Ph.D., M.D., is a professor in the Department of Philosophy, Rice University, and professor emeritus, department of medicine, Baylor College of Medicine, Houston, TX.

Alfonso Llano Escobar, S.J., Ph.D., is the former Director and founder of the Bioethics Centro of Javerian University – Pontificia Universidade Javeriana (Bogotá – Colombia). He is also founder of FELAIBE – Latin American Federation of Bioethics Institutions.

Corina Bontempo Duca de Freitas, Ph.D., M.D., is the former executive secretary of the National Commission for Research Involving Human Beings/Ministry of Health.

Dirce Guilhem, Ph.D., is Chair of the Department of Health Sciences at the University of Brasília. She is currently director of the *Latin American Forum of Committees Ethics in Investigation and Health* (*Flaceis*) and has written *Escravas do risco: bioética, mulheres e Aids* [*Slaves of Risk: Bioethics, Women and Aids* – Editora UnB/Finatec, Brasília, 2005].

Diego Grácia Guillén, Ph.D., is the Chair of History of Medicine and Medical Ethics at the Medical School of Universidad Complutense de Madrid (Spain). He has a consulting role with the Bioethics Unit of the Pan-American Health Organization – World Health Organization (Santiago, Chile). He is the author of several reference works on bioethics, among them *Fundamentos de la bioética* (*The Foundations of Bioethics* – 1989); *Procedimientos de decisión en ética clínica* (*Decision Procedures in Clinical Ethics* – 1991); *Contribución de las humanidades médicas a la formación del médico* (*The Contribution of Medical Humanities to Doctors' Training* – 2006).

William Saad Hossne, Ph.D., is Professor Emeritus at the State University of São Paulo in Botucatu's (UNESP) medical school. He has been coordinator of the Masters of Bioethics *stricto sensu* at Saint Camillus University Center (Centro Universitário São Camilo) in São Paulo (SP) since 2004. He is a former president and co-founder of the Brazilian Society of Bioethics, as well as former president of the National Commission for Research Involving Human Beings/Ministry of Health, and has authored many articles in the field of research ethics.

Gerardo Jiménez-Sánchez, Ph.D., M.D., is an affiliate member of the Institute of Genetic Medicine, Johns Hopkins University, Baltimore, USA. He is Professor of Genomic Medicine at the UNAM and Resident Investigator of the Mexican Health Foundation (FUNSALUD).

José Roque Junges, S.J., Ph.D., is Professor of Bioethics in the post-graduate courses at the Universidade do Vale do Rio dos Sinos (São Leopoldo, RS). He is a member of the Board of Directors of the Brazilian Society of Bioethics. He has authored several books, including *Bioetica: perspectives e desafios* (2005) and *Bioética: hermeneutica e casuística* (2006).

Miguel Kottow, Ph.D., is a professor in the Department of Philosophy at the College of Philosophy and Humanities, the University of Chile (Santiago). He is the author of many papers and books in bioethics, including *Bases conceituais da bioética: enfoque latino-americano* (*Conceptual Bases of Bioethics: A Latin American Approach* – Gaia, São Paulo, 2006).

César Francisco Lara-Álvarez, Ph.D., was awarded a fellowship from the Fogarty National Institutes of Health (NIH) – USA. He is Director of Educational Programs at the National Institute of Genomic Medicine, México, and coordinator of the Ethical, Legal and Social Issues Research Center of Genomic Medicine. He is also a professor in the Bioethics Master Program, IPN, Mexico City.

Germán Alberto Calderón Legarda, Ph.D., is the former Director of the Institute of Bioethics of the Universidade Javeriana de Bogotá (Colômbia). He works in bioethics with an emphasis in the areas of ethics, human rights, and justice.

Hubert Lepargneur, Ph.D., is the former Editor-in-Chief of the journal *O Mundo da Saúde*, published by Centro Universitário São Camilo (São Paulo). He is the author of many books in the field of bioethics, including *O lugar atual da morte* (1993), *Antropologia do sofrimento* (1996), and *Bioética: novo conceito: a caminho de um consenso* (1996).

Fernando Lolas Stepke, Ph.D., is a professor at the University of Chile and Director of the Bioethics Program of the Pan-American Health Organization (Santiago, Chile). He has authored and edited several books, among them *Bioethics and Medicine: aspects of a relation* (*Bioética y medicina: aspectos de una relación* – Biblioteca Americana, Santiago, 2002) and *Beyond the Body: the narrative construction of health* (*Más allá del cuerpo: la construcción narrativa de la salud* – Editorial Andres Bello, Santiago, 1997).

José Alberto Mainetti, Ph.D., is President of the Doctor José Mainetti Foundation in Bonnet (Buenos Aires, Argentina) and director and professor of the Institute of Bioethics and Medical Humanities, Doctor José Mainetti Foundation for the Progress of Medicine in La Plata (Argentina). He is one of the founders of FELAIBE. He organized, with Juan Carlos Tealdi, the *Second World Congress of Bioethics*, held in Buenos Aires in 1994.

Walter Osswald, Ph.D., is a former director of the Institute of Bioethics, Portuguese Catholic University (Porto) and a former president of the World Association of Catholic Doctors. He has authored and edited many works in the area of medical and bioethical ethics, including *Direitos do homem e biomedicina* (Ed.) (*Man's Rights and Biomedicine* – Universidade Católica Editora, Porto, 2003) and *Um fio de Ética* (*A Stream of Ethics* – Gráfica de Coimbra, Coimbra, 2004).

Marta Lucia Perez, B.A., develops works linked to the Chair of Medical Philosophy of the College of Medical Sciences of the National Universidad of La Plata, Argentina.

Leo Pessini, Ph.D., is researcher and professor in the *stricto sensu* master course in bioethics of São Camilo University Center, and vice-president of the Society of Bioethics of São Paulo (2006–2008). He was a member of the organizing committee of the Fourth World Congress of Bioethics in Brasília (2002). He has authored many books in the areas of bioethics and moral theology, including *Distanásia: até quando prolongar a vida* (Dysthanasia: Until when to extend life? – Ed. Loyola, São Paulo, 2001), *Eutanásia: por que abreviar a vida* (Euthanasia: why shorten life? – Ed. Loyola, São Paulo, 2004), co-author of *Humanização e cuidados paliativos* (*Humanization and Palliative Care* – Ed. Loyola, São Paulo, 2005) and *Problemas atuais de bioética* (*Current Problems of Bioethics* – São Paulo, Loyola, 8th ed., 2007).

Katya Rodríguez, Ph.D., teaches research ethics at the Universidad Central del Ecuador (Quito). She is a member of FELAIBE – Federación Latino Americana de Instituciones de Bioética.

Leonides Santos y Vargas, Ph.D., is the director of the Institute for Bioethics and the Humanities, Universidad de Puerto Rico, Medical Sciences Campus.

José Ramón Acosta Sariego, M.D., M.A., is an expert in public health and holds the Chair of Bioethics at the Medical University of La Habana. He is the scientific editor of *Bioética: Desde uma perspectiva cubana* (*Bioethics from a Cuban Perspective* – Publicaciones acuario, Centro Félix Varela, La Habana, 1997). He is a pioneer of bioethics education in Cuba.

Ludwig Schmidt H., Ph.D., is Associate Professor of Bioethics at the Universidad Católica Andrés Bello (UCAB) Caracas, Venezuela. He is vice-president of the National Center for Bioethics and one of the founders of the Venezuelan Bioethics Society. He serves on the Editorial Board of the online journal *Bioética Latino Americana.*

Marco Segre, M.D., Ph.D., Researcher and Professor. Department of Forensic Medicine, Medical Ethics and Social and Work Medicine, University of São Paulo, Brazil.

Lucilda Selli, Ph.D., Professor of Bioethics in undergraduate and post-graduate courses at the Universidade do Vale do Rio dos Sinos (São Leopoldo – RS). She is the author of *Bioética e enfermagem* (2006). Died on May, 25, 2009.

José Eduardo de Siqueira, M.D., Ph.D., is professor of Clinical Medicine and Bioethics at the State University of Londrina (Universidade Estadual de Londrina, Paraná, Brazil), former president of the Brazilian Society of Bioethics, member of the commission on Terminally ill and Palliative Care for the Federal Council of Medicine of Brazil.

Miguel Angel Suazo, M.D., M.A., studied at the Autonomous University of Santo Domingo (Dominican Republic). He attended a Master's of Bioethics course at the University of Chile – Pan-American Health Organization (1998–2000). Currently, he is Dean of the Technological Institute of Santo Domingo (Intec), Director of the Intec Center of Bioethics, and coordinator for its bioethics specialization course.

Núria Terribas, J.D., is a lawyer and legal researcher. She has been director of the Borja Institute of Bioethics (IBB) since 1999, when Francesc Abel's term ended. She also teaches at IBB and co-ordinates the Master's of Bioethics program. Since 1995 she has been editor of the journal, *Bioética y Debat* (*Bioethics and Debate*), and is a legal consultant in commissions for the Governo Autônomo da Catalunha (Autonomous Government of Catalonia) on bioethical matters.

Claude Vergès, M.D., M.A., is a pediatric pulmonologist. She is also president of the Ethics Committee at the Hospital Del Nino and Professor of Medical Ethics and Bioethics for the Faculty of Medicine at the University of Panama.

Roberto Llanos Zuloaga, M.D., is a psychiatrist and psychotherapist. He is Head of the Department of Psychotherapy of the Ricardo Palma Clinic. He is the founder and current president of the Peruvian Association of Bioethics, and teacher and coordinator of the doctorate in psychology at the University of the Sacred Heart. He is an Invited Professor of Bioethics at San Marcos National University and Caetano Heredia University.

Translators

Jennifer A. Bulcock is a graduate student in the Department of Philosophy, Rice University, Houston, TX. She is also co-managing editor of the *Journal of Medicine and Philosophy* and *Christian Bioethics*.

Adail Sobral, Ph.D., is a Brazilian translator of English, French, Portuguese, and Spanish, mainly in human sciences, philosophy, and health fields. He has authored books about discourse and translation, has served as a translator for *O Mundo da Saúde* (*The World of Health*), published by São Camilo University Center), and the English language reviewer of the journal, *Applied Cancer Research*, published by A. C. Camargo Cancer Hospital.

Maria Stela Gonçalves, M.A., is a Brazilian translator of Spanish, French, Portuguese, and English, mainly in the area of human sciences and health. She is a self-employed translator – Adail Transervices Ltd. São Paulo, Brazil.

Introduction

Leo Pessini and Christian de Paul de Barchifontaine

Every new book has a history of its origin, sometimes marked by rigorous planning, such as dissertations and theses, and other times born simply from some moment of inspiration. *Ibero-American Bioethics: History and Perspectives* appeared due to a lively accidental discussion during a flight between São Paulo and Foz do Iguaçu, with our friend in bioethical endeavor, H. Tristram Engelhardt, Jr., when he came to Brazil to participate in the Fifth Brazilian Bioethics Congress in Foz do Iguaçu (PR) in 2005. We were invited to contribute and with Fernando Lolas Stepke were chosen to be editors of a volume of essays written by the pioneers responsible for the introduction and spread of bioethics in Latin America, the Caribbean, and the Iberian peninsula.

In the letter we sent to all the collaborators when announcing the objective of this new project, we said that bioethics emerged, four decades ago (1970–2010), as a new area of education and ethical sensitivity devoted to preserving and caring for human life, even cosmic–ecological life, before the extraordinary techno-scientific advances in the life and health sciences. Every part of the world has its peculiar history in terms of the development of bioethics, formed by different pioneering personalities and cultural contexts, as well as by the specific circumstances of each country. Our project aims to present essays by researchers responsible for the emergence of bioethics in their respective countries, telling in first person their first insights as well as experiences of and contributions to the development of bioethics. The hope is to have a critical historical account of the debates, controversies, and concerns of a bioethics that forged its own identity in Latin America as well as in the Iberian peninsula. In order to reach a wider audience, *Ibero-American Bioethics: History and Perspectives* is being published in three languages: English, Spanish, and Portuguese.

This work is a result of four years of intensive work, contacts, and dialogues, via telephone, internet, written correspondence, and meetings, with supporters of bioethics scattered throughout Latin America, the Caribbean, and the Iberian peninsula. We opted for adopting the "Ibero-America" category as a general inclusive geographical expression of the contributions from the pioneers of bioethics in these regions of the world. Our research perspective was to be maximally open and inclusive to allow the participation of the highest number of countries. Certainly, it is our desire in some future edition to include more countries that have a history of their own developments in the field of bioethics. We believe the participation of 17 countries in this book is a great victory and signals that our objective was reached. The accounts here presented, in their diverse points of view, offer a picture of the greatest accomplishments in and future perspectives of bioethics in this important, but often overlooked, region of the world.

This work has been divided into five sections. In the first we have *reflections from the Latin-American context*. Here we present the historical context of Hispano-American bioethics (Diego Gracia Guillén), the discourses of bioethics in Latin America and references made to bioethics in Argentina (José Alberto Mainetti), an overview of the development of bioethics in the Ibero-American cultural realm (James Drane), bioethics in Latin America and Colombia (Alfonso Llano Escobar, S.J.), and lastly an account of the important role of the Pan-American Health Organization (Fernando Lolas Stepke). In the second section, there are *reflections from pioneering voices* of different countries: Argentina (José Alberto Mainetti and Marta Lucia Perez), Bolivia (Javier Luna Orosco Eduardo), Brazil (Leo Pessini and Christian de Paul de Barchifontaine), Chile (Miguel Kottow), Costa Rica (Daniel Bustos-Montero), Cuba (José Ramón Acosta Sariego), Dominican Republic (Miguel Angel Suazo), Ecuador (Katya Rodríguez), Mexico (Gerardo Jiménez-Sánchez, Cesara Francisco Lara-Álvarez, and Alberto Arellano-Méndez), Panama (Claude Vergès), Paraguay (Marta Ascurra), Peru (Roberto Llanos Zuloaga), Portugal (Jorge Biscaia and Walter Osswald), Puerto Rico (Leonides Santos y Vargas), Spain (Francesc Abel and Núria Terribas), and Venezuela (Ludwig Schmidt H.). In the third section, to demonstrate the scope of bioethics in the region, we address five *specific issues*: bioethics and religion in Latin America (Márcio Fabri dos Anjos), bioethics and women in Latin America (Debora Diniz and Dirce Guilhem), bioethics and environmental concerns (José Roque Junges and Lucilda Selli), issues of human vulnerability (José Eduardo de Siqueira and Marco Segre), and research ethics involving human subjects (William Saad Hossne and Corina Bontempo Duca de Freitas). In the fourth section, we ask ourselves what sort of future awaits us in bioethics by considering the lessons that can be learned from the Hispano-American historical context (Hubert Lepargneur), providing a critical assessment of the development of bioethics in Latin American (Germán Calderón Legarda), and identifying general questions for the future (Leo Pessini and Christian de Paul de Barchifontaine). The volume concludes with a postscript (Jennifer A. Bulcock) that acknowledges the important contributions made by the authors of this volume in preserving the history of the development of bioethics in the Spanish and Portuguese cultural domains.

This work is offered not merely to demonstrate the ever-increasing output of bioethical literature in our countries, but also to serve as a foundational historical reference for those who – in the present as well as the future – research and study various topics related to the history of the development of bioethics in Ibero-America. In the 1990s there were already some initial efforts to publish a historical picture of bioethics in the Latin American context. We remember, among other publications: a special edition of the *Boletin de la Oficina Sanitaria*

Pan-Americana[1] (Bulletin of Pan-American Health Organization – PAHO) in 1990; two texts by the editors published in the journals, *Saúde em Debate* and *O Mundo da Saúde*, in the year 1995 (Pessini 1995a–c); and a special thematic issue of the *Journal of Medicine and Philosophy* published in 1996 (Drane 1996).

The beginning of 2008 was marked by the publication of the *Diccionário latino-americano de bioética* (*Latin-American Dictionary of Bioethics*), an event of signal importance for the history of Ibero-American bioethics. This project, conducted under the auspices of the Latin-American and Caribbean Network of Bioethics under UNESCO, had as its editor-in-chief the Argentinian philosopher, Juan Carlos Tealdi. Tealdi states in the introduction to the *Diccionário* that the objective is "to think about bioethics from the various disciplines and moral visions that serve as a meeting point for critical and normative reflections related to Latin American life and those living here" (Tealdi 2008, p. xxvii). The *Diccionário*, published by the National University of Colombia, compasses 685 pages with 249 entries by 184 authors drawn from 16 countries of this region. From this point forward, anyone wanting to study bioethics in Latin America must take this important text into account.

It is in this current decade, the first decade of the new millennium, that significant advances in bioethical education have been made, with specialization and Master's degrees, publications and commissions, either in the field of human research or in consulting roles created by governments. Partial as they are, their very existence demonstrates the need for a volume like this.

Our most sincere gratitude is extended to all those who worked with us – "friends of the cause of bioethics." They allowed us to make this dream become a reality.

---

[1]PAHO/WHO published a special issue dedicated to Bioethics in their official Bulletin in 1990, four years before PAHO's "Special Regional Bioethics Program." The issue presents several translated papers by authors from the USA, Canada, and Europe. In Latin America we have data on the development of bioethics in Argentina, Brazil, Colombia, Chile, Mexico, and Peru, clearly from the perspective of bioethics based on medical ethics.

IBERO-AMERICAN BIOETHICS: History and Perspectives is a landmark work, collecting the voices of those who participated in the founding and development of bioethics in Latin America, the Caribbean, and the Iberian Peninsula. The volume offers the reader a cluster of perspectives on the various births of bioethics in this region. The essays in part are irreplaceable first-person voices that give an account of how bioethics took shape within the Spanish and Portuguese cultures both in Europe and in the Americas. As such, the volume is a collection of primary sources, otherwise not available in English, that presents historical panoramas and explores the new perspectives born of the different phases of bioethics in Ibero-America – from its assimilation of bioethics to the creation of its own authentic voices. The volume also encompasses critical reflections from this region on the quite different ways in which its local bioethics have taken shape. As such, this volume also offers an introduction into the quite different concerns that frame and direct bioethics in the cultural context of Ibero-America.

The book gives a rich, deep, broad, and pluralist presentation of Ibero-American bioethics and its contribution to the international phenomenon of bioethics. It is a volume for all readers interested in bioethics, Ibero-American studies, and international approaches to health care policy.

References

Drane JF (ed) (1996) J Med Philos 21.6

Pessini L (1995a) O desenvolvimento da bioética na América Latina. Saúde em Debate 47:57–66

Pessini L (1995b) O desenvolvimento da bioética na América Latina – algumas considerações – Parte I. O Mundo da Saúde 19:84–91

Pessini L (1995c) O desenvolvimento da bioética na América Latina – algumas considerações – Parte II. O Mundo da Saúde 19:116–119

Tealdi JC (2008) Introducción. In: Tealdi JC (ed) Diccionário latinoamericano de bioética, pp xxiii–xxviii. UNESCO, Paris

Part I
Reflections from the Latin American Context

Chapter 1
The Historical Setting of Latin American Bioethics

Diego Grácia Guillén

1.1 Introduction

Bioethics has been and continues to be an American movement. It would be difficult to successfully transfer its propositions, unchanged, to other countries, even to those with very similar economic, social, and cultural conditions, such as European countries in general and those of Latin or Mediterranean Europe in particular (Drane 1988; Gracia 1993, pp. 97–107). The differences are compounded when a culture does not share Western roots, such as in Japan (Bai et al. 1987, pp. 18–20), China (Qiu 1993, pp. 108–125), or Nigeria (Gbadegesin 1993, pp. 257–262). One's inability to universally apply the American principles to different cultures highlights the importance of trans-cultural studies and the history of peoples that need to be appreciated. Outside of cultural and historical context the ethics of a people or an epoch and their bioethics cannot be understood. In this paper, I propose to study the historical setting of Latin American bioethics. This is necessary because the culture of these peoples stems not only from the Anglo-Saxon but also from a Latin and Mediterranean tradition, from which it has derived highly specific characteristics. In what follows, I will offer a brief review of the history of these peoples and then define the ethical features of the main periods of that history.

1.2 The Pre-Columbian Age and the Time of Discoveries: The Ethics of the Gift

Most primitive cultures seem to share a religious view of life and the world (Laín-Entralgo 1961). The pre-Columbian cultures of the American hemisphere are no exception to this rule. Despite their rich variety, they all see the world and the

D.G. Guillén
Universidad Complutense de Madrid, Facultad de Medicina, Maldonado 48 28006, Madrid, ES
e-mail: dgracia@fcs.es

L. Pessini et al. (eds.), *Ibero-American Bioethics: History and Perspectives*,
Philosophy and Medicine 106, DOI 10.1007/978-1-4020-9350-0_1,

events of life as a complex system of powers, some good and some evil, which express and symbolize the good and bad relations of mortals with divinity and of divinity with mortals. As a result, natural phenomena and the events of life are always seen as "gifts" of divinity or as "debts" incurred to it. The dialectic of the gift–debt is particularly clear in the case of disease. Health is a gift of the divinity, a sign of divine pleasure, while disease is a punishment for sins, or is inflicted by malign spirits. This type of interpretation is encountered in virtually every pre-Columbian culture (Guerra 1971, 1990, p. 233), and we have highly valuable literary examples of it, particularly from the Maya (Rivera 1986, pp. 22, 28–29; Sáenz de Santa María 1989).

This mythic-magical and religious interpretation of the world did not dissipate with the coming of the Spaniards to America in 1492: first, because indigenous people remained attached to their beliefs and, second, because the Spaniards brought with them an equally strong reliance on providence. The Christian religion, however, was certainly different from any seen before in the New World.

A reading of the letters from Christopher Columbus to the King of Spain (Colón 1989) or of those from the voyage of Amerigo Vespucci (Vespucci 1986) is sufficient to show that Columbus saw his discovery as a divine "gift" vouchsafed to him and the Spanish sovereigns. Favorable events continued to be seen as gifts and unfavorable events as reverses brought on by the hardheartedness of the conquistadors or the American indigenes. The discovery of the new continent was considered in any case a marvelous gift. The fact of having come upon America unexpectedly, "by chance," convinced Columbus that it was a gift from heaven. So began a providentialist interpretation of America that would have incalculable consequences (Xirau 1973). One of the first was the "mythification" of the American Indian and his society. Columbus' letters refer over and over to what could be called the American "white legend": Indians living in a "state of nature" with neither laws nor government, with a sexual morality quite different from that of medieval Europe.

The "mythification" of America was so broad that Columbus and the early discoverers saw an entire utopia that led them to locate an earthly paradise in the southern part of the American hemisphere (in an account of his third voyage, Columbus said that it lay in the southern hemisphere, below the equinoctial line (Colón 1989, p. 216)). This subject resonated extensively in the medical literature, for the earthly paradise had to be, by definition, the most beautiful and healthful of all places (Cisneros 1618, p. 99 et seq.). This myth of paradise and of the natural goodness of its inhabitants led to the creation of European literature about the myth of the "noble savage," who lived in what then came to be called a "state of nature." Without this antecedent, modern political doctrine from Thomas Hobbes and John Locke to Jean-Jacques Rousseau and Immanuel Kant would make no sense. Only after it could a distinction be drawn between a "state of nature" and a "civil state," from which the features of the "social contract" were derived (Douchet 1971).

1.3 The Ethical Problem of the Conquest: The Ethics of Despotism

Although the relations between the Spaniards and the Indians were excellent at the outset, they soon deteriorated. Liberty and peaceful coexistence gradually gave way to coercion and force. The famous sermon of brother Antonio de Montesinos on the island of Hispaniola in 1511 was the first public statement of the changed state of affairs (Hanke 1988, pp. 29–35; Pereña 1992, p. 20ff). The thesis of the noble savage was gradually replaced by that of the evil savage, to be treated almost as an irrational being. The use of force became systematic to bring them to the true faith and into the service of the King of Spain. This attitude intensified after 1519 with the conquest of Mexico by Hernán Cortés. In Cortés's harangue to his troops before they embarked for Mexico, nothing remained of the earlier utopia of the naturally good and gentle Indian. Quite the reverse: Cortés saw the Indian as a perverse being who must be won over, if necessary by force, to civilization and Christian morality (Pereña 1992, p. 46). Peaceful coexistence was thus followed by military conquest, and the white legend was succeeded by the "black legend" (Molina 1991). The Indian was no longer a noble savage but a "dirty dog" to be subjugated and enslaved. He lived in a state of nature, but that state was bestiality, the *bellum omnium contra omnes* of Thomas Hobbes.

The conquistadors came to believe that the Indians must be subdued by force, and not for their own good but for that of the conquistadors and Spain. The ethic of the gift was succeeded by the ethic of despotism and tyranny. All of classical philosophy has accepted without discussion, at least since Aristotle, that the slave must be governed for the convenience not of the slave but of the master (Aristotle, *Politics* 1278b, pp. 33–35). This act Aristotle called "despotism" when done by the master of a house, and "tyranny" when done by a monarch (Aristotle 1295a). Both forms differ, argues the philosopher, from the government of one's children, in which the father seeks not his own benefit (as in despotic and tyrannical relationships) but the benefit of the governed (Aristotle 1278b 35–40). The latter is paternalism. From 1510 on there can be no doubt that the ethic of the American conquest became clearly despotic. It could not be correctly termed tyrannical, for after 1526 the Spanish crown attempted to prevent the degradation of the Indian community (Pereña 1992, p. 40), but neither was it paternalistic. The ethic consolidated in these years was clearly a despotic one.

According to Francisco de Vitoria, Peru had been conquered (1531–1532) by despotism, and he referred contemptuously to the despots who ruled over the Inca Indians as "*peruleros*," against whom he inveighed in 1534: "I am not frightened or embarrassed by the things that come to my hands except the tricks of benefices and things of the Indies, the very mention of which freezes the blood in my body" (Vitoria 1967, p. 135). The letter is dated November 8, 1534, and is one long tirade of invective against the conquistadors of Peru: "Of those of Peru, *timeo* [I fear] that they are the kind *qui volunt divites fieri* [who want to become rich]. And of some it has been said that *impossibile est divitem intrare in regnum caelorum*" [it is impossible for the rich to enter the kingdom of heaven] (Vitoria 1967, p. 138). Vitoria says he "does not understand the justice of that war" (Vitoria, loc. cit.), for "from what I understood from those who were at the recent battle with Tabalipa, neither Tabalipa nor his people had ever done any wrong to the Christians or anything else that would justify making war on them" (Vitoria, loc. cit.). In his view, "there was no cause for war other than to rob them ... and I believe that the other conquests since have been even more wicked" (Vitoria, loc. cit.); besides, Indians "think the Spaniards tyrannize them and make war on them unjustly" (Vitoria, loc. cit.). Vitoria's point is that "war, especially against vassals, must be started and waged for the good of the vassals and not of the prince" (Vitoria, loc. cit.). The former is paternalism, while the latter is despotism. Vitoria believes that the *peruleros* are behaving despotically (for their own benefit), and so rob the Indians of all their wealth: "I do not see how they can rob and despoil the unfortunates they have vanquished of all their goods" (Vitoria, loc. cit.).

He argues that

> There is only one way to justify the cruelty of the conquistadors; that is, to regard the Indians not as people, but as apes ... In truth, if the Indians are not men, but apes, *non sunt capaces injuriae* [they are incapable of suffering injury]. But if they are men, and our fellows, and therefore vassals of the emperor, *non video quomodo* [I do not see how] to excuse any conquistador of ultimate impiety and tyranny, nor do I know what so great service they render His Majesty in ruining his vassals (Vitoria 1967, pp. 138–139).

The acts of the conquistadors are so unjustifiable that Vitoria writes:

> If I wished for the archbishopric of Toledo, which is vacant, and they were to give it me if I subscribed or affirmed the innocence of these *peruleros*, I would surely not dare to: May my tongue and my hand wither ere I say or write such a thing so inhuman and alien to all Christianity. Let them do what they will and leave us in peace (Vitoria 1967, p. 139).

Vitoria's judgment agrees with that expressed by Bartolomé de Las Casas in his polemical works, especially the *Brevisima relación de la destrucción de las Indias* (1542) (A Very Short Report on the Indies Destruction). Against him Ginés de Sepúlveda, a great Aristotelian and official chronicler of Emperor Charles V, maintained in his book *Democrates Secundus* (1544) that the despotism in the Americas was ethically correct. From their confrontation in Valladolid (1550–1551) (Pagden 1982) at least one clear idea emerged: the despotic treatment of the Indians must give way to another that is more humane and would treat them not as animals or slaves but as sons and daughters. The despotism of the Conquest was to be succeeded by the paternalism of the colonial age.

What consequences did the ethic of despotism have for the lives of the American Indians? The denunciations of Bartolomé de Las Casas attest well to the destruction and death wrought by this policy:

> At this time the clergy of Santo Domingo had already noted the sad life and harsh captivity suffered by the native people of this island and how they were being consumed thereby; the Spaniards who owned them being no more concerned than if they had useless

> animals, and sorry when they died only because they had such need of them in the gold mines and other profitable ventures; nor did they for all that, use those that were left with more compassion or mitigation of the rigor and harshness with which they were used to oppressing and exhausting them. And in all this there were Spaniards who were better and worse, for some were of utmost cruelty, with neither pity nor mercy, having regard only to their own enrichment with the blood of those unfortunate wretches, while others were less cruel, and some it may be supposed must have grieved at their misery and anguish, but all, the ones and the others, tacitly or expressly put their own private material interests before the health and lives and salvation of the unfortunates (Las Casas 1961, p. 174).

1.4 The Colonial Age: The Ethics of Paternalism

The colonial age departed both from the optimism of the "noble savage" and from the pessimism of the "dirty dog." The ideology of this third phase lay in between: the Indian was free, but was seen as a minor, as a small child in need of supervision. This could already be seen in the Laws of Burgos of 1512 (Molina 1991, p. 87), but became accepted as standard in the New Laws of the Indies of 1542. As Luciano Pereña has written, these Laws are the outcome of the theoretical work done by Vitoria, Covarrubias, Soto, and Cano, of the school of Salamanca (Pereña 1992, p. 172).

Paternalism is the solution proposed by Las Casas in his books. Vitoria, in his *Relectio de Indis* of 1539, does not accept the proposition that the Indians are irrational beings by nature. Nor does he accept Aristotle's thesis to the effect that "there are those who are by nature slaves" (Vitoria 1967, pp. 13–14). Although, in his opinion, the Indians are very similar to animals, he does not think them "mindless or idiots":

> They are actually not idiots, but have, in their own way, the use of reason. It is evident that there is a certain order in their affairs: they have properly ordered cities, well-defined marriages, magistrates, lords, laws, professors, industries, trade; all of which requires the use of reason. They also have a kind of religion and do not err about things that are evident to others, which betoken the use of reason. God and nature do not abandon them regarding what is necessary to the species; and the principal thing in man is reason, and useless is the potentiality that is not reduced to an act. Moreover, they may have been so many thousands of years, through no fault of their own, outside the state of salvation, for they were born in sin and are without baptism, and may not have the use of reason to inquire into what is needful for salvation. From which I believe that the fact that they seem to us such idiots and dullards derives in most part from their poor and barbarous education, for among us, too, we see many men of the countryside who are little removed from the brute animals (Vitoria 1967, pp. 29–30).

After this, Vitoria replies to the counterargument that denied rationality in Indians based on the authority of Aristotle. What is truly consistent with Aristotle's thought, he says, is "that there is in them a natural need to be ruled over and governed by others, and it is very beneficial to them to be subject to others, as children need to be subject to their parents and a woman to her husband" (Vitoria 1967, p. 31; cf. Aristotle, *Politics* 1259a, b). Here, we see clearly the paternalism of Vitoria's solution.

Vitoria, however, is not untroubled by doubts. These doubts lead him to view this argument as merely probable, but for that very reason valid as a guide to practical conduct (it should not be forgotten that the Salamancan school that started with Vitoria gave rise to the moral doctrine of probablism). Here is a highly significant passage:

> There is another point that could not be affirmed with surely but can indeed be discussed and appears legitimate to some. I would venture neither to approve nor to condemn it absolutely. This point is: *Those barbarians, though they may not be, as has been said, entirely incompetent, are so little removed from the mentally retarded that they seem not capable of establishing or administering a legitimate republic within human and political limits.* Hence they have no proper laws, or magistrates, and do not even have enough capacity to govern the family. Indeed they are without not just liberal but also mechanical sciences and arts, and a diligent agriculture, artisans and many other amenities that are even necessary for human life.
>
> It could then be said that for the utility of them all the kings of Spain may take upon themselves the administration and government of those barbarians, appoint to them ministers and governors for their peoples, and even give them new princes so long as it is clear that this is conducive to their well-being.
>
> It would be difficult to persuade oneself of all this because if all were incapable, there is no doubt that it would only be permissible and most advisable, but even princes would be in the obligation of doing this just as if they were entirely children. And there appears to be the same reason for so dealing with those barbarians as with the mindless, for they can do little or no more to govern themselves than the mentally deficient. And they are almost as the very wild beasts, for they use foods no more prepared and not much better than they. Thus they could similarly be entrusted to the tutelage of men more intelligent than themselves.
>
> And this thesis is confirmed with some appearance of truth or likelihood. For if perchance all the adults of those regions were to perish and leave only the children and the adolescents with some use of reason, but still within the years of childhood and puberty, it seems clear that princes could take them in charge and govern them while they were in that state. If this is granted, it seems true that it is not to be denied that the same could be done with the parents of the barbarians, assuming the mental incapacity ascribed to them by those who have been there, which they say is much greater than that of adolescent children in other nations.
>
> And in truth this conduct could even be founded on the precept of charity, for they are our fellow men and we are obliged to do what is good for them. I accept this (as I have said) without affirming it absolutely and, moreover, on condition that it is done for the good and utility of them and not as a pretext for profit to the Spaniards. For herein lies all the danger to souls and their eternal salvation. This argument may also be supported by what was said before, that they are serfs by nature. And such these barbarians do appear to be, and it is partly for this reason that they could be governed as serfs (Vitoria 1967, pp. 97–98).

These passages convey Vitoria's mind-set very well and therewith the mentality underlying the *Laws of the Indies*. Indians are men, not animals, and hence merit our respect; but they are barbarian men, to be protected like children. Vitoria proposes that we behave paternalistically toward them and avoid tyranny. He therefore inveighs against the excesses of the conquistadors, and in a letter to Father Arcos says "*non video quomodo* (I do not see how) ... to excuse these conquistadors of ultimate impiety and tyranny" (Vitoria 1967, p. 139).

José de Acosta is another great theoretician of paternalistic protection of the Indians. In his work *De procuranda indorum salute* (1576), he defines the Indians as "barbarians" and asserts, "By the definition of prestigious writers, barbarians are those who shrink from right reason and the habitual practice of men (*qui a recta ratione et hominum communi consuetudine abhorrent*). This is why the most illustrious writers emphasize the incapacity of barbarians, their ferocity, including their techniques and works, which show how far they are from the usual practice of other men and how little wisdom and rational activity they have" (Acosta 1984, p. 61). This is the mind-set that presides over all the Spanish colonization: the Indians are barbarians and hence have physical strength, but not rational or spiritual vigor and are by nature in need of tutelage. They are like the artisans in Plato's *Republic,* whereas the guardians and governors are the Spaniards.

José de Acosta distinguishes three levels of barbarism, from least to most. The least is that of the East Indies. The peoples of the West Indies are at the second and third levels. At the second level are the Mexicans and Peruvians, and almost all the other American peoples are at the third. And, Jose de Acosta adds:

> All these men or half-men must be given human instruction that they may learn to be men and become educated like children. And if with flattery they let themselves be improved, so much the better; if they do not, they must not be left to their fate: if they stubbornly resist their own regeneration and talk nonsense against their own teachers and physicians, they must be compelled by force and some convenient pressure must be exerted on them that they do not raise obstacles to the Gospel, and they must be made to fulfill their obligations; and it will be well to force them to move from the jungle to the human comity of the city, and to enter, however reluctantly, into the kingdom of heaven (Acosta 1984, p. 69).

De Acosta does not hesitate to apply to the American Indians the hard words in the book of the *Wisdom of Solomon* on the Canaanites: "knowing that they came of evil stock, that they had been wicked from birth, and would never change their way of being. Their whole nation was cursed from the beginning" (Wisdom, 12:10–11). And, de Acosta adds, "There are therefore individuals afflicted by a congenital and hereditary malice, so to speak; their way of thinking is so stubborn and perversely deep-rooted that it is almost impossible to extirpate.... This is, then, the first and principal cause of why in these regions so little fruit is to be expected from so much effort: they are a cursed race, almost beyond divine help and destined for perdition" (Acosta 1984, p. 89). Similar passages could easily be found (see, for example, Acosta 1984, pp. 139, 141, 143 and 145).

In these and many similar expressions, José de Acosta is not justifying the despotism of the conquistadors. Quite the contrary, what he proposes as an alternative to despotism is paternalism. So he writes immediately thereafter the following passage:

> I mention all this not to approve in any way of the "tyrannical" power and cruelty (so removed from the teachings of Christ) that have been used with the peoples of the Indies, or because I think they are to be commanded like serfs, or because I do not abhor and condemn with all my energy the crimes of the scoundrels and the greed of those who convert the goods, work and sweat of those wretches to their sole benefit, taking most iniquitous advantage of their dull-wittedness (Acosta 1984, p. 147).

This is the mentality with which decent Spaniards sought to govern the American colonies from about 1550 until independence. The Indians were protected like children rather than treated as slaves (which was prohibited by law). This does not mean that slavery did not exist. In fact, the traffic in African slaves to America took place precisely because of the demand of the most burdensome tasks which only slaves carried out. Negroes were not considered in the "Leyes de Indias" (Legislation for Indians) and therefore could be treated as slaves according to the medieval legislation which Alfonso X recapitulated in the *Partidas*. Consequently, colonial society was stratified into an authentic caste system in which the Spaniards occupied the top level, then came the American Spaniards or *Criollos*, then the *Mestizos* (a mixture of European and Indian), after them the *Mulatos* (a mixture of European and African) and then the Zambos (a mixture of Indian and African), then the Indian and finally at the bottom the Negro slaves. Paternalistic treatment never reached the last level.

In the medical sphere, this caste system had both good and bad consequences. One good consequence was the categorical prohibition under the New Laws of 1542 of inhuman and degrading labor. It was forbidden to make Indians carry burdens on their backs, with the sole exceptions imposed by the absence of beasts of burden or of roads, and only as moderate tasks voluntarily undertaken and never compelled, and without detriment to the health, the lives, and the preservation of the Indians, and always in exchange for payment accepted by them freely and voluntarily (Pereña 1992, p. 166). Mistreatment and abuse were also forbidden, and severe punishment awaited whoever killed or wounded any Indian. The bad consequence was undiluted paternalism. What was good for the Indian was defined by the Spaniard or the *Criollo*, not by the Indian himself. What was done was that which the Spaniard or the *Criollo* thought was good for the Indian and in most cases was merely what was good for the Spaniard or the *Criollo*.

Far from solving existing problems, belief in the natural inferiority of Indians and the necessity of guiding them only compounded problems. This is obvious in the area of health care. Seeing themselves looked down upon and rejected by white and *criollo* society, Indians took refuge in their own traditions and reverted to the faith medicine of their forebears. Western medicine reached them not through physicians and surgeons but through missionaries, who carried out important health initiatives for evangelization, founding hospitals for the lower classes and educating people in health matters.

In conclusion, then, we may say that during the centuries of the colonial age the Indians were accorded some civil rights (e.g., the right to life and to humane treatment in the sense of the integrity of one's person), but these civil rights never turned into political rights, and the Indians remained in a state of social relegation. This moved them to withdraw into their ancient traditions, which reduced their health care largely to their old faith-healing practices. The paternalism of the colonial age protected their lives but also segregated them socially, prevented the betterment of their condition, and barred them from the benefits of Western medicine.

The European residents in America and the *Criollos*, however, did benefit from the Western medical practices that the Spaniards brought to the New World. The sixteenth century was a century of great splendor in Spanish medicine, which had clear effects on American medicine (Guerra 1972, p. 346). Schools of medicine were opened in the leading universities (Mexico: 1555, Lima: 1634, Guatemala: 1681, Quito: 1693, Bogotá: 1715, Havana: 1726, Caracas: 1727 etc.), which produced physicians trained to European standards. In addition, with the promulgation of the *New Laws of the Indies* in 1542, medical practice passed under the control of the Tribunal del Protomedicato (Examining Board of Physicians), which began to function in 1570. Thereafter, Hispano-American medicine flourished increasingly and uninterruptedly until the end of the eighteenth century.

In this way, different forms of medical care were established in Indian society, each corresponding to the different castes. The physicians from the universities tended to the health needs of the highest class, made up of the nobility and the governors from Spain. They also cared for *criollos* with money. Surgeons and barbers took care of the *mestizos* and *mulatos* and these castes also employed the techniques of folk medicine. Some Indians benefited from the Western medicine provided by missionaries, but most were taken care of by folk doctors. The African slaves used their own folk medicine as well. All of the above-mentioned medicines were paternalistic, but each in a different way. European medicine regarded the patient as a child or a moral invalid and hence as incapable of deciding on matters of one's own body. Indians were in a different situation, for they were regarded as children even when they were healthy, and hence were subject to paternalism in every area of life. It may also be said that the Indian was seen and treated, in all cases and without exception, like a patient. The white and *criollo* were treated paternalistically only when they were sick, but for the Indian and *mestizo*, paternalistic treatment was the rule and affected every aspect of life. Their racial condition was regarded and treated as if it were a disease. This is particularly clear with Negroes whose race and skin color condemned them to something worse than paternalism, i.e., to despotism and tyranny.

1.5 The Age of Independence: The Vicissitudes of Ethnic Autonomy in Latin America

During the centuries of the colonial age, American society consisted of several strata: the highest, consisting of the European governors, the middle stratum, made up mostly of *criollos*, and the third and lowest consisting of the indigenes. With time, it was seen that the first two had clearly opposing interests, for there was no necessary identity between the interest of the crown, represented by the European governors, and the interest of the settlers themselves. This was the wellspring of the internal struggles for political power that began in the colonies during the nineteenth century. The occasion for revolt was created by the French invasion of Spain and the imprisonment of the Spanish monarch, Ferdinand VII, in 1808. As in Spain, so in America: local and vice-royal "*juntas*" (boards of governors) were formed and assumed political control of the colonial cities and territories. These *juntas* were made up of *criollos*, who by this means acquired effective power against Spanish authorities in the colonies. This process took place between 1808 and 1810 and was consolidated years later, between 1820 and 1824, in the form of autonomous political authority independent of the Spanish Crown. The process was influenced by the *Declaration of Independence* of the British colonies in North America in 1776, the French revolution of 1789 and, in general, the intellectual climate of the French Enlightenment. The great Hispano-American revolutionaries (e.g., Antonio Nariño, Francisco Miranda, Simón Bolívar, etc.) were scions of the wealthy, cultivated *criollo* bourgeoisie who, having studied in Europe, were acquainted with liberal ideology and realized the importance of the new doctrine of human rights for democratic politics. In 1793 Nariño translated and printed in Bogotá the *Declaration of the Rights of Man,* which the French constituent assembly had promulgated shortly before in 1789. It is interesting to note that, similar to Spain – where many of the members of the Cortes who in 1812 proclaimed the first *Liberal Constitution* were physicians – a very high proportion of the leaders of the independence movements of the new American nations were also physicians (Guerra 1975, pp. 23–51). The fact that medicine was one of the most esteemed professions by the new *criollo* bourgeoisie had considerable importance.

The constitutions of the new American countries were drawn up on the models of those of the United States (1776), France (1789), and Spain (1812). This means that they started from the assertion of popular sovereignty and from the recognition in all human beings of certain inborn and inalienable rights referred to as civil and political rights. Against the old model of the paternalist state, the new model asserted that all human beings are adults and autonomous, that is, persons with rights that none may violate (Sánchez Agesta 1987). The place of paternalism in the old model was now occupied by the idea of autonomy. All citizens, including Indians, were considered autonomous and were to be treated as equals in the new democratic state.

From a formal standpoint this constituted an indisputable step forward, and yet in other ways it was distinctly retrogressive. In this stage the Indian actually made no gains in prestige or social standing, but remained completely outside the social dynamics in these countries. Indeed, being no longer protected by the structures of the old paternalist state, Indians were left utterly defenseless against the economic and social interests of the *criollo* bourgeoisie. Wars of persecution of the Indians were undertaken in several Hispano-American countries in the second half of the nineteenth century, some of which nearly exterminated the Indians.

The revolution allowed the *criollo* bourgeoisie to organize itself on new lines of conduct very similar to those of Europe and the United States. When the Spanish colonies became independent, a bipolar social structure emerged even more clearly in the new American countries: a bourgeoisie of European and first-world patterns and customs, and an extensive underclass closely attached to Indian traditions and of a clearly third-world caste.

This social structure had major consequences for health. From the early days of independence the bourgeoisie enjoyed health care very similar to that of the advanced countries of the West, while the health care of the needy classes was seriously deficient. In Latin-American countries, an exercise of civil and political rights was impossible where these were not accompanied by economic, social, and cultural rights. Among civil and political rights are the right to life and to humane treatment or personal integrity and the right to freedom or autonomy. There can be no doubt that People of good economic and social status can secure their rights without the help of the state. But without state help those of very humble economic and social stations cannot secure the so-called economic, social, and cultural rights, which include the right to health care. Put differently, in these cases the civil and political rights and specifically the rights to integrity and to autonomy remain merely formal instead of actual rights. The real exercise of these rights requires basic conditions that unfortunately are absent in large sectors of Latin American society.

Typical of the health care systems in developing countries, major cities in Ibero-America have very well-equipped high-tech health facilities that serve the sector of the population that can pay, but for all others medical care is quite primitive. In these countries the most important bioethical problems are those relating to justice and the allocation of scarce resources. Many sectors of the population have not yet benefited from the advanced technology of health care or from the movement of patient emancipation. Therefore, in those sectors, issues of autonomy are not of the highest priority, although they are raised in the wealthier sectors whose citizens turn towards the high-technology centers in the large cities. In developing countries, society is divided into two groups separated by a wide gulf: the bourgeoisie on the one hand, and the majority of the general population on the other. The result is two completely different health care systems, one that falls prey to the problems of Western medicine and the other that does not (Gracia 1990, pp. 281–282). In many developing nations in Latin America, social security covers the health care of most people (Chile, Costa Rica, Panama, Venezuela, Mexico, and so forth), but the health care provided is tertiary or high-tech care that co-exists with a poorly developed primary care system; this system fails to address malnutrition, bad drinking water and sewer systems, deficiencies in health education and personal hygiene, unemployment, and marginalization.

This is why the bioethical problems and sensibilities of present-day Latin-American societies differ greatly, depending on the social level under consideration. The bourgeoisie receives Western-type medical care, similar to that provided in developed countries, and therefore the same moral issues arise that demand the interest of the developed countries: patient autonomy, informed consent, rejection of paternalism, problems of assisted reproduction, prenatal diagnosis, organ transplants, etc. At this level Latin-American bioethics could be described as similar to that of any part of the developed world.

But if the problems of bioethics are addressed from the standpoint of the needy, who are the majority of the population in these countries, the all-absorbing autonomy concerns of the first world are without meaning. The issue of informed consent is unimportant in a setting of deep poverty, where the most pressing problem is obtaining food and even survival. The concerns related to tertiary care, which have motivated the development of bioethics in developed countries, do not extend to primary care. At this level of care, the primary concerns are those with direct significance to justice and harmlessness and do not include issues of autonomy, etc.

The ethical problems related to these two principles (harmlessness and justice) have not been well developed in recent decades. In my opinion, contact with the reality of Latin American life can offer an ideal occasion to encourage their study. We must not forget that these are the problems that beset developing countries, which today is the reality of most of mankind.

Post Script – History in First Person

From Anthropology to Bioethics

I would like to speak of my own contributions to the movement of bioethics in the region of Ibero-America. I studied philosophy in the first half of the 1960s and medicine during the other half, specializing in psychiatry. This is when I became interested in the history of medicine, completing my doctoral dissertation in 1973 on the history of Spanish psychiatry. After that, I did postdoctoral studies on medical anthropology in Germany, following the style and method of the School of Heidelberg. I returned to Spain in 1978 and accepted the History of Medicine chair at Madrid's Complutense University just vacated by my mentor Pedro Laín Entralgo, upon his retirement.

I first discovered bioethics in 1975. Following Laín's method, I had tried to approach medicine from two different and complementary angles: historical and philosophical. Medical anthropology was the intersection of these methods.

Nevertheless, after years of intense work in that field, I felt immensely frustrated because the analysis of all issues was invariably too theoretical and abstract, with no practical applications. This is what made it so meaningful to find the newly developed and growing field in the United States under the neologism of *bioethics*. What surprised me most was the profoundly practical character of the then new field, being always interested in the search for practical solutions to ethical problems. Its conceptual scaffolding was probably inferior to that of the Germans' medical anthropology but its applicability, its utility, was much greater. This made me focus on bioethics, to which I have devoted myself practically full-time since the early 1980s.

Rediscovering the History of Ethics

My first research project was a revision of the history of medical ethics, following a rather unorthodox method. Instead of looking at who physicians *had been* or what they *had done*, my interest was to know the history of what physicians *had wanted to be* or believed they *had to be*. The sources of this study were the ethical texts themselves, which do not reveal the reality, but rather the *idealism* of the medical profession.

This work consumed an amount of time and effort that I could not have imagined when I started. In fact, I dedicated the first half of the 1980s to this work, and the product was the first part of my 1989 book, *Foundations of Bioethics* (Gracia 1989).

When analyzing the medical ethics tradition, I realized that all of them adhered to the same logic and exposed the same ethical ideal: the Hippocratic *beau ideal*. My primary hypothesis was that medical ethics had evolved internally, and that it would be possible, therefore, to find those turning points that would benchmark different phases, or even different ethics. But the sources rebelled against this idea, convincing me that there had been one medical ethics tradition throughout history, since Hippocrates. Changes had originated outside medicine and were invariably received as external threats by the medical establishment.

Another finding was that there were three lineages to medical ethics: the medical, from the Hippocratic Tradition; the juridical, reflecting modernity; and the philosophical and political, drawn from antiquity and the Greek Tradition. To my surprise, the first tradition revolved around the principle of beneficence, the second around the principle of autonomy, and the third around justice. These were, curiously, the same principles identified by The Belmont Report. The confluence of those three traditions had happened very recently, in the second half of the twentieth century, and had caused countless conflicts. Nonetheless, my conclusion was that this convergence and conflict had synthesized into bioethics as an independent discipline by the 1970s.

My American Experience and Return to Fundamentals

With those findings fresh in *my* mind, I felt the need to visit the main bioethics and medical humanities centers in the United States at that time. I visited them all in the company of James F. Drane, who had just spent a year in Madrid writing a book, *Becoming a Good Doctor* (Drane 1988), strongly inspired by the works of Laín Entralgo.

Back in Spain, I believed that I had a clear picture of what was going on in America and what I should do in my country. I could not be satisfied with simply importing American bioethics. We belong to different cultures, with different philosophical traditions and values. It was necessary to do something more difficult, but also more fruitful: to rethink, redo, recreate everything from scratch, drawing from the American experience but also taking into account European traditions.

American bioethics had achieved something until then unimaginable, which was to have practical utility, solving conflicts and helping practitioners better handle the clinical relationship. This was a nonnegotiable outcome for any project in the clinical sphere. On the other hand, American bioethicists had been able to free clinical ethics from theology and from jurisprudence while staying on good terms with both disciplines. To my European mentality, however, American bioethics suffered from a deficient philosophical foundation; it gave disproportionate weight to conflict resolution at the expense of foundational considerations. This was understandable, given the empiricist and pragmatic American tradition, but difficult to understand and incorporate into European rationalism. To address these challenges, I devoted the second half of the 1980s to working on the foundations of bioethics.

The fruit of that effort was the second part of my book, *Fundamentos de bioética* (*Foundations of Bioethics*). There I analyzed the main doctrines that have given birth to medical ethics in Western history and proposed a model that tried to incorporate the wisdom of that historical process. I built that model upon the teachings of my mentor in philosophy, the late Xavier Zubiri, who was concerned with the inseparability of sensitivity and intellect in human reason, in what Fie called "sentient intelligence." I also maintained that it was not possible to construct a philosophical foundation for bioethics without proposing a method of decision making. Corresponding methods were therefore included with each foundational theory.

This cycle, devoted to the history and foundations of bioethics, ended in 1990, with *Primum non nocere*, a discourse I gave upon my admission to the Spanish Royal Academy of Medicine (Gracia 1990a).

Clinical Ethics

My plan for the 1990s was to study the concrete problems faced by clinical ethics in order to publish *Clinical Bioethics* (*Bioética Clínica*). This was a natural continuation of *Foundations of Bioethics*. The first step was to analyze the clinical decision-making methodologies, which resulted in the book *Clinical Ethics Decision-Making Procedures* (*Procedimientos de Decisión en Etica Clínica*) (Gracia 1991), where I discussed the then current methodologies and proposed another based on the four principle approach. (*Clinical Bioethics*, incidentally, was never published.)

During the 1990s I became incredibly busy publishing articles on clinical ethics issues. The production was so robust, and yet so specialized, that it was impossible to collect it in a systematic volume. Thanks to the insistence of friends and colleagues, most of those published articles were collected in a four-volume collection, *Ethics and Life: Studies on Bioethics*, published in 1998 (Gracia 1998).

After my deep immersion in clinical ethics and its specific problems in the 1990s, I became even more aware of how much bioethics, as it is understood in Europe – and in Latin America – demands sound philosophical foundations. Thus, with the new millennium, I felt the compelling need to go back to the beginning and rethink the foundations of bioethics. I believe that the most characteristic feature of the past century's ethical thinking has been its attempts to go beyond the classic dichotomy between deontology and teleology, toward what is properly called the "ethics of responsibility." This is the ethics that I consider most capable. Today I am working on a new book, *Ethics of Responsibility*, which I hope will be my final contribution to the foundations of bioethics.

An ethics of responsibility needs a decision-making method. Over the years I have become convinced that this method is based on *deliberation*. One of the most urgent tasks of bioethics is to understand the history and basis of deliberation, in such a way that it can be taught and applied. This will be another book, called *Moral Responsibility*.

Teaching Bioethics: Spain and Latin America

My work in bioethics has not been carried out by myself alone, nor has it been restricted to the confines of my office. It has been carried out in the classroom, working hundreds of hours with students and doctors in innumerable courses in the medical humanities both at the medical school and postgraduate levels.

European regulations require that each country defines a number of core courses in the curricula of all medical schools. In Spain, bioethics was included in that core category, and my school, Complutense University, made it obligatory for all students to take two bioethics courses: Bioethics and Pain Management. This is the good news.

What is not so good is that bioethics was included in the second year of the medical curriculum. In our 6-year program that is too premature, because second-year students have had no clinical experience. It is a shame that in the clinical years the students do not have the chance to take a course on clinical ethics. I hope to fill this gap with a textbook of clinical ethics, which has a provisional title of *Facts, Values, Duties: Bioethics Textbook for Clinicians.*

In 1988, my department at the Complutense University organized a Master's program in Bioethics, which is still being offered. The first half of the 2-year curriculum is dedicated to the foundations of bioethics; the second year focuses on clinical ethics and decision-making methods. Inevitably, this curriculum traces my own personal voyage into bioethics. For more than a decade, the *Instituto Nacional de la Salud* (INSALUD) – the governmental agency that runs the Spanish national health care system – formed around our graduates Committees for Ethical Assistance (*Comités de ética asistencial*). The more than 300 Complutense graduates now hold key positions in public and private hospitals, government agencies, and IRBs, and constitute the next generation of my country's bioethics leadership. Graduates have created the very active *Asociación de Bioética Fundamental y Clínica*, which organizes a popular yearly congress and has published more than 11 books authored by its members. In 1996, in a joint effort with the Pan-American Health Organization (PAHO), the Master's program was offered in Santiago, Chile, where PAHO had recently opened a Regional Program of Bioethics for Latin America and the Caribbean. The curriculum has the same format and contents as that in Madrid, but the 600 hours of instruction is concentrated over two intensive 8-week retreats. Students and faculty live on campus during those weeks, which makes these courses a uniquely rich academic and vital experience, not least because of some puzzlingly different visions and sensitivities among students from different parts of Latin America, which – on another level – sometimes resemble the cultural gaps between American and European bioethics. Two groups of students graduated from the Latin American Master's program in Santiago between 1996 and 1999, another completed the course in the Dominican Republic in 2001, and yet another one graduated in Lima, Peru, in 2003.

Looking to the Future

I will perhaps never know if my contributions to Spanish bioethics were large or small. At any rate, I believe they have strengthened the independent identity of Spanish bioethics, which remains vulnerable to being overshadowed by religion and the law.

Religious organizations, particularly the most conservative ones, have embraced bioethics as one of their pastoral missions. The result is incessant activity, although the quality of these activities is academically rather uneven. Nonetheless, their campaigns strictly follow Vatican directives. We bioethicists have had to defend our identity and freedom of thought. At times this has been difficult, but this defense has proven fruitful.

The other struggle has occurred between bioethicists and the law. It would be difficult to imagine that bioethics was safe in a country that has more lawyers than Germany and France combined. Jurists, naturally, do have a role in this field, but that is limited to health law. The problem is that – in a very Mediterranean way – jurists tend to identify ethics with the law and reduce morality to legality. The problem for Spanish bioethics is that many jurists call this approach *bioethics.*

Perhaps these tensions come from the fact that, although bioethics is a new arena, it enjoys a positive reputation and prestige in Spain. It thus attracts many people, some of whom are moved by their own agenda. But after so many years, bioethics still has to elbow its way forward. But if bioethics has so many suitors, it must mean that our efforts are worthwhile. I am generally satisfied with what I have done. But I also have to confess to my mistakes.

I was wrong when I insisted that bioethics had to be hosted by the departments of history of medicine in Spanish medical schools. And it took me too long to realize my mistake. My thesis was that bioethics had to stay together with its epistemologically closest disciplines. I believed that history of medicine had that closeness with bioethics, as both were social rather than natural sciences. Spanish philosopher José Ortega y Gasset considered that those sciences should be called "humanities." And by following Ortega, I was wrong.

Social sciences deal with culture and values, but not with values in themselves, but rather with values as *facts.* This is why they are so specific and so limited. Ortega was wrong. Humanities cannot be identified with social sciences simply because humanities are not sciences. They do not even want to be sciences. Ethics has always been part of philosophy, not part of any science.

I am convinced today that bioethics should be studied – and taught – in specific academic divisions of medical humanities, which should be equidistant from both the departments of social and biomedical sciences. It is necessary that the medical humanities, and bioethics as its main branch, have their own life and autonomy. And their own, dedicated faculty. This way, society will judge bioethics and bioethicists by their works.

When that happens, we will know whether bioethics and bioethicists have truly provided a response to the real problems of Spanish medicine. And if we fail, we will have no one else to blame, for as Don Quixote said, "Everyone is the son of his works" (Cervantes 1990, p. 119).

References

Acosta J (1984) De procuranda Indorum salute [1590]. Pereña L (ed) Consejo Superior de Investigaciones Científicas, Madrid

Aristotle (1984) Politics (trans.) Jowett B. In Barnes J (ed) The complete works of Aristotle. The revised Oxford translation, Princeton University Press, New Jersey, pp. 1986–2129

Bai K, Shirai Y, Ishii M (1987) In Japan, consensus has limits. Hastings center report. Special Supplement, 17.3, 18–20
Cervantes SM (1990) Don Quijote de la Mancha. Cátedra, Madrid, p. 119
Cisneros D (1618) Sitio, naturaleza y propiedades de la Ciudad de México, México
Colón C (1989) Textos y documentos completos. Relaciones de viajes, cartas y memoriales, Consuelo Varela (ed) Alianza Editorial, Madrid
Sáenz de Santa María C (ed) (1989) Popol Vuh. Historia 16, Madrid
Douchet M (1971) Antropologie et histoire au siecle des lumieres. Maspero, Paris
Drane JF (1988) Becoming a good doctor: The place of virtue and character in medical ethics. Sheet and Ward, Kansas City
Gbadegesin S (1993) Bioethics and culture: An African perspective. Bioethics 7:257–262
Gracia D (1989) Fundamentos de Bioética. Eudema, Madrid
Gracia D (1990a) Primum Non Nocere: El princípio de no-maleficiencia como fundamento de la ética médica. Real Academia Nacional de Medicina, Madrid
Gracia D (1990b) I Problemi Etici Della Medicina Nell´area Linguistica Spagnola. In: Viafora C (ed) Vent´anni di Bioetica. Fondazione Lanza/Gregoriana Libreria Editrice, Padova
Gracia D (1991) 12. Procedimientos de Decisión en Etica Clínica. Eudema, Madrid
Gracia D (1993) The intellectual basis of bioethics in southern European countries. Bioethics 7:97–107
Gracia D (1998) *Etica y Vida: Estudios de Bicética.* This edition was prepared by my friend Germán Marquínez Argote, who selected, ordered, and edited the content of all four volumes. El Buho, Santafé de Bogotá
Guerra F (1971) The pre-Columbian mind. Seminal Press, London
Guerra F (1972) Medicina colonial en Hispanoamérica. In: Laín Entralgo P (ed) Historia universal de la medicina, vol 4. Salvat, Barcelona, pp 346–355
Guerra F (1975) El médico político. Afrodisio Aguado, Madrid
Guerra F (1990) La medicina precolombina. Ediciones de Cultura Hispánica, Madrid
Hanke L (1988) La lucha por la justicia en la conquista de América. Madrid, Istmo
Laín-Entralgo P (1961) Enfermedad y pecado. Toray, Barcelona
Las Casas B (1961) Historia de las Indias. Rivadeneyra, Madrid
Molina M (1991) La leyenda negra. Nerea, Madrid
Pagden A (1982) The fall of natural man. The American Indian and the origins of comparative ethnology. Cambridge University Press
Pereña L (1992) La idea de justicia en la conquista de América. Mapfre, Madrid
Qiu R-Z (1993) What has bioethics to offer the developing countries? Bioethics 7:108–125
Rivera M (ed) (1986) Chilam Balam de Chumayel. Historia 16, Madrid
Sánchez Agesta L (1987) La democracia em Hispanoamérica. Rialp, Madrid
Vespucci A (1986) Cartas de viaje. Alianza, Madrid
Vitoria F (1967) Relectio de Indis [1539]. Pereña L, Perez Prendes JM (eds) Consejo Superior de Investigaciones Científicas, Madrid
Xirau R (ed) (1973) Idea y querella de la Nueva España. Alianza, Madrid

Chapter 2
The Discourses of Bioethics in Latin America

José Alberto Mainetti

2.1 Introduction

Bioethics was born in the United States, and over time was adopted by (and adapted to) other countries. Among the countries accepting bioethics were those in Latin America, the name given to a linguistic and cultural community encompassing South America, Central America, Mexico, and part of the Caribbean. Because bioethics is a discipline whose discourse flourished in a North American cultural tradition, it is natural to compare Latin American and North American biomedical ethics. Latin American bioethics has evolved over a period of 30 years, in three decade-long stages commencing in the 1970s: reception, assimilation, and re-creation. As a pioneer of the process by which bioethics was institutionalized in Argentina, I cannot avoid some personal reference to my own experience, as a testifying witness (Mainetti 1987, 1990, 1995, 1996). Such an autobiographical narrative about the emergence of bioethics in Latin America can be justified by the comment of a well-known American bioethicist who said: "Identifying the origin of bioethics in the United States is a matter of some considerable controversy. But the Latin American bioethics story is to a large degree the story of one man." (Drane 1996, pp. 557–569).

2.2 Reception of Bioethics in the 1970s: Argentina's Pioneering Role in the Reception of Bioethics in Latin America

The 1970s were the reception stage for bioethics in Latin America. "Reception" should not be understood as a formal introduction of the discipline, since in the 1970s the term "bioethics" was not in use, even in the United States. Instead, "reception"

J.A. Mainetti
Instituto de Bioetica y Humanidades Médicas, y 18, La Plata, Buenos Aires AR
e-mail: elabe@netverk.com.ar

L. Pessini et al. (eds.), *Ibero-American Bioethics: History and Perspectives*, Philosophy and Medicine 106, DOI 10.1007/978-1-4020-9350-0_2,

refers to how the cultural and historical situation in the region made possible, or impeded, the inception of bioethics. The 1970s were characterized by reaction, either resistance or rejection, to this new movement by those who adhered to a traditional civic and professional ethos. As a liberal and secular morality, bioethics promoted patient autonomy, introducing into medicine the idea of the patient as a moral subject and emphasizing the patient's role as a rational and free agent, whose decisions are central to the therapeutic relationship. These ideas were alien to the old medical ethics still reigning in Latin America. At that time, Latin American medical ethics remained confessional, following the moral doctrine and authority of Roman Catholicism, and paternalistic. Physicians' practices were in accord with Max Weber's "domination role," in which the physician's authority is paramount and the patient's role is to submit to the physician's authority (Macklin and Luna 1996, pp. 140–153).

Initially, bioethics was perceived primarily as "made in the USA," an American approach appropriate to an American style of medicine and health care. American ideas, moreover, were bound to meet resistance because Marxist, anti-American attitudes were deeply entrenched in Latin America. Bioethics could not simply be transplanted into the Latin American context without taking into account cultural and political differences; consequently, the meaning of "bioethics" would have to change and adapt to those particular societies.

The first Latin American bioethics program was established in Argentina at the Institute for Medical Humanities of the José María Mainetti Foundation (1969). Dr. José Alberto Mainetti founded the Institute in 1972 and played an important role in the early bioethics activities in the region. Later, educational programs were developed through a Latin American School for Bioethics, under the direction of Juan Carlos Tealdi. Over the years, many scholars from the United States have participated in this project. The center has published since 1970 the journal *Chiron* and has produced several monographs on medical ethics (Figueroa and Fuenzalida 1996, pp. 611–627).

This institute fostered Latin American bioethical studies, under the influence of the Spanish School of the History of Medicine, led by Pedro Laín Entralgo, the father of Latin American medical humanism. Laín Entralgo's history of medicine provides a way towards a theory of medicine based on philosophical medical anthropology, which is inspired by European existential and hermeneutic philosophy. This intellectual movement created favorable conditions for the reception of the American medical humanities movement in Latin American bioethics.

The first decade of the Argentinean Institute for Medical Humanities recorded the reception stage of these disciplines, spurred in part by personal and institutional intercourse initiated with physician and philosopher H. Tristram Engelhardt, Jr., who was then at the Institute for Medical Humanities at the University of Texas Medical Branch in Galveston, and the physician bioethicist Edmund Pellegrino, who was Director of the influential Institute of Human Values in Medicine, based in Washington, DC. This medical humanities connection explains why Argentina and Spain were the first countries to establish bioethics in Latin America and Europe, respectively.

The medical humanities movement, in search of medical humanism, was much in tune with Lain Entralgo's medical anthropology, whose school of thought was joined by many Latin American scholars (Escobar 1996, pp. 651–657). The reception of bioethics as part of the theoretical perspective of the medical humanities therefore denotes a critical attitude, in the sense of challenging hidden assumptions and value judgments in both medicine and bioethics. During the 1970s, "postmodern medicine" emerged as a critique of positivistic medical reasoning. This criticism was far-reaching and affected the object, method, and end of medicine itself. That is, medicine was no longer a "normal science" in the Kuhnian sense but was in the midst of a moral revolution. Critical literature about medicine emerged, including Ivan Illich's famous *Medical Nemesis* (Illich 1976), Ian Kennedy's iconoclastic Reith Lectures, *The Unmasking of Medicine* (Kennedy 1981), and the critical social analysis of capitalist medical power by American writers like Vicent Navarro (Navarro 1975, pp. 65–94; see also Chapter 39).

"Postmodern medicine" owes its relativism to its increasingly comprehensive, interpretive, and evaluative nature – in short, to its reflexivity. The philosophy of medicine encompasses medical anthropology, epistemology, and axiology. The latter study would include bioethics in both its clinical and public health aspects. In this way, in Latin America we approached bioethics as the new humanist medical paradigm, and primarily an ethics "implied in" rather than "applied to" medicine, that is, an ethics derived from the intrinsic axiology of the medical profession. Thus, in contrast to the American development of bioethics, which involved physicians, theologians, philosophers, and lawyers, the Latin American protagonists of the discipline were mainly physicians and other health care professionals.

2.3 Assimilation of Bioethics in the 1980s

Assimilation marks the second stage in the development of bioethics in Latin America. The academic discipline and public discourse became institutionalized throughout the region and in this respect followed the American model. With the restoration of democracy and the introduction of new medical technologies in Latin America, such as critical care, transplantation, and assisted reproduction, public and academic interest in bioethics expanded in the 1980s. Assimilation reflected American bioethics in two ways: first, increasing malpractice litigation in medical cases and the movement for patients' rights imitated factors that led to the birth of bioethics in the United States; second, with the restoration of democracy came a renewed interest in moral and political philosophy, as well as ideological pluralism and consensus formation, which were then applied to medicine and became key components of the new bioethics, as in the United States (Lolas 2000a,b).

In 1980, the Mainetti Foundation launched a second stage of the institutionalization of bioethics in two academic settings: the medical school and the philosophy department at the nearby La Plata National University. The post-graduate chair of medical humanities provided the opportunity for reflection on a philosophy of medicine as a post-Flexnerian philosophy of the art of healing, rather than a reductionist model. Flexner's model involved the old positivist medical paradigm of medicine restricted to applied natural sciences. Latin American bioethics rejected this approach and turned to a new humanist medical paradigm that employed the social sciences and humanities to develop a theory and practice of medicine. In the 1980s, we continued to assimilate bioethics into the present philosophy of medicine. The chair of philosophical anthropology introduced bioethics as a cultural phenomenon, that is, the conception of a biological revolution that transformed human nature, and a new civic morality about health care.

The late 1980s witnessed the blooming of bioethics centers, institutes, and professionals around the region. The Colombian Institute of Bioethical Studies (Instituto Colombiano de Estudios Bioéticos) (Bogotá, Colombia) was founded in 1985, encouraged by the remarkable teaching of Alfonso Llano Escobar, S.J., from the Universidad Javeriana. In Venezuela, Dr. Augusto León C. wrote a classical text on medical ethics in 1975 and wrote the article on bioethics in Latin America in the first edition of the *Encyclopedia of Bioethics* (León 1978, 3, IV, C, pp. 1005–1007). The Universidad Católica de Chile created a bioethics unit in the School of Medicine in 1988, and several physicians participated in this program, notably Alejandro Serani and Manuel Lavados. The Pontificia Universidad Católica de Rio Grande do Sul, in Porto Alegre, Brazil, established a post-graduate program in bioethics in 1988, headed by Joaquim Clotet, a philosopher from Barcelona, Spain.

A radical stage of bioethics assimilation followed the critical reception stage in Latin America. Latin American bioethics' radical nature goes beyond philosophy of medicine to become a philosophy of culture and technology, moving from metamedicine to metaethics in seeking a fundamental questioning of techno-science. The novelty and seriousness of the problems concerning life today shape a bioethical crisis of the technological era. In this vital and normative crisis three new themes appear to be interwoven: (a) ecological catastrophe; (b) biological revolution; and (c) the medicalization of life. Bioethics became possible as a result of far-reaching changes in our understanding of the human condition and our increasing ability to transform the human body. From its very beginning, the Latin American road to bioethics has been a quest for humanity in the sense of a search for the basis of bioethics in philosophical anthropology centered in the new capacity to alter the body and to create an alternative morality (Drane 1996, pp. 557–569; Drane 1999, pp. 109–121).

2.4 The Re-creation of Bioethics in the 1990s

In the 1990s, a Latin American bioethics recreated itself in ways that incorporated the region's own intellectual and moral traditions. In most countries of the region, the bioethics movement was organized into three areas, academic (scientific research and higher education), health care (clinical and public health consultation, as in hospital ethics committees), and health policy (advisory services and recommendations to public authorities on normative and regulative issues). Concurrently with each nationwide bioethics network, regional associations have developed and propelled the Latin American bioethics movement forward. As a result, a distinctive regional ethical identity has developed in the Latin American bioethical model.

Founded in 1990, the Latin American School of Bioethics (ELABE) of the Mainetti Foundation was the first initiative of academic work in our area of cultural influence. It was established as a training program to create human resources for leadership within the country of the participant's origin, while providing a forum for cultural and scientific exchange throughout the region. The International Course of Bioethics of ELABE during the 1990s was chaired by prominent professors from the leading international centers of the discipline. The Centro Oncológico de Excelencia (Mainetti Foundation) launched the Federación Latinoamericana de Bioética in December 1991.

In 1990, James Drane of the United States was commissioned by the Pan American Health Organization (PAHO) to visit several countries in Latin America and to produce a report that reviewed the development of bioethics in Latin America. This influential report proposed several steps for the further regional development of the discipline (Drane and Fuenzalida 1991, pp. 325–338). In the same year, PAHO published a special issue on bioethics, edited by Susan Scholle Connor and Hernán Fuenzalida-Puelma, formally introducing bioethics in Latin America (Scholle Connor and Fuenzalida 1990). This is the first collection in which early authors in the field addressed diverse topics and developed different perspectives on the discipline. Finally, PAHO, a pioneer among international health organizations, created the Regional Program on Bioethics in 1994, with headquarters in Santiago, Chile, but whose activities were decentralized in order to serve all the member countries of PAHO. This program, designed to be a comprehensive policy in bioethics and its associate disciplines, is in a new stage, under the leadership of the outstanding scholar, Fernando Lolas Stepke (Programa Regional de Bioética 2000).

The re-creation stage reveals a third feature of Latin American bioethics: its global concern. Bioethics is encyclopedic by definition, etymologically "ethics of life" (and "life of ethics"), but not semantically circumscribed to the technological bios and the liberal ethos characteristic of the North American model. In contrast, the Latin American model emphasizes a human bios and a communitarian ethos. That is why bioethics is now more of a political movement or social reform movement than an academic discipline restricted to the domain of health care (see, e.g., Navarro 1975, Chapter 40). In Latin American bioethics, the principles of solidarity and justice play the central role that autonomy plays in North American bioethics. Thus, Latin American health policies embrace universal access to health care and stress distributive justice and equity in medical resources allocation.

This is not the place for a survey of bioethical developments in different Latin American countries, or for a review of the bioethical problems peculiar to the region (Mainetti et al. 1992, pp. 83–96; Tealdi et al. 1995, pp. 113–135). Bioethics has become a field of new challenges in Latin America. An apparent uniformity hides a rich, heterogeneous set of activities. Not only European and Christian influences, but also indigenous intellectual traditions are very important in the development of Latin American bioethics. It does not have its own philosophy, as Anglo-American bioethics is perceived to have, but it does have its own literature and narrative style. The particular historical setting, cultural ethos, and social reality of Latin America could infuse new life into the global bioethics community. In this sense, a symptom of the new times is the fact that the Second Congress of the International Association of Bioethics took place in Buenos Aires, Argentina, in 1994, and the Sixth Congress was held in Brasilia, Brazil, in 2002. A "new Brazilian bioethics" or "hard bioethics" has begun to flourish in recent years under the inspiration of the country's contradictory social reality, which explores alternative perspectives to traditional bioethical currents (Garrafa 2000, pp. 177–182).

2.5 Conclusion

This chapter has provided an account of the development of the incorporation of bioethics in Latin America over the past three decades, depicting this development in terms of three stages: reception, assimilation, and re-creation. Bioethics first arrived as a foreigner and underwent a cultural transformation. Transplanted to a land that was not its "natural" habitat, bioethics in Latin America has now taken on its own distinctive character and voice and has become a strong intellectual and political enterprise (Lolas 1994, pp. 28–30; Lolas 1998).

In comparison to the North American style of bioethics, Latin American bioethics takes a more theoretical and philosophical approach. As a search for a critical, radical, and global bioethics, Latin American bioethics represents a global, "post-bioethical" age (Drane 1988, pp. 53–64; Spinsanti 1995, pp. 167–176). Although Latin American bioethics is far from being a unified theoretical system or a single coherent perspective, it represents the *ethica spes* (ethical hope) of the new millennium.

References

Drane JF (1988) Universal medical ethics. Quirón 29 (2 June):53–64

Drane JF (1996) Bioethical perspectives from Ibero-America. J Med Philos 21(6):557–569

Drane JF (1999) Complejo bioético: Pigmalión, Narciso y Knock. Acta psiquiátrica y psicológica de América Latina 45(2):109–121

Drane JF, Fuenzalida H (1991) Medical ethics in Latin America: a new interest and commitment. Kennedy Inst Ethics J 1(4):325–338

Escobar Triana J (1996) Humanistic and social education for physicians: the experience of the Colombian school of medicine. J Med Philos 21(6):651–657

Figueroa PR, Fuenzalida H (1996) Bioethics in Ibero-America and the Caribbean. J Med Philos 21(6):611–627

Garrafa V (2000) A bioethical radiography of Brazil. Acta Bioética VI.1:177–182

Illich I (1976) Limits to medicine: medical nemesis – the expropriation of health. Marion Boyars, London

Kennedy I (1981) The unmasking of medicine. Allen and Unwin, London

León C, Augusto (1978) Latin America in the twentieth century. In Warren R (ed) Encyclopedia of bioethics, vol 3. Macmillan, New York, pp 1005–1007

Lolas Stepke F (1994) El discurso bioético. Una anécdota personal. Quirón 25:(December 4), 28–30
Lolas Stepke F (1998) Bioética. Editorial Universitaria, Santiago de Chile
Lolas Stepke F (2000a) Bioética y antropología médica. Mediterráneo, Santiago
Lolas Stepke F (2000b) Bioethics and the culture of life: a contribution to peace. Bioética Informa 6 (January 19). Programa Regional de Bioética, OPS/OMS, pp 8–11
Macklin R, Luna F (1996) Bioethics in Argentina: a country report. Bioethics 10(2):140–153
Mainetti JA (1987) Bioethical problems in the developing world: a view from Latin America. Unitas. A Q Arts Sci 60 (2 June):238–248
Mainetti JA (1990) Out of America: the scholastic and mundane bioethical scene in Argentina. Symposium Transcultural dimensions of medical ethics, co-sponsored by Fidia Research Foundation and Georgetown University Center for the Advanced Study of Ethics. National Academy of Sciences, Washington, DC, April 26–27
Mainetti JA (1995) Medical ethics, history of the Americas: Latin America. In: Reich WT (ed) Encyclopedia of bioethics. Macmillan, New York, pp 1639–1644
Mainetti JA (1996) In search of bioethics: a personal postscript. J Med Philos 21(6):671–679
Mainetti JA, Pis Diez G, Tealdi JC (1992) Bioethics in Latin America. In: Lustig A (ed) Bioethics yearbook, vol 2, Regional development in bioethics: 1989–1991. Kluwer Academic, Dordrecht, pp 83–96
Navarro V (1975) The political economy of health care. Int J Health Serv 5:65–94
Programa Regional de Bioética OPS/OMS (2000) Instituciones y centros especializados en bioética en América Latina y el Caribe. Santiago de Chile
Scholle Connor S, Fuenzalida H (1990) Bioethics. Issues and perspectives. Pan American Health Organization, Washington
Spinsanti S (1995) La bioetica. Biografie per una disciplina. Franco Angeli, Milan. Chap. 16: José Alberto Mainetti: simboli dell' antichità classica in America Latina, pp 167–176
Tealdi JC, Pis Diez G, Esquisabel O (1995) Bioethics in Latin America: 1991–1993. In: Andrew L (ed) Bioethics yearbook, vol. 4, Regional development in bioethics: 1991–1993. Kluwer Academic, Dordrecht, pp 113–135

Chapter 3
A Personal History of Bioethics in Latin America: The Current Challenge to the Medical Profession and the Influence of Pharmaceutical Companies

James Drane

3.1 The Beginnings of Bioethics

In the 1960s, Dan Callahan and I traveled around the world together. At that time, Dan was the editor of *Commonweal*, a national Catholic journal of religion and politics based in New York. I was at Yale University on a fellowship after having been suspended from the priesthood for writing an article advocating change in the Church's teachings on birth control. Dan was doing research on public policies on abortion in different cultures. I was studying different public policies on birth control. Both of us were writing books on these topics. What I remember most about our time together was that he missed his wife and children, and that he kept wondering whether he could leave his job at *Commonweal* in order to start an institute for the study of ethical problems raised by contemporary medicine.

Issues of ethics in medicine were very much in the public consciousness after World War II (WWII). First, there were the shocking ethical failures of Nazi physicians, revealed at the Nuremberg trials. Following the war, the US government invested enormous amounts of money in medical research. The ethical issues embedded in all the different research projects were supposedly handled by an Episcopal priest ethicist, John Fletcher, who was an employee at the National Institutes of Health (NIH), but he had too little authority, and the research projects were more numerous than any one person could monitor effectively.

Fruits of the enormous government investment, in the form of new treatments and new technologies, were arriving in clinical practice in a constant stream. Every new development raised its own specific ethical problems. Older ethical issues associated with the beginning and the end of life, which went back to before the

J. Drane
Director of the Russell Roth Bioethics Center of Edinboro University (Pennsylvania, U.S.A.).
Advisor of the Pan-American Health Organization - Program of Bioethics
e-mail: jdrane@edinboro.edu

L. Pessini et al. (eds.), *Ibero-American Bioethics: History and Perspectives*, Philosophy and Medicine 106, DOI 10.1007/978-1-4020-9350-0_3,

Second World War period, became more and more prominent. For example, Dr. John Rock developed the birth control pill, which raised ethical questions about its use and about legal controls on the sale of contraceptives.

Procreational issues like abortion and birth control were widely discussed in the media, in federal and state legislatures, and in the courts. The general trend was to remove legal restrictions. The debate was intense and legislators were looking for ethical insight. Doctors working in clinical medicine also needed help with ethical issues, once the post-war technologies arrived at the bedside. Many of the new technologies made it possible to extend a patient's dying and created questions about medicine's role process.

Finally, there were the more philosophical questions about the nature of the medical profession and the ends of medicine. By the 1960s, ethical problems existed everywhere in medicine, which called for serious study, direction for medical practitioners, and effective public policies.

Dan and I talked about these questions all during our travels together. About the proliferation of ethical problems created by contemporary scientific medicine, there was no doubt. The doubt was whether or not financial help could be found to establish an institute for the study of the ethical problems in medicine. Could he find enough grant money to start a medical ethics institute? This was the big question.

When we got back from this trip, he did two things. First, Dan finished his book on abortion, which had an important impact on Supreme Court judges when they made the *Roe v. Wade* decision. Second, he received the financial help he needed, left his position at *Commonweal* and started the Hastings Center. This was 1969. The establishment of this first medical ethics institute marked an important step toward the establishment of a new academic discipline that came to be called *bioethics*. The term bioethics is attributed to Van Rensselaer Potter in his book, *Bioethics: Bridge to the Future* (Potter 1971).

Today, the idea of medicine as separate from bioethics, in the sense of formal and systematic attention to ethical issues, is unimaginable. The new bioethics was much broader and more complex than traditional medical ethics. Once established, it spread quickly around the world, and today it is one of the defining disciplines of our age. No one could presume to understand the medieval culture without seriously studying theology, and in the future no one will be able to understand today's medical culture without studying bioethics. The discipline of bioethics defines us because medicine and health for us today are what religion and salvation were for western people of the Middle Ages. Disease, illness, surgeries, experiments, aging, enhancements, genetics, etc., preoccupy us and identify us. Ethical questions are bound up with every aspect of contemporary medicine. Professional associations like the World Health Organization (WHO), Pan American Health Organization (PAHO), American Medical Association (AMA), and similar medical associations in every country have to be concerned about ethical standards for medical research and medical practice.

Ethics has been joined to Western medicine from its Hippocratic beginnings. In fact, the classical philosophical ethics of Aristotle was medically based in the sense of being based on nature, i.e., the same physiology and biology that defined medicine. This bond between medicine and ethics continues into contemporary scientific medicine. Contemporary scientific medicine is German medicine, which links medicine with laboratory science. By the end of the nineteenth and early twentieth centuries, professional medical associations and German government authorities had developed ethical rules for medical research and medical practice.[1] We know, however, how quickly and how thoroughly these ethical norms were ignored by Nazi physicians who substituted a belief in eugenics for the classical background commitment to love and care expressed in the Hippocratic code.

In Nuremberg, after WWII, separate trials were conducted to address the crimes against humanity committed by so many physicians. The judges at Nuremberg formulated their own ethical code for medical research. Actually, this Nuremberg code was not all that different from the German government regulations so blatantly ignored by Nazi physicians. What facilitated the Nazi ethical violations was not the absence of ethical rules and regulations, but the absence of continued surveillance on the part of professional organizations, continued professional monitoring of medical activities, and continued emphasis on the ethical components of professional medicine. Withdrawal on the part of government and professional organizations from hands-on involvement with the ethical dimensions of medicine made possible the ethical violations which were condemned at Nuremberg. This is a lesson that cannot be forgotten without running the danger of having something similar happen all over again.

After WWII, the Nuremberg code was followed by ethical directives issued by the US government, the World Medical Association, the American Medical Association, and the Declaration of Helsinki. It was widely assumed that Nuremberg marked the end of ethical violations in medical research and medical practice. In the 1960s, there were many articles on medical research published in the United States, but great attention was not paid to the topic of ethics because it was assumed that the Nuremberg code and subsequent regulations had provided more than adequate direction for avoiding new ethical problems. Besides, the gross ethical violations committed by the Nazi physicians, people thought, could not happen in America.

Then in 1966, Henry K. Beecher, professor of anesthesia at Harvard University, dropped a bomb. In the *New England Journal of Medicine*, he published an article that detailed information about over 20 research projects that violated all the above-mentioned ethical standards (Beecher 1966). The similarity between these ethical failures in medicine and Nazi ethical failures was shocking. The ethical violations revealed by Dr. Beecher were done on the most vulnerable of patients, with government money, and presumably by good American physicians.

Rules and norms and codes had been in place for some time. One thing that was not in place was effective in-site monitoring of the research taking place everywhere. Many of the research subjects were patients who had gone to their doctors for help

[1] I am referring here to the Directive on Human Experimentation issued by the Prussian Minister of the Religious, Educational, and Medical Affairs in 1900. Then in 1931, the Reich Minister of the Interior published a circular that issued clear and concrete ethical rules for research with human subjects. These were even more specific and more far-reaching than the first Nuremberg and Helsinki directives.

and were turned into research subjects without being informed or giving consent. The established ethical controls did not work, because doctors and researchers had so many personal incentives to pursue what they believed to be important scientific objectives. The classical ethical virtues of a good doctor, as well as the ethical rules of ancient and modern codes, were both simply ignored.

Dr. Henry Beecher's revelations of ethical failures signaled the need for extensive reform in medical education and medical practice. This fomented a call for more supervision both by the government and by professional medical organizations. Dan Callahan's idea of an institute for the study of ethical issues in medical research and clinical practice seemed a very appropriate next step.

3.2 The Role of the Pan-American Health Organization

The WHO had expressed its commitment to ethics in medicine in the preamble of its constitution. The PAHO had done the same thing much earlier and had established an ethics committee at the Washington office to examine all research projects taking place within its region. Dr. George Alleyne, who later became the director of PAHO, was the head of the institutional ethics committee at PAHO for many years. During his years as director (1995–2003), he continued to emphasize ethics within PAHO.

Dr. Carlile Macedo, during his tenure as director of PAHO (1983–1995), had recognized that the review of research projects at PAHO's Washington office was not adequate to guarantee the required respect for human subjects. Under his administration, a conference on bioethics was organized in Latin America. Bioethics publications, originating from PAHO's Washington office, were distributed in all Latin American countries. But even this was not enough. Latin Americans needed to be trained in the new discipline of bioethics and then organized into official Institutional Review Board committees in order to monitor research activities on site. This need required a giant new involvement with bioethics on the part of PAHO. Rather than have bioethics essentially as a Washington-based project, the decision was made to train bioethicists in every country in Latin America and the Caribbean in order to make sure that medical research and medical education and medical practice were all involved with the new discipline of bioethics.

What led to the decision to amplify PAHO's bioethics projects was an ethical failure that bore a heavy cost. Certain American pharmaceutical companies wanted to move trials required for drug approval outside of the United States. In poorer countries of Latin America it was easier to recruit subjects for drug testing. It was also easier to avoid the restrictions imposed by the US government and professional medical associations. When some of the drug testing caused severely damaging consequences for the (mostly female) subjects, even death in some instances, PAHO was blamed for the failures. This created a crisis within PAHO. One change that followed from the crisis was a decision to create ethical monitoring committees in each country in order to provide in-place and hands-on oversight of medical research with human subjects. I came on board at PAHO in order to help with this project.

It was a series of subversions of medical ethics by pharmaceutical firms in order to advance their own economic interests that created the need to bring bioethics to Latin America in a more aggressive way. After all that has been done since then, all the educational programs that have taken place, all the new courses in bioethics at the medical schools, etc., the threat that first brought bioethics to Latin America has not been eliminated. Much has been done, but much remains to be done. There will be a bond between my generation of bioethicists and the younger generation now doing this work. We will be bonded by the values that we share, as well as by the need to address the threat to professional medicine that is still with us.

I worked with the bioethics project at PAHO during the 1980s. In the early 1990s, I traveled throughout the region to identify persons willing to be trained to work in this field. I worked with PAHO offices in each country, visited government officials, university hospitals, and medical schools in order to inform interested persons of PAHO's plan to promote bioethics. What I communicated in my contacts was the urgent need for an in-place functioning bioethics throughout the region in order to address both the ethical problems in clinical practice and the ethical problems in medical research. I also communicated my personal conviction that a Latin American bioethics would have to be developed in order to expand, enrich, and in some cases correct the North American and European perspectives. This project marked the beginning of bioethics in Latin America that was promoted and sponsored by the powerful medical organization (PAHO) responsible for the character and quality of medicine in the region.[2]

One thing is sure; in the years ahead, bioethics is not going to decline in importance or recede from the front-line concerns of professional organizations like PAHO. It cannot do so because today there are even greater dangers to the medical profession than were posed by the earlier ethical failures. Different academic congresses and seminars on ethics in medical research have been held over the years and have demonstrated the continuing need for PAHO support and for other independently sponsored bioethics programs. The bioethics issues and the need for ongoing attention to bioethics now go far beyond the area of medical research. Today the very soul of the medical profession is in danger.

Henry Beecher is one of the giants of medical ethics. He pushed governments and health organizations and research associations to develop ethical rules and policies, especially in the area of informed consent. But he did more than that. In the book he wrote in the late 1960s, he made the point that, as important as objective ethical rules are in medicine, they will never be enough to bring about truly ethical medicine. In his final major work, he made the point that only able, informed, compassionate, and responsible medical professionals can ensure that medicine meets its ethical objectives (Beecher 1970). The Latin American bioethics project

[2]For another version of the history of Ibero-American bioethics, cf. Drane (1966).

originating from PAHO aspired to create effective monitoring of research, and then to help create medical professionals who are committed to the high ethical ideals of professional medicine.[3]

3.3 An Ongoing Bioethics Project

During my travels throughout Latin America, I visited with medical school faculties and with medical association officials in order to promote a Latin American bioethics. I found many physicians who were interested in the new discipline, and I found persons who were already doing what I was trying to promote. In Argentina, I knew of a program in medical humanities that had been in place for years under the direction of Dr. Jose Alberto Mainetti. Dr. Mainetti and I had been educated in medical ethics by the same Spanish intellectuals.[4] Jose Alberto provided important help for the design of a PAHO bioethics project throughout Latin America. With his ideas, and the ideas of staff members at the legal offices at PAHO, and with ideas provided by medical professionals in all the different countries, a Latin American Bioethics Project was put into place. It was based in Santiago, Chile. It represented a collaborative effort by PAHO, the University of Chile, and the Chilean Federal Government.

My personal academic background included Catholic theology studied at the Gregorian University in Rome, and philosophy and ethics studied at the University of Madrid. Later, I studied medicine and did a residency in psychiatry with Karl Menninger in Topeka, Kansas. Because of my theology background, I was familiar with Latin American theologians. During my travels, I visited with theologians who enjoyed international recognition and had a particular interest in social justice, including the issue of justice in health care. I also made contact with several important Catholic hierarchs (e.g., Cardinal Evaristo Arns). For me it was important to develop a social justice perspective in bioethics, which in the United States and Europe was at best only a marginal concern. The Catholic universities and medical schools I visited already had medical ethics components, which they were very disposed to enlarge. Within a few years, with the help of an already in-place medical ethics base, a new Latin American discipline of bioethics was established and immediately started its own development.

In 1994, I spoke at the inauguration ceremony for the Pan-American Bioethics Program in Santiago. Eduardo Frei, then president of Chile, attended, as well as the president of the University of Chile, the director of PAHO, and many other distinguished guests. Ten years later, in 2004, I gave an address at the University of Chile in which I tried to describe how far we had come in the development of

[3] Some years later a book of mine was published in the United States that addressed the same topic of virtue and character in medical ethics. Cf. Drane (1988). This book was translated into Spanish and made available in Latin America. Cf. Drane (1993).

[4] I am referring to Jose Luis Aranguren and Pedro Lain Entralgo.

bioethics, and how far we still had to go. The bioethics that many had worked so hard to get established in Latin America could decline in importance. Indeed, it could fail unless certain ongoing dangers were recognized. In that talk I tried to refer to important aspects of the medical profession that I think are under threat and that bioethics must address. In fact, they may be under more threat today than they were in 2004.

Violations of medical research standards by pharmaceutical firms had generated PAHO's original bioethics campaign and my personal involvement with bioethics in Latin America. These have not been eliminated. Over the years, we found that there were physicians working in clinical medicine that had turned themselves into salesmen for certain drug companies and promoters for certain drugs. In the 1980s, there was a threat to the profession of medicine coming from drug companies, and it remains a threat after all that has been done during this first period of Latin American bioethics. A bond between first generation bioethicists like myself and those who are now carrying the bioethics banner is a common concern about the influence of an aggressively capitalistic pharmaceutical industry on the profession of medicine, the practice of medicine, and the personal ethics of physicians.

3.4 The Medical Profession

Let me tap into my seminary background and do a little Latin etymology. The term *professional* comes from the deponent verb, *profiteor, profiteri, professus sum*. It means to vow publicly, to make a public promise, to declare publicly a commitment. A professional is one who makes a public commitment to do good for others: to *bene facere*, to beneficence. The three historical professions in Western civilization are Law, Priesthood, and Medicine. By examining medical history, we can gain insight into the meaning of a profession and into its important ethical components. With this background preparation, we can then look at the contemporary situation of medicine and see the challenge facing the classical medical profession and the new discipline of bioethics.

A professional is one who makes a public promise to provide services that are considered crucial in a decent society. A professional is defined by the following characteristics:

1. Professions provide essential public services for the good of others.
2. To aspire to do professional public service is considered a vocation, a calling rather than just a job.
3. Prolonged specialized university training is a pre-requisite for entering a profession. The university-based education includes both theoretical understanding and practical training.
4. Control over entering a profession is through licensing; one must have a proper license to practice a profession.
5. License and admission boards are made up of members of the profession.

6. Laws having to do with a profession are ideally influenced by the profession.
7. Those who pay for professional services do not control or have authority over what is provided.
8. Professions enjoy autonomy in the provision of services.
9. Professions compose their own ethical codes and the ethical standards of practice.
10. Professions operate according to objective ethical rules and with subjective virtuous attitudes in practitioners.

All the characteristics of a profession deserve attention. Autonomy, high levels of education, the setting of its own ethical standards, all deserve special attention today. They are particularly constitutive of a profession, and today they are under serious threat. Society grants professional privileges in exchange for a professional's university preparation and a publicly declared altruistic ethic, versus a superficial academic formation and a selfish or self-serving personal ethic. Society grants individual autonomy, public respect, and a decent remuneration in exchange for being a good person and doing what is best for others.

The autonomy traditionally granted by society to medical professionals today is threatened. There are increasing pressures from different sources to control what physicians do. More and more frequently, physicians are treated like employees rather than like independent professionals.

The autonomy, respect, and monetary benefits historically enjoyed by the medical professional were never total. Society grants these benefits to professionals, and society monitors the way professionals carry out their promises. Are they truly providing needed services to others, or are they serving other interests? This is a question continually asked by society.

Monitoring of professions at the most concrete level, i.e., at the level in closest contact with actual medical practice, is not done by government officials. Governments do not have police just to watch over the behavior of medical professionals. Ethical monitoring is done by fellow professionals, medical associations, and professional medical organizations. The AMA oversees medical research and medical practices inside the United States. Internationally, World Medical Associations are responsible for maintaining ethical standards in medical research and clinical practice. Medical associations are the first line of ethics monitoring agents. If they do not perform this essential ethical monitoring and do not make sure an altruistic ethic is maintained in medicine, we have a situation similar to what took place in Germany during the 1930s.

Without maintaining a strong commitment to traditional ethical standards and contemporary bioethical principles, medicine loses its professional character and physicians slide toward employee status. The quickest way to undermine medicine as a profession is to ignore or downplay bioethics and professional ethical obligations. Every ethical failure in medical research or clinical practice invites outside control, and with enough outside control the profession of medicine is gone.

Without a strong and evolving discipline of bioethics and continuing involvement with bioethics on the part of professional medical associations, the future of the profession of medicine is dim. The involvement of professional associations must be substantial; perhaps the proper word is aggressive. The national and international professional associations cannot fulfill their ethical responsibilities by window-dressing-type programs in bioethics, any more than medical schools can fulfill their ethical responsibilities toward medical students by having them recite the Hippocratic Oath at graduation. A serious responsibility requires a serious commitment.

There is overwhelming evidence that the privileges so defining of a profession today are threatened. More and more physicians in the United States., Europe, and Latin America are workers in a health care industry. Obedience to orders from administrators of health care businesses or government officials, rather than autonomy, increasingly defines day-to-day medical practice.

The biggest threat today to a medical profession, however, comes from the pharmaceutical industry. Pharmaceutical firms are increasingly in control of more and more aspects of medical education and medical practice. This is true both in state-run and free-market health care systems. Bioethics came to Latin America because of concern about unethical treatment of medical research subjects. Bioethics today has to continue to be concerned with the pharmaceutical industry's influence on both medical research and medical practice. This is true in Latin America, the United States, and wherever contemporary scientific medicine is practiced.

3.5 The Pharmaceutical Industry's Influence

The pharmaceutical industry continues to increase its control over medical research. Its influence is enormous for determining which new drugs receive attention and which drugs are approved. Now, once a drug is on the market, the pharmaceutical industry moves to educate physicians. Education that historically and by definition is university-based and under control of the profession is gradually being moved by giant pharmas from academic settings to business settings.

Continuing medical education is necessary to retain professional medical competence. A certain number of hours of continuing education are required to retain a medical license. Meetings authorized to provide the continuing education credits for physicians are increasingly organized by pharmaceutical firms. They do the advertising for continuing education conferences. They pay the speakers and choose the topics to be addressed. Many of the speakers are employees of pharma firms, but even those who are not know who contracts them to speak and who pays them. For what once was independent and university-based, the continuing medical education system is now strongly influenced if not controlled by the pharmaceutical industry.

Day-to-day education about drug therapy takes place in doctors' offices and is provided by pharmaceutical salespersons. The salespersons (many of whom are attractive women) are trained to sell, i.e., to convince physicians to use their company's medication rather than other competitive products. Selling could be based on objective scientific communication, but that is not what is taking place. The sales representatives are schooled in ways to manipulate physicians rather than ways to provide objective scientific information. Salespersons are taught how to convince rather than how to educate. Most salespersons lack the educational background to be teachers of biological science. Physicians get free drug samples to pass out to their patients, but they do not get updated objective education about medications.

Even the approval system for medications is strongly influenced by the pharma industry, and consequently most of the new drugs approved are not new therapies. Rather, they are most often imitations of already available drugs (Angell 2004). This means that the system put into place to provide physicians with ongoing education about medications has actually been turned into a stage where actors compete to sell products. For good reason, salespersons bring gifts to physicians and invite them and their families to dinners and other types of entertainment. Salespersons who refuse to be manipulators and insist on being honest about the information they communicate first are warned, then downgraded, and finally they are fired.[5]

Sometimes, manipulation of physicians becomes even more direct. In Latin American countries, I found that some physicians were directly paid to use certain medications. In some instances I found that medical "research" was being paid for to show positive data and get new publicity for already-approved medications. Patients were often turned into "research subjects" without their informed consent. The most basic professional ethical principles of beneficence and truthfulness and respect were being violated for economic gain. Some physicians and some pharmaceutical companies cooperated to undermine the foundations of the medical profession. The subversion of ethics by large pharmas, which in the 1980s required PAHO to be involved with the promotion of bioethics, turned out to be much more extensive than originally thought.

A most recent reflection of the corruptive influence of large pharmaceutical companies on the ethical core of the medical profession is a fine paid by Pfizer for ethical violations. This pharmaceutical giant agreed to pay 2.3 billion to settle criminal and civil allegations of illegal marketing of a painkiller, Bextra (now withdrawn). 2.3 billion is the largest fine in history. The federal government's responsibility to protect patients from the dangers of inappropriate drug use was undermined by Pfizer's promotion of drugs for unapproved use. Patients were seriously damaged by company promotion tactics to doctors. This was Pfizer's forth fine for illegal marketing since 2002. The company not only engaged in criminal activities but did so over and over again. The illegal marketing of Bextra was engaged in while the company was paying other fines and promising to reform its practices. Pfizer's general counsel said once again that the company had reformed. From 2002 to 2009, company executives planned and carried out illegal marketing schemes. The illegal marketing of Bextra followed similarly harmful marketing practices for an epilepsy drug, Neurontin. The fine for this illegal activity was 430 million.

Sales representatives were trained to miseducate the doctors whom they visited. The miseducation was supported by gifts to the doctors, meals, invitations to resorts, money for attending meetings and other illegal incentives. For protection, patients are now advised to ask doctors who are prescribing medications, whether the drug is

[5] I have interviewed sales representatives of large pharmas who provided the evidence for the above statement.

F.D.A approved for their condition. The next likely government move will be to begin prosecution of doctors doing the off-label prescribing.

One remedy for healing a continuing education system controlled by pharmaceutical companies would be to insist that physicians focus on mainline medical literature and on education coming from the major medical journals. But even the area of professional education has not been immune from pharmaceutical industry influence.

Pharmaceutical firms employ persons just to write articles on their drugs. Then they pay academic physicians to "author" the articles and send them to journals for publication. Some "authors" re-do the material, others may slightly alter a text, and some just send the company article for publication. The percentage of articles in medical journals that are "manufactured" differs in different journals, but the fact that professional literature in some instances is being manufactured testifies to a manipulation even of the science of medicine. Pharmaceutical companies pay to manufacture articles, to influence the content of educational programs, and finally to have their salespersons teach doctors how to practice medicine using their products.

The issue of equity and justice in access to health care is one that needs special attention in Latin American bioethics. Current drug prices place health care beyond the reach of millions of poor people. One explanation for the ever-increasing cost of prescription medications came from an unusual source: Dr. Peter Rost, a former vice president of marketing at Pfizer.[6] Interviewed by a television journalist, Dr. Rost talked about the fact that drug companies are the cause of the continuing inflation of drug prices. People need the drugs. They will sacrifice any other purchase, even food, to pay for medications. Therefore, the strategy of the companies is to keep jacking up prices. Most recently, major pharmaceutical firms have adopted a strategy of charging thousands of dollars for a single dose of critically needed medications. In many cases, the pill is not even a new drug, but rather a new version of an older drug, usually for something serious like cancer. The pharmaceutical industries are taking advantage of patients in desperate situations and then charging thousands of dollars for a small particle of hope. If patients are desperate to hold on to life, not only will they exhaust savings on a helpful drug, but also these patients are not likely to initiate suits, thereby saving the drug company even more money. *Abraxane* is a "last hope" drug for patients with advanced breast cancer which costs $4,200 a dose. The drug company expects to make one billion dollars a year in annual sales.

The new drugs and many more like them exemplify a medicine only for the rich. The pharma industry is creating a contemporary medicine that ignores not just poor patients, but the very essence of the medical profession, which is a commitment to providing help to all patients in need. These new pills, focused on rich patients, not only take advantage of the desperate, but also undermine medical insurance programs and government health care systems. Governments cannot afford the cost of these medicines; neither can employers who provide health insurance for their workers.

Cancer drugs worldwide soon are expected to cost 55 billion dollars a year. Who can pay such a cost? Pharmaceutical companies threaten poor patients, the image

[6] Rost interviewed in CBS, 60 minutes, June 2005.

of physicians, and the whole medical profession. Social justice in health care, historically a focus of Latin American theologians, today is one of the most important issues in bioethics. Bioethics is concerned with many different aspects of contemporary medicine, but the pharmaceutical industry's behavior is one aspect that cannot be ignored. Its ethical misconduct launched the bioethics program in Latin America, and its threatening behaviors are still a cause of concern.

Justice and equity concerns in contemporary medicine certainly affect Latin American patients and professional medical practice in Latin America. It is an aspect of contemporary medicine that Latin American thinkers with deeply rooted interests in social justice must address. As important as these developments are for bioethics, they are not given anywhere near the attention which they deserve.

Why did Dr. Rost make his shocking revelations about how drug companies operate? "Everyday, Americans die," he said, "because they cannot pay for life-saving medications." The same is true of patients in Latin America. His reasons were a reflection of his professional consciousness. In his case, the traditional professional medical ethics, and the basic bioethics principle of doing good for patients, kicked in. This basic ethical principle of beneficence does not play a role in the conduct of most pharmaceutical companies. More and more of the most vulnerable patients are being abandoned. Is there any wonder that the large pharmas spend billions of dollars on ads that try to offset their bad public image? The ads emphasize the ethical values that should be promoted but are so often ignored that many ordinary people with infirmities are furious.

It was money that drove medicine and medical practitioners in ancient Greece. The Hippocratic healers not only developed a scientific approach to medical treatment but also developed a truly professional ethics committed to doing what was beneficial to the patient and avoiding whatever might be harmful. The Hippocratics distinguished themselves by their science and by their ethics. They separated themselves from those healers who were driven to manipulate the sick for money. Roughly 2500 years later we can see the same division in today's medical world. It creates a demand for the development of a distinctly Latin American bioethics, focused on social justice.

3.6 Conclusion

Who can make sure that bioethics remains vital throughout Latin America? Who can protect the integrity of medical professionals and the solidity of medical science? Who can protect the subjects of research and keep medicine focused on those most in need? Who can help physicians to keep their public promises? Who can make sure that medical education and medical research retain their integrity? Unless professional medical associations advocate for solid medical science and safe ethical research and patient-centered medical practice and social justice in health care systems, a noble medical profession will be in serious danger. There are serious challenges ahead for the discipline of bioethics in Latin America.

The discipline of bioethics was sent to Latin America in response to large pharma violations of basic bioethical standards. Patients (mostly female) were turned into research subjects and some of them died. Pan American Health Organization leaders accepted responsibility for the violations and in response organized a program designed to bring the discipline of bioethics to every nation in Latin America and the Caribbean. With sound leadership, good effects were made to come from bad acts. The spread of bioethics throughout Latin America is not a good that can now simply be left in place. Bioethics must continue to be taught and applied at every level of contemporary medicine. The bioethics project initiated by PAHO continues. The reasons that brought bioethics to Latin America have not disappeared. They plead for continued development of the discipline.

Dan Callahan did not invent bioethics, and Henry Beecher did not invent research ethics. They did not impose an outside set of concerns upon medicine. Both of these men recognized the ethical issues embedded in contemporary medicine, and they took action to address them. Imagine the number of persons who had contact with the same realities but did not see, or saw and chose not to act. And imagine the social and personal damage this may have caused.

At some point, persons who had an opportunity to be involved in the emergence of bioethics in Latin America have to step aside and pass on the work to others. If I played a role at the beginning, I am grateful to those who gave me this opportunity. Those of us working in bioethics during different periods are all related. We share certain experiences. We aspire to similar goals. We participate in a unique community of bioethics that stretches around the world.

I hope that there is life after our short stay here on this planet. I hope, too, that those of us who worked together in medicine and ethics will get to enjoy the presence of God, who communicated in creation the foundations of a universal ethics and in revelation the importance of compassion for those who are ill.

References

Beecher HK (1966) Ethical and clinical research. N Engl J Med 274(24):1354–1360
Angell M (2004) The truth about drug companies. Random House, New York
Beecher HK (1970) Research and the individual. Little Brown, Boston, MA
Drane JF (1966) Bioethical perspectives from Ibero-America. J Med Philos 21:557–559
Drane JF (1988) Becoming a good doctor. Sheed and Ward, Kansas City
Drane JF (2003) More Humane Medicine: A Liberal Catholics Bioethics, Edinboro University Presss
Drane JF (1993) Cómo ser un buen médico. San Pablo, Santafè de Bogotà
Drane JF (2003) Medicina Más Humana: Una Bioética Católica Liberal. San Pablo.
Drane JF (2009) Finding Relief from Suffering and Depression: The Role f Understanding and Faith. St. Paul's Press
Potter VR (1971) Bioethics: bridge to the future. Prentice-Hall, Englewood Cliffs, NJ

Chapter 4
Bioethics in Latin America and Colombia[1]

Alfonso Llano Escobar, S.J.

4.1 The Subject in Its Context

Bioethics was born in the United States, in the second half of the twentieth century, as a typically North American product, concretely as a "new ethics," with North American characteristics and meant to solve North American problems.

Bioethics was not born as a single bioethics. Already in its origin we find two interpretations – very different from each other – that would later multiply. The first is the one of Van Rensselaer Potter (1971), presented in his book, *Bioethics, Bridge to the Future*; he coined the word "bioethics," developing the idea of a new discipline and a world movement in favor of life and the environment, which were in danger. He conceives of bioethics "in a situation of emergence, as a dialogue between two cultures or knowledge modalities, scientific knowledge and ethical knowledge, with a view to the survival of Man and the planet Earth" (Potter 1971).

A.L. Escobar, S.J.
Jesuit theologian. Former-director and founder of the Center of Bioethics of Javerian University (Bogota, Colombia). Founder of Latin American Federation of Bioethics Institutions
e-mail: cenalbe@javeriana.edu.co

[1] To our knowledge, there are, for historical reasons, at least four Americas, very different in extension and culture, despite having in common the name "America." Florencio Galindo arrived at that conclusion in his valuable study, *El fenómeno de las sectas fundamentalistas. La conquista evangélica de América Latina*. He says:

There are actually four Americas, each one representing historically a territory, an experience, a style, a way of being; four Americas that have, through different ways, their own manner of expression, their culture: Indo-Spanish America, with a surface of 14,000,000 km^2; Portuguese America (Brazil), 8,500,000 km^2, English or Anglo-Saxon America (USA), 9,300,000 km^2, and Anglo-French America (Canada), with 9,000,000 km^2. Only the first has to do with Columbus; the history of the others started years, and even centuries, later (Galindo 1994, p. 95).

In this study, we refer to the Indo-Spanish and Portuguese Americas, those we generally call Latin America – to which are added the Caribbean countries. The name 'America' "is applied for the first time to the New World in the Cosmographiae Introductio, in Saint-Dieu (Vosges, Lorena, France), April 25, 1507, due to an exaggerated gratitude to the Italian cartographer Américo Vespucci: text of the poet Matthias Ringmann; attached map, of Lorena cartographer Martin Waldseemüller" (Galindo 1994, p. 95).

L. Pessini et al. (eds.), *Ibero-American Bioethics: History and Perspectives*, Philosophy and Medicine 106, DOI 10.1007/978-1-4020-9350-0_4,

The second interpretation is the one of The Kennedy Institute of Ethics, Georgetown University, Washington, D.C. The same year that Potter published his book and presented his proposal for a new discipline, Georgetown formalized and institutionalized bioethics by giving it academic support and understanding it as a medical macro-ethics, a trend that would prevail in the following decades (1970–2000) in the United States.

Bioethics was born in a scientific context (McArdle Laboratory)[2] and in a secular frame[3] – that is to say, nonreligious – in an attempt to make humane the fast growing new biotechnology and to allow patients to be heard as persons (Ramsey 1970),[4] for practical effects, in decision-making circumstances related to their treatment.

4.2 The Impact of Bioethics on the Contemporary Universal Culture

4.2.1 Characteristics

Possibly no other area of study or human knowledge, in the recent history of universal culture, other than bioethics has:

1. Developed so quickly
2. Changed so greatly the way individuals who study it see and deal with current reality
3. Included more fields of interest, not only of professionals, but also of average cultured individuals
4. Been called to have a greater influence in public life
5. Faithfully characterized and reflected the contemporary world.

4.2.2 Bio-Ethics

The two essential components of bioethics, bios and ethos, are perhaps the two themes of greatest interest and attraction to humanity at current. Let us examine these themes:

---

[2] McArdle Laboratory, Department of Oncology, University of Wisconsin.

[3] The secular context, that is, non-religious, wants to emphasize that this new ethics is not developed by representatives of some religion; and more than this, we cannot even say that bioethics has been developed, because one of the characteristics of the new ethics, or bioethics, is to be not completely developed, and if possible it will never arrive at this. It is a continuous work, especially in the universities. Without trying to lock it up in four walls of a definition, it could serve as orientation of the proposal, slightly reformulated, offered by the unit of bioethics of OPS, Chile: "Bioethics is the creative use of interdisciplinary dialogue in order to formulate, to articulate and, as much as possible, to decide on some of the problems that evoke current society to research and intervene in life, health and the environment."

[4] See "The Patient as Person" by Paul Ramsey, a Methodist priest (1970), a landmark work on the emergence of this new discipline.

1. BIOS: Consider some terms and expressions that have become topics of our life: the cult of the body, physique, yoga, aerobics, sex, eros, life, love, health, right to life, clinics, hospitals and health centers, UCIs, cells, human genomes, biotechnologies, biology, genetics, fetuses, tourism, trips, pleasure, happiness, freedom, and autonomy, among others. These terms, and their corresponding concepts, have become words and facts that arouse a passionate interest in all human beings.
2. ETHOS: In recent years ethics has become a universal, interesting, and worthwhile term of study, defining human behavior as morally good or bad. It is, however, a more adequate term for a secular, independent, and pluralistic society, than that of a "moral" (a term more common in past times) society.

4.3 The First Stage of Bioethics in Latin America: "The Transplant"

We will now discuss the origin and development of Latin American bioethics, according to our limited and modest knowledge and using the previously presented data to contextualize our analysis. We will give some general information about the origin of Bioethics in Latin America, without examining each country individually.

4.3.1 Antecedents

Given the unusual development of Bioethics, first in Argentina and subsequently in Colombia, Chile, Mexico, Brazil, and other Latin American countries, Bioethics was transplanted throughout Latin America, without consideration of the differences between the different countries and their peoples – without questioning whether this "plant" would give fruits in disparate countries, or, put differently, whether this new "medicine" was apt to cure the diverse problems or evils of these various populations. Here, we will talk about the birth and development of Bioethics in Ibero-America, that is, Latin America plus Brazil and the Caribbean Islands.

We warn that cultural, political, and even religious differences – in regard to poverty, underdevelopment, violence, political instability, religion, and so forth – outnumber the commonalities of these 25 or 30 countries. We will try to point out some historical data on the birth and development of Bioethics in Latin America and also to emphasize its strengths and weaknesses. Our study will be as objective as possible, offering updated information to erudite and non-erudite Latin American bioethicists including: on the one hand, data and reflections that make us aware of the strengths of continental Bioethics, as well as how to adapt and improve them, and, on the other hand, a brief panorama of their weaknesses and limitations and how to correct and surpass them as efficiently as possible.

An antecedent of Bioethics in Latin America worthy of consideration is the teaching of medical ethics and deontology promoted by the Pan-American Federation of

Medical Colleges and Schools (FEPAFEM) in the numerous medical schools of the different countries. Such teachings made medical ethics the primary concern of Bioethics, which became the dominant trend in the beginning years.

Bioethics as such was not known in Latin American countries in the first decade of its emergence in the United States (1970–1980), outside of the development of humanities and ethics and some references to it in the medical classrooms of Argentina, Colombia, and Venezuela.

The first stage of Latin American Bioethics, 1980–1990, is characterized by the phenomenon of a "transplant" of North American Bioethics to some countries in Latin America. This stage will be the focus of the following section.

4.3.2 A Contrast Between Two Cultures[5]

The typical problems of Latin America in the nineteenth and twentieth centuries differed greatly from those of the United States. Latin America consisted of 27 States that just achieved independence from Spain or Portugal, with the persistence of poverty, underdevelopment, and the domination of political and economic minorities that exploited individuals and the indigenous ethnic groups, preventing the establishment of true democracies. Simultaneously, scientific and technological developments were limited, due to a lack of human and financial resources.

Catholic morality (the source of medical ethics) directed private and public life in almost all Latin American States. Secularization was slow and difficult in some countries (e.g., Mexico, Uruguay, and Chile), while accelerated and delayed in others (e.g., Colombia). It brought the reduction of the public and private authority of the Catholic Church and the morality that it preached; yet, this morality was not replaced by a civil ethics (De Roux 1992) able to restrain either the abuses of politicians and rich landowners or the squandering of natural wealth and environmental resources.

4.3.3 Bioethics Revolution

Mainetti observed that the bioethics revolution consisted of *bios*, the "technoization" of life, and of *ethos*, the secularization of the moral. Together they constituted historical change resulting from bio-technological progress in the United States and the liberal and secular character of Protestant ethics. Further, these two facts deeply conflicted with "the pre-technical" culture; and the religious morality of Latin American countries (Mainetti 1998).

---

[5]This perspective is inspired by the introduction of Dr. José Alberto Mainetti's paper published in the second edition of "Bioethics in Latin America" (Mainetti 1998).

It is worth noting that when "transplanting" North American Bioethics – medical, principlist, utilitarian – to our countries, no one considered this conflict of values. This oversight can explain the many difficulties experienced in the first stages of acceptance, study and dissemination of Bioethics in Latin America.

More concretely, it is no surprise that the transplant of North American Bioethics, which was preoccupied with humanizing an advanced biotechnology inspired by Anglo-Saxon ethics, to countries which were little developed (both technologically and culturally) and strongly influenced by the Catholic morale, and influenced by a paternalistic and Hippocratic medical tradition, faced serious difficulties. To mention some:

1. Bioethics did not raise interest in the beginning.
2. There was no understanding of why and when one should begin to study it.
3. One did not know how to use it or when to apply it.
4. Bioethics began to be known and studied only as a new medical ethics, as were the cases in Argentina and Venezuela and, partly, Colombia.
5. States and universities ignored it.

It is no surprise that Mainetti wrote, in reference to this first stage, that: "the institutionalization of Bioethics, the creation of research centers and chairs in the university, committees of ethics in hospitals, national commissions of Bioethics, etc. are up to now – 1990 – not significant, and of course neither are the three main functions of bioethical studies programmatically fulfilled: education, welfare and politics" (Mainetti 1998, p. 4).

4.4 The Transplant and Development of Bioethics in Latin America

4.4.1 Argentina: Institute of Medical Humanities and ELABE

The Argentine physician, José Alberto Mainetti, a great humanist and a member of the Foundation Jose Maria Mainetti (in the locality of Gonnet, near the city of La Plata, Argentina), has the merit of having initiated the movement for the humanization of medicine that preceded the "transplant" of bioethics from the United States to Latin America in the 1970s and 1980s.

Mainetti, inspired by another great humanist, Dr. Pedro Laín Entralgo, founded the Institute of Medical Humanities in 1972, also located in Gonnet, which soon spread its humanistic ideals to the Southern Cone of Latin America through conferences, courses, and the *Chiron* Journal. At the beginning of the 1980s, Mainetti visited the Kennedy Institute of Ethics at the Georgetown University, in Washington, D.C., and began to invite esteemed bioethicists from the Kennedy Institute to attend conferences at his Institute of Humanities: specifically, Edmund Pellegrino, H. Tristram Engelhardt, Jr., James Drane, and others.

Later, at the end of the 1980s, Juan Carlos Tealdi, with the endorsement of Mainetti, founded the Latin American School of Bioethics (ELABE); the school, with the collaboration of bioethicists from the Kennedy Institute of Ethics, organized and taught for several years a 2-month-long educational program in bioethics. This program contributed significantly to the formation of present-day bioethics in Southern Cone countries.

4.4.2 Colombia Begins to Work

In the decade between 1970 and 1980, without bioethics being publicly known, a movement for the humanization of medicine, motivated by the great humanists of Bogotá and Medellin, began in Colombia, causing new medical schools to appear. These new schools absorbed the overflow of students from State medical schools and echoed the famous (1968) university revolts of Europe. These humanists, when founding the medical schools, made an effort to go beyond science, to contribute to the integral formation of the future Galen. It is worth mentioning a few involved individuals of great stature, including: Fernando Sanchez Torres, Jaime Escobar Triana, Juan Mendoza Vega, and many others.

During the humanization process of medicine, the Colombian Association of Medical Schools (more widely known in Colombia by its abbreviation ASCOFAME, a FEPAFEM branch) not only contributed notably to the design and implementation of educational programs in medical ethics at the schools, but also emphasized the importance of properly educating all medical students. In this contribution, Dr. Abel Dueñas Padrón, the director for many years, deserves an honorable mention.

Already in the years of 1980–1990 (and without special connection with Argentina), Professor Fernando Sanchez Torres, who had been dean of medicine and president of the National University of Colombia, along with a group of several professionals from differing branches, founded in December 1985 the Colombian Institute of Bioethical Studies (ICEB). The Institute established a seminar of bioethical studies that is still offered to date.

4.5 The Second Stage: Consolidation of Bioethics in Latin America

The second stage, 1990–2000, is characterized by an intense development of bioethics in all Latin American and Caribbean countries, which was brought about by three factors. First, the publication of an issue of the Bulletin of PAHO that soon appeared in book form, wholly dedicated to bioethics, at the beginning of the 1990s, which gave formal presence to bioethics in all Latin American countries. Second, the foundation of the Latin American Federation of Bioethics Institutions (FELAIBE) helped to organize the first centers of bioethics in several Latin American countries, and identified in each country a leader of bioethics for promoting the discipline. Third, the PAHO in Santiago, Chile, founded the Regional Program of Bioethics. Let us say a word, at least, about each one of these historical landmarks.

4.5.1 The Bulletin of PAHO

In 1991, Susan Scholle Connor and Hernán Fuenzalida-Puelma, from PAHO, in Washington, D.C., published the Bulletin of the Pan-American Health Organization, with a series of articles that appeared first in magazine form, and then in book form, on diverse topics of bioethics, written by authorities on the matter, and whose importance and broad dissemination formally introduced Latin America to bioethics.

Copies of this Bulletin – soon followed by copies of the book – arrived in the cities and on the corners of the Continent, and were almost literally devoured by doctors and health professionals interested in making a first approach to such a novel discipline. Soon, bioethicists from the United States were invited to participate in conferences about the subject.

4.5.2 Latin American Federation of Bioethics Institutions (FELAIBE)

In 1990, Fr. Alfonso Llano Escobar, S.J., working for the Colombian Association of Medical Faculties (ASCOFAME), founded the National Center of Bioethics (Centro Nacional de Bioética – Cenalbe), which was devoted to the study and diffusion of bioethics inside and outside of Colombia. Recently, Cenalbe (which is today linked to the Institute of Bioethics of the Pontifical Javerian University), contributed to the foundation of the Colombian National Association of Bioethics (Asociación Nacional Colombiana de Bioética – ANALBE) and to the establishment of the Intersectorial Bioethics Commission, created by a Presidential Decree in June 2001.

Years before, in 1991, Cenalbe had decided to found a Latin American Federation of Bioethics Institutions (FELAIBE) to promote the foundation of institutes and centers of bioethics in all Latin American countries. In order to make FELAIBE known, Cenalbe organized, from its foundation, forums and meetings in several countries of the Latin American Continent and the Caribbean.

Given the fast growth of bioethics in these countries, FELAIBE began to organize Latin American Congresses of Bioethics in 1995 to promote the knowledge and diffusion of bioethics, with great success. The first was in Sao Paulo, Brazil, in 1995; the second in Bogotá, Colombia, in 1998, with the presence of 1,500 people; the third in the city of Panama, in 2000; the fourth in Puerto Rico, in 2003. FELAIBE also publishes a quarterly Bulletin, named BIO-VINCULO (Bio-Link) that tracks the different bioethical activities in Latin America.

Cenalbe, affiliated to FELAIBE, also has the merit of having established the Programs of Specialization in Bioethics in 1995, the first of which was elaborated and taught by Cenalbe in the University of El Bosque, in Bogotá. Now there are graduate and undergraduate courses offered in the cities of Bogotá, Cali, and Medellín. At present, the University of El Bosque boasts a Doctorate program in bioethics, the first of its kind in the country; and Colombia offers the most graduate courses of any Latin America country.

4.5.3 *The Regional Program of Bioethics, PAHO*

Another decisive fact that has contributed to the development of bioethics in Latin America and the Caribbean has been, at the end of 1994 and in the city of Santiago, Chile, the foundation of the Regional Program of Bioethics, from the Pan-American Health Organization (PAHO) in close collaboration with the University of Chile.

We report with pleasure that the Regional Program of Bioethics has contributed much to a solid diffusion of bioethics in all Latin American countries. Besides conceptual and economic support to multiple activities organized by different countries, the Regional Program (Unit of Bioethics for Latin America, PAHO) offers to professionals from different sciences, since 1996, a Masters in Bioethics, directed by Professor Diego Gracia Guillén. The Masters program, now in its fifth class, is given in Cuyo, Argentina, and constitutes a true landmark in the solid and deepening study of bioethics in Latin America. For the previous 12 years (1998–2009), the Regional Program or Unit of Bioethics of PAHO has been under the direction of a true "scholar," Professor Fernando Lolas Stepke.

4.6 A Brief Summary

Two sporadic and independent, although very valuable, events laid out the first stage of bioethics in Latin America. That is, from 1980 to 1990, a "transplant" of bioethics from the United States to Latin America occurred, marked by: (1) the Latin American School of Bioethics (Escuela Latinoamericana de Bioética – ELABE), in La Plata, Argentina, and (2) the Colombian Institute of Bioethical Studies (Instituto Colombiano de Estudios Bioéticos – ICEB), in Bogotá, Colombia, founded in 1985.

The second stage, the establishment and broad diffusion of bioethics in almost all the countries of Latin America, was due to three remarkable occurrences:

1. The publication of the Bulletin of PAHO on Bioethics was widely disseminated in Latin America as a journal and later in 1990 as a book.
2. The foundation of the Latin American Federation of Bioethics Institutions (FELAIBE).
3. The establishment of the Regional Program of Bioethics, of PAHO, in Santiago, Chile.

Let us examine, although superficially, the remarkable responses given by some Latin American countries to the three factors we just mentioned.

4.7 The Fast Dissemination of Bioethics in Latin America

From its inception in 1991, FELAIBE's president spent the following years visiting the main countries of Latin America, publicizing bioethics and inviting people to found centers and institutes of bioethics. In each country visited, he identified individual leaders who had attended the forums and annual assemblies of FELAIBE and urged them to take charge of the study and dissemination of bioethics in one's own country. The first was held in Gonnet, Argentina, in December, 1991; the second in Villa de Leyva, Colombia; the third in Lima, Peru; the fourth in Guanajuato, Mexico; the fifth in Sao Paulo, Brazil, where, in 1995, the simple forum of previous years became the First Latin American Congress of Bioethics.

4.7.1 Pros and Cons

To be honest, we must confess that bioethics in Latin America has achieved great advances and merits, but it is also reasonably accompanied by some faults and deficiencies. Beginning with the faults, we must recognize that there are the following:

1. Minor disorder and lack of unification of human and economic resources.
2. Some improvisation: one repeats, omits, suspends a work, a center, a journal, and so forth.
3. A lack of self-identity: We tend to mimic the bioethics of other countries, especially the United States and Spain, without trying to develop an adequate Latin American bioethics, with foundations, tendencies, subjects, and problems of our own.
4. Lack of interest in bioethics on the part of some States. Latin America predominates in what we would call "private" or "particular" bioethics, cultivated in committees, commissions, centers, institutes, publications, undergraduate and graduate programs, among others; everything is organized to a large extent by the universities and hospitals. But the States, occupied by urgent and serious problems of public, political, and economic order, are not able to give attention and financing to the legislation and establishment of the National Commission or Council of Bioethics. There is more "political" or "public" bioethics in the United States and Europe than in our Latin American and Caribbean States.

Among the merits, it is fair to recognize that:

1. In spite of the limited economic and scientific resources, bioethics has been developed widely in almost all the countries of the Latin American Continent.
2. In different Latin American countries, graduate courses and degree programs have been organized in bioethics.

We would like to emphasize the presence in each Latin American country of one or two remarkable leaders who, through forums, courses, publications and other venues, have promoted bioethics. Let us mention some esteemed bioethicists, mainly the pioneers:

Mexico:	Professor Manuél Velasco Suárez (deceased), Dr. Fernando Cano
Costa Rica:	Dr. Hernán Collado
Guatemala:	Dr. Carlos Lara Roche

Panama:	Drs. Eduardo Sousa-Lennox and Luis Picard
Cuba:	Drs. José Acosta and Daniel Piedra
Puerto Rico:	Drs. Jorge Ferrer and Elena Lugo
Venezuela:	Drs. Augusto León and Alfredo Castillo Vallery
Ecuador:	Drs. Emilio Cerezo and Mary de Martínez
Peru:	Roberto Llanos
Chile:	Drs. Fernando Lolas Stepke and Alejandro Serani
Paraguay:	Dr. Alberto León
Uruguay:	Dr. Omar Franca
Bolivia:	Dr. Miguel Manzanera
Brazil:	Drs. Volnei Garrafa, José Eduardo de Siqueira, Leo Pessini
Colombia:	Drs. Jaime Escobar Triana, Fernando Sánchez Torres, Alfonso Llano Escobar
Dominican Republic:	Dr. Andrés Peralta

I offer my apologies to many other renowned bioethicists whose names are not mentioned here.

Virtually all Latin American countries are organizing different bioethical activities for the end of this decade, to mention some: congresses, forums, panels, activity days or weeks, hospital committees, institutes and centers, forums, journals, books, undergraduate and graduate courses and especially National Associations of Bioethics. So today, virtually all the countries of Latin America promote all, or almost all, of the activities we have just mentioned.

4.8 An Explanatory Note

The present work has a second part that will not be presented due to the limits of space. It is a collection of data according to a scale of parameters from almost all 27 Latin American countries. I had the good fortune to coordinate a team of 5 investigators who, over 20 months, worked seriously at accumulating data and interviewing bioethicists from the different Latin American countries, with the purpose of gathering information for the Data Center of the Institute of Bioethics – Cenalbe of Javerian University of Bogotá. The parameters, criteria, and questions that were followed in the interviews and the requests of data by electronic mail were the following:

1. When and how did bioethics begin in your country?
2. Who was (were) the leader(s) of the movement?
3. What centers or institutes have been created?
4. What are the main publications, works, journals, books?
5. Can you say there are specific grounds or a special trend in bioethics in your country?
6. What forums, congresses, or dedicated days have been promoted?
7. What are the main bioethics strengths and weaknesses in your country?

References

De Roux F (1992) Fundamentos de una ética ciudadana. Quirama 15:132–156

Galindo F (1994) El fenómeno de las sectas fundamentalistas. La conquista evangélica de América Latina. Verbo Divino, Navarra, Spain

Mainetti A (1998) Bioethics in Latin America. In: Reich W (ed) Encyclopedia of bioethics, 2nd edn. Macmillan, London, pp 132–156

Potter VR (1971) Bioethics, bridge to the future. Prentice Hall, New York

Ramsey, Paul (1971) The Patient as Person. Explorations in medical ethics, Yale University Press, Yale

Chapter 5
The Pan American Health Organization and Latin American Bioethics

Fernando Lolas Stepke

5.1 The University of Chile and the PAHO Bioethics Program

In a paper published in 1990 (Lolas 1990), I delineated the situation of Chilean biomedical ethics, its main issues, and its potential developments. At the time, Chile was under military rule, and professional associations had lost ethical oversight of their associates. Additionally, medical schools devoted no more than 6% of their academic hours to teaching the humanistic and ethical aspects of medicine, and bioethics as such did not appear in curricula, publication titles, or associations.

However, during the 1990s, a strong movement began. The University of Chile established a bioethics commission in 1991, which was formalized in 1992 and organized a meeting entitled the "Institutionalization of Bioethics" that same year. In 1993, the Interdisciplinary Center for the Study of Bioethics was formally established and began work compiling existing information and forming strategic alliances with other institutions (Lolas 1998). Among the institutions selected, the Pan American Health Organization (PAHO) proved to be the most important. Its prestige among health care workers, the wide scope of its activities, and the commitment of its authorities were particularly important for establishing a fruitful association.

5.2 The Involvement of PAHO

In 1994, the PAHO and the regional office of the World Health Organization (WHO), in association with the University of Chile and the Chilean Government, created a regional bioethics program. Its purpose was to serve the needs of the countries and territories of the Americas and the Caribbean by providing the necessary

F.L. Stepke
MD, Psychiatry, University of Chile. Full Professor - Medical College - University of Chile
Director of the Bioethics Program of the Pan-American Health Organization and the Interdisciplinary Center for Bioethics Studies (University of Chile).
e-mail: lolas@chi.ops-oms.org

L. Pessini et al. (eds.), *Ibero-American Bioethics: History and Perspectives*, Philosophy and Medicine 106, DOI 10.1007/978-1-4020-9350-0_5,

assistance to stimulate reform in their health care systems, to improve their scientific infrastructure, and to provide essential medical and sanitary services for their populations (Lolas 2004).[1] Additionally, the PAHO initiative was contemporaneous with the establishment of UNESCO's International Bioethics Commission, created for the purpose of addressing the challenges posed by genomic research and the advancement of knowledge in the biological sciences. In 2002, a unit was created at the WHO Headquarters in Geneva to serve as a counterpart to the PAHO program, whose responsibilities included ethics, trade, and human rights.

5.3 Education and Training

During the first years of the program, funding was obtained for programs aimed at training a cadre of professionals conversant in bioethics within the Americas and the Caribbean. Advanced programs were established at the diplomate and Master's levels in several universities, and short courses were also delivered or sponsored in more than 25 countries, allowing for the exposure of more than 300 professionals to bioethical concepts and practices. Professor Diego Gracia of the Complutense University in Madrid, Spain, assisted in the establishment of the Master's programs at the University of Chile, the Technological Institute of Santo Domingo, the San Marcos University in Lima, Perú, and the National University of Cuyo, Argentina. In addition, program staff participated in educational activities at other institutions and developed a series of seminars devoted to bioethics and meant to serve the needs of professionals from all over the continent.[2] Educational materials were also prepared and distributed, including several books now widely used for teaching purposes.[3] As an addition to the virtual health library developed by the Biblioteca Regional de Medicina and BIREME, located in Sao Paulo, Brazil, a virtual library dedicated to bioethics was created.

During this initial period, the legitimization of bioethics within the context of an international service organization was also challenged. Some critics indicated that bioethics should be regarded as a luxury and, to some extent, an irrelevant concern in comparison with other, more pressing, health care needs. Therefore, it was necessary to demonstrate the practical application of bioethics and its relevance for actual needs. In this vein, it should be observed that bioethics deals with the quality of services and excellence in research, both essential components of patient satisfaction and the correct prioritization of policies. The improvements to undergraduate training and the incorporation of bioethics into the curriculum of different professional fields, including medicine, nursing, and select areas of the biological and environmental sciences, also evidence this people-centered approach.

---

[1] The contributions of James Drane and Hernán Fuenzalida in establishing this program should be noted (Drane and Fuenzalida 1991).

[2] A synopsis of the reports of these activities is available at the Web site: www.paho.org/bioetica.

[3] A complete list of publications can be found at http://www.paho.org/bioetica.

5.4 Research and Advocacy

Aside from training professionals, the program also responded to the demands of groups and organizations for information and advocacy. Program staff answered questions and gave opinions on matters of public policy, in addition to advising the implementation of ethical guidelines. It also began publishing a quarterly newsletter[4] and a scholarly journal,[5] which, in a few years' time, became standard reading for Latin American and Caribbean scholars and practitioners. As part of its dispersion initiative, bioethical cases were also presented in the form of illustrated stories (comics) for young audiences, to be used in the classroom and other settings.

A special program on bioethics and oral health was established under the sponsorship of an NIH-Fogarty International Center funded grant, which produced a newsletter,[6] additional publications, special meetings, and studies focusing on the role of bioethics in the curriculum of dental schools. The program also contributed to translating international guidelines and organizing seminars on its content, tailored to different audiences, which proved instrumental for bringing individuals together from different backgrounds and orientations to disseminate the material.

Shortly after its establishment, the PAHO bioethics program began collecting data on persons and institutions. Comprehensive databases on training opportunities, research projects, and publications were assembled, and surveys were published regarding biomedical publications, funding agencies, codes of ethics, and relevant legislation. In addition, an international advisory board of renowned bioethicists and the contributions of PAHO representatives within the countries helped to establish the guiding principles of the bioethics program.

With a limited budget but efficient fundraising actions and the cooperation of the University of Chile and the Chilean government, the PAHO bioethics program positioned itself as a referent, not only in the region relevant to the PAHO, but also in other parts of the world. The relevant issues of priority for the program included the creation of ethics committees in the areas of research and clinical care, the establishment of national bioethics commissions, and professional trainings. These efforts contributed to the better administration of resources, a broader concept of quality care (including ethical principles), an increased satisfaction among health care practitioners and researchers, and the provision of better information of general interest to the public. Bioethics seeks to answer those questions prompted by the application of science and technology in human affairs by employing dialogue as a means to challenge beliefs, dogma, and opinions and to arrive at ethically sustainable solutions. The program and its activities have emphasized the importance of this

---

[4] Bioética Informa, ISSN 0717-6112.

[5] Acta Bioethica, ISSN 0717-5906, continuation in 2000 of Cuadernos del Programa Regional de Bioética.

[6] Salud Oral y Bioética, ISSN 0718-2392.

Table 5.1 Summary of Activities and Products of the PAHO Bioethics Program

Courses	Publications	Interventions	Alliances	Other activities
Training	Scholarly journal	Response to inquiries	Academic institutions	Advocacy
				Surveys
	Newsletter		Other agencies	Data bases
Specialization	Books	Establishment of ethics committees	Industry	Public dissemination of information
Curriculum development				

dialogical process and the participation of all stakeholders in health-related decisions. Some of the activities and products of the PAHO bioethics program are presented in Table 5.1.

In the Americas and the Caribbean, bioethical practices and deliberations are particularly important. In some countries, the high inequity of access to health care, the continued threat of corruption, and poverty that affects almost half of the population continue to be issues. Furthermore, political instability and the pervasive influence of transnational capital affect the continuity of governmental decisions. Health care professionals and researchers also tend to experience frustration and anger at not having enough resources to fulfill their roles.

Significant developments in these countries have occurred; however, their intensity and salience have varied from country to country. Nonetheless, bioethics has become a standard word and institutions commonly request advice pertaining to bioethical issues. A good measure of the impact of PAHO and other agencies is the establishment of ethics committees and national bioethics commissions. Additional products of the bioethical sensibility brought about by the program are better research practices and cooperation, although these remain hard to assess.

The bioethics program is responsible for monitoring the quality of Latin American and Caribbean academic activities, establishing new educational and research programs, promoting the creation of facilities, and assisting interested parties in preparing research proposals for international funding agencies. Additionally, the meetings of the International Advisory Board, established by former PAHO Director, Sir George Alleyne, have served to address a number of significant bioethical issues (e.g., Lolas 2000; Lolas and Agar 2002; Lolas and Quezada 2003).

5.5 Future Challenges

The pioneering efforts of the PAHO have successfully demonstrated a practical need for bioethics and have also responded to this need appropriately.

In the interest of continuing to fulfill its role, PAHO should strengthen its character as a knowledge-based organization that not only fosters the acquisition and application of relevant information but also considers the moral implications of knowledge and efficient action. This can be achieved with the establishment of a program meant to address these issues and comprised of respected practitioners, irrespective of their country of origin, their academic affiliation, or their profession. The relationship between PAHO representatives and the bioethics program, which serves to provide specialized assistance to a majority of countries, is a good example of a concerted effort to develop country-focused action. PAHO has successfully responded to the needs of the countries within the region of the Americas and the Caribbean (Lolas 1999). However, to evaluate its public service mission in bioethics and its influence on research and health care, some considerations are necessary.

By establishing bioethics as a legitimate field of intellectual activity, meant to provide guidance for proper action, the risk of creating a group of people requiring recognition and convinced of their own superiority in matters of moral judgment is high. At this point in its development, it appears unwise to professionalize the field of bioethics. The focus should remain on training professionals to engage in bioethical deliberation and the dissemination of bioethical principles among various populations. However, in the future, advanced scholarship will be indispensable for providing unique contributions to the field and stimulating further development. True experts do not conflate ethical deliberation and political indoctrination and understand the basic need for tolerance and dialogue, which is essential to bioethics. They do not engage in demagogic claims about originality and imperialism and strive to bring fresh insights into perennial problems.

Educating the population is also part of the bioethical enterprise. Since its fundament is dialogue, individuals should acquire the skills necessary to engage in dialogue. This implies a concerted effort on the part of experts, academic institutions, self-help groups, and public services. A well-educated community is better informed and confident about its own resources, does not have unrealistic demands of its service providers, and develops a sense of solidarity that is a precondition for a good quality of life.

The bioethics program of PAHO should receive support in accord with the evolution of the field. However, its presence in the moral debate is justified on several grounds. First, radical groups may use bioethics to sustain their arguments or disseminate particular beliefs. Second, industry may find arguments for aggressive interventions rendering economic gains. Third, governments may employ bioethical discourse for legitimizing inappropriate or authoritarian practices. And, as a response to these concerns, PAHO, as a specialized cooperation agency, is able to guarantee expert neutrality in matters of common interest to minorities and majorities, therefore reducing the danger of misusing moral arguments for economic or political aims.

The primary challenge is to work for the common good of the people of the Americas and the Caribbean, free from economic or ideological constraints, while engendering confidence and respect from the people by remedying practices of discrimination and exclusion. In matters of health, everyone counts and the aim continues to be: "Health for all, by all, with all".

References

Drane JF, Fuenzalida H (1991) Medical ethics in Latin America: a new interest and commitment. Kennedy Inst Ethics J 1(4):325–338
Lolas F (1990) Bioethics in Chile: present and future status. In Scholle Connor S, Fuenzalida-Puelma H (eds) Bioethics: issues and perspectives. Pan American Health Organization, Washington, DC, pp 150–154
Lolas F (1998) Bioética en la Universidad de Chile, Anales de la Universidad de Chile, Sexta Serie, 8, 13–18
Lolas F (1999) La bioética en el contexto de los programas globales de salud, Revista Panamericana de Salud Pública, Washington, 6.1, 65–68
Lolas F (ed) (2000) Bioética y cuidado de la salud. Equidad, calidad, derechos. Santiago de Chile Programa Regional de Bioética, Organización Panamericana de la Salud, Santiago de Chile
Lolas F (ed) (2004) Diálogo y cooperación en salud. Diez años de bioética en la OPS. Unidad de Bioética OPS/OMS, Santiago de Chile
Lolas F, Agar L (eds) (2002) Interfaces between bioethics and the empirical social sciences. Programa Regional de Bioética, Organización Panamericana de la Salud, Santiago de Chile
Lolas F, Quezada A (eds) (2003) Pautas éticas de investigación en sujetos humanos: nuevas perspectivas. Programa Regional de Bioética, Organización Panamericana de la Salud, Santiago de Chile

Part II
Reflections from Pioneering Voices

Chapter 6
References to Bioethics in Argentina[1]

José Alberto Mainetti and Marta Lucia Perez

6.1 Introduction

The present survey of Argentinean bioethics institutions is not exhaustive but illustrates its present development in the country. Thus, it mentions the main academic institutions (study, research, and teaching centers), assistance or welfare institutions (ethics committees, commissions, and boards), and public policy institutions (legislation and jurisprudence). It also mentions a few national publications on bioethics and web sites maintained by institutions and organizations.

6.2 Study Centers

The first antecedents that shape the development of bioethics in Argentina are, namely, the Institute of Medical Humanities (Instituto de Humanidades Médicas) of the Mainetti Foundation and its continuity in the homonymous University Chair and the Latin American School of Bioethics (Escuela Latinoamericana de Bioética – ELABE). The culture of the discipline now covers the national map almost completely. Among the study centers, we emphasize the professional associations, the university chairs and other institutes and programs listed below.

J.A. Mainetti
Ph.D. Medicine, Philosophy. President of Fundação Dr. José M. Mainetti para o Progresso da Medicina (Foundation Dr. José M. Mainetti for the Progress of Medicine), Buenos Aires - Argentina
e-mail: elabe@netverk.com.ar

M.L. Perez
Has an undergraduate degree in Medical Philosophy. Associated to the Medical Philosophy discipline of the College of Medical Science of Universidad Nacional de La Plata, Argentina
e-mail: elabe@netverk.com.ar

[1] We would like to thank Drs. Pedro F. Hooft, Juan Carlos Tealdi and Eduardo L. Tinant for the information.

L. Pessini et al. (eds.), *Ibero-American Bioethics: History and Perspectives*, Philosophy and Medicine 106, DOI 10.1007/978-1-4020-9350-0_6,

6.2.1 Professional Associations

Asociación Argentina de Bioética [Argentinean Bioethics Association]
Asociación Argentina de Investigaciones Éticas [Argentinean Association for Ethical Research]
Bio & Sur, Asociación de Bioética y Derechos Humanos (Bs. As.) [Association of Bioethics and Human Rights]
Latin American Federation of Bioethics Institutions (FELAIBE)
Argentinean Academy of Ethics in Medicine

6.2.2 University Chairs

Graduate Chair of Medical Humanities (Medical Sciences School, Universidad Nacional de La Plata, 1980)
Medical Philosophy (School of Medical Sciences, Universidad Nacional de La Plata, 2006)
Academic Unit of Bioethics, Medical School of Universidad de Buenos Aires
Master's Course in Bioethics of the Medical School of the Universidad Nacional de Córdoba
Master's Course in Bioethics of the Pontifical Catholic University of Argentina
Biomedical Ethics (Universidad del Salvador)
Master's Course in Bioethics of the Medical School of the National University of Cujo
Master's Course in Biomedical Ethics, Catholic University of Argentina
Master's Course in Applied Ethics – Bioethics, Universidad de Lanús
Master's Course in Applied Ethics – Bioethics, School of Philosophy (Universidad de Buenos Aires)
Master's Course in Legal Bioethics (School of Legal and Social Sciences, Universidad Nacional de La Plata)

6.2.3 Programs and Institutes

Institute of Bioethics and Medical Humanities (Mainetti Foundation)
Institute of Biomedical Ethics (School of Health Sciences, Pontifical Catholic University of Argentina, Buenos Aires)
Institute of Bioethics (Universidad Católica de La Plata)
Institute of Bioethics (Universidade do Museu Social da Argentina – UMSA)
Thematic Interdisciplinary Program in Bioethics (Universidad Nacional de Mar del Plata)
Proyecto Bioética [Bioethics Project] (Facultad Latinoamericana de Ciencias Sociales, FLACSO-Argentina)
Program of Bioethics, Fraternitas Foundation, Rosario, Santa Fe

Centro Cuyano de Estudos Bioéticos (Center of Bioethical Studies, Cuyo)
Centro de Investigaciones Bioéticas (Center of Bioethical Research), Universidad Nacional del Sur
Bioethics Center – Universidad Católica de Córdoba
Biomedical Study Center, Universidad CAECE, Buenos Aires
Centro de Investigaciones de Filosofía Jurídica y Filosofía Social [Research Center of Legal Philosophy and Social Philosophy], Universidad Nacional de Rosario
Center of Bioethics of the University Juan Agustín Maza
Ethics Research Center "Rizieri Frondizi", Universidad de Lanús
Department of Bioethics (School of Biomedical Sciences, Universidad Austral)

6.3 Ethics Committees, Commissions, and Boards

The Mainetti Foundation should also be included in the antecedents of Argentinean ethics, as the first mention of them was in an article by José A. Mainetti in the journal *Chiron* (1984, 15:2/4, 5–8), entitled "Philosophers at the Hospital: Hospital Ethics Committees" ("Filósofos al hospital: los comités hospitalarios de ética"), followed years later by another article by Juan Carlos Tealdi and José Alberto Mainetti, "Hospital Ethics Committees" ("Comités Hospitalarios de Ética") (PAHO Bulletin 1990; 24:410–18).

In the last article mentioned, ethics committees were identified from: the Hospital of Clinics of Buenos Aires, the Service of Neonatology of the Italian Hospital of Buenos Aires, the Oncology Excellence Center of the Mainetti Foundation, the Emilio Civit Hospital de Mendoza, and the Francisco Muñiz Infectious Diseases Hospital of Buenos Aires. The Latin American School of Bioethics of the Mainetti Foundation supported the non-governmental initiative of the Regional Network of Ethics Committees (1990), whose activities strengthened the objective of cooperation within the network – including bioethics committees and specialists from different Latin American countries. Until 1999, the network had the institutional support of the Mainetti Foundation, and in the year 2000 that support was offered by the Bio & Sur Bioethics and Human Rights Association. Finally, in the 1990s, three national bioethics commissions were created – one by the Secretary of Science and Technique of the Presidency and two by the Ministry of National Health – but all of them turned out to be frustrated attempts. Although a national system of biomedical research review committees does not yet exist in Argentina, a new proposal for the establishment of the Council of Ethics and Human Rights for Biomedical Research has been proposed by the Secretary of Human Rights of the Ministry of Justice and Human Rights.

Below is a list of current Argentinean references according to EULABOR (Latin American and European Ethical Regulation Systems of Biomedical Research: Comparative Analysis of their Pertinence and Application for Human Subjects Protection) (Eulabor, WP2, Argentina, P6): Ethical Review of Biomedical Research in Argentina (Revisión Ética de la Investigación Biomédica en Argentina).

This regulates the creation of ethics committees and commissions, as well as the protection of research subjects, data privacy, and patients' rights:

República Argentina, Ministerio de Salud, Disposición 3916/85, "Normas para solicitar autorizaciones para realizar investigación en Farmacología Clínica"
República Argentina, Ley 24.742/96, Poder Ejecutivo Nacional, crea los Comités Hospitalarios de Ética
República Argentina, Decreto del Poder Ejecutivo Nacional 426 – 1998, Crea la Comisión Nacional de Ética Biomédica
República Argentina, Ley 25.326 (Regl. Art. 43ª C.N.) sobre Protección de Datos Personales y Habeas Data
Republica Argentina, Administración Nacional de Medicamentos, Alimentos y Tecnología, Disposición 5330/97, de Buenas Prácticas de Farmacología de Investigación Clínica
Provincia de Buenos Aires, Ley 11.044/91 sobre Protección de Personas que participan en Investigaciones Biomédicas
Gobierno de La Ciudad de Buenos Aires, Resolución 2575/SS/01, crea Foro AD-HOC en Bioética
Provincia de Río Negro, Ley 3076/97, sobre Derechos de los pacientes
Provincia de Río Negro, Ley 3028/96, sobre Regulación de la Investigación Clínica
Provincia de Tucumán, Ley 6952/99, sobre Derechos de los Pacientes
Provincia de Catamarca, Ley 5057/01, sobre Creación del Comité de Ética de la Investigación
Provincia de Chaco, Ley 4781/00, sobre Consejo Provincial de Bioética
Provincia de Jujuy Ley 5009/97, sobre Consejo Provincial de Bioética

6.4 Public Policies

In Argentina, as in most parts of the world, there is a political agenda regarding the moral sensitivity caused by the biomedical revolution and its manipulation of life (both human and other) through the invention of new reproductive technologies and those technologies meant to affect the dying process. An ethics of life (or a life ethics) requires the provision of adequate moral deliberation within a democratic and pluralistic society by bioethics. Mentioned below are examples of legislation and jurisprudence which reflects the normative standards of Argentinean biopolicy throughout the last decade.

For the period 1989–1993, see the text by José A. Mainetti, Gustavo Pis Diez, Juan Carlos Tealdi, "Bioethics in Latin America: 1989–1991" (in *Bioethics Yearbook – Regional Developments in Bioethics: 1989–1991* [vol. 2, pp. 83–96, 1992]. Kluwer Academic Publishers, Dordrecht). See also the text by Juan Carlos Tealdi, Gustavo Pis Diez, and Oscar Esquizabel, "Bioethics in Latin America: 1991–1993" (in B. Andrew Lustig [ed.], *Bioethics Yearbook* [vol. 4, 113–135, 1995], Kluwer Academic Publishers, Dordrecht).

6.4.1 Conventions on Human Rights Included in the National Constitution (Art. 75, Items 22 and 23, Ref. 1994)

Universal Declaration of Human Rights of the United Nations – 1948
American Declaration of the Rights and Duties of Man – 1948
American Convention on Human Rights – 1969 ("Pact of San Jose da Costa Rica" (approved by Act 23,054))
International Pact of Economic, Social and Cultural Rights (and General Observation 14/2000 of PIDESC Committee: "The Right to the Benefit of the Highest Possible Level of Health")
International Pact on Civil and Political Rights and its Facultative Protocol (Act 23, 313)
International Convention on the Elimination of All Forms of Discrimination against Women (Act 23, 179)
Convention on the Rights of Children (Act 23, 849) and other conventions on human rights with constitutional status (art. 75, items 22 and 23, and sub-items, CN)

6.4.2 Other Argentinean Legal Norms

Exercise of Medicine and Activities of Collaboration (17.132), Obligatory Medical Program (PMO), Determination of the Moment of Person's Death (21, 541 – art. 21 – ref. 23, 464, DEC reg. 3011), National System of Health Insurance (23.661), Genetic Data Bank (23.511), Prevention and Fight against HIV/AIDS (23.798), Regime of Organs and Anatomical Material Transplants (24.193), System of Basic Benefits of Integral Attention in Favor of Deficient People (24.901), Sexual Health and Responsible Procreation (25.673), Basic Law of Health of the Independent City of Buenos Aires (153), Pregnancies Incompatible with Life (1044, CABA), Research in Human Beings (11,044, PBA), etc.

N.B.: To consult publications about provincial Acts or decisions of the Buenos Aires Legislature, see e.g. Mainetti and Tealdi, "Bioética e investigación en salud", and Hooft, "Comentario a la ley 11.044", ed. Cámara de Diputados, La Plata, 1991; id. "Transgénicos. Biotecnología en el agro", ed. Cámara de Senadores, La Plata, 2000).

6.4.3 Relevant Judicial Decisions

CSJN (National Supreme Court) statements, especially in cases: "Bahamondez" (1993), "B.R.E. v. Policía Federal Argentina" (1996), "Campodónico de Beviacqua" (2000), "T.S. v. Gob. Ciudad de Bs.As. s/anencefalia" (2001), "Portal de Belén" (2002), "Vázquez Ferrá" (2003); see also other national and provincial courts and magistrates, esp. "bioethical" decisions of Mar del Plata's justice Pedro Federico Hooft, from the year 1991 (v. Revistas *El Derecho, La Ley, La Ley Buenos Aires,*

Lexis Nexos-Jurisprudencia Argentina). See also Foreign Jurisprudence (esp. decisions of North American courts in the matters of a right to life, vegetative state, vital support treatment interruption, and euthanasia).

6.5 Relevant Publications of Bioethics

Relevant publications in matters of bioethics by Argentinean authors are considerable, both in quantity and quality, and have been stimulated by the introduction of bioethics into higher education (especially within medical, legal, theological, and philosophical disciplines). The consolidation of the relationship between bioethics and the medical humanities as a main concern of Mainetti Foundation translates in a publishing activity of works aimed at promoting a deepening of Bioethical studies. The journal *Chiron*, with its 36 volumes to date, and a series of books by the same publishing house, are undeniable testimonies of the presence of humanist thought in medicine within the second half of the last century. Below, some general publications within bioethics are presented.

6.5.1 *Books*

Fracapani de Cuitiño M (1999) Liliana Giannacari de Mathus, Alberto Bochatey, Celia Bordin: *Bioética*. Bs. As, Sus instituciones, Lumen

Luna F e Salles A (1995) Decisiones de vida, muerte, eutanasia, aborto y otros temas de ética médica. Editorial Sudamericana, Bs. As

Zanier T et al. (1990) Estado Actual y perspectivas de la Bioética en la Argentina, no Boletín de la Oficina Sanitaria Panamericana, vol 108, 5–6, Mayo y Junio de 1990. Número Especial de Bioética

Outomuro D (2004) manual de fundamentos de bioética, Ed. Magíster, Bs. As

Estévez A (2002) Bioética. De la cuestión nominal a la cuestión del concepto, Editorial de la Universidad Nacional del Sur, Bahía Blanca

Pérez de Nucci AM (1998) Bioética themática, Ediciones Universidad Católica de Santiago del Estero, Santiago del Estero, República Argentina

von Engelhardt D, Mainetti JA, Cataldi AR, Meyer L (2004) Bioética y humanidades médicas, Academia Argentina de Ética en Medicina, Editorial Biblos, Bs. As

Federico Hooft P (1999) Bioética y derechos humanos. Temas y casos, Desalma, Bs. As

Tinant EL (2004) Antología para una bioética jurídica, La Ley, Bs. As

Manzini JL (1997) Bioética paliativa. Quirón, La Plata

Guillermo BL (Organizador) (2002) Bioética y bioderecho. Cuestiones actuales, Eudeba, Bs. As

Salvador DB e, Monyerski N (Organizadores) (2004) Bioética y derecho, Rubonival – Culzoni, Bs.As

Andorno R (1998) Bioética y dignidad de la persona. Tecnos, Madrid

Maliandi R (1984) Cultura y conflicto. Investigaciones éticas y antropológicas, Biblios, Bs. As

Fernández G e, Cecchetto S (Organizadores) (2003) Transgénicos en América Latina: el retorno de Hernán Cortés, Suárez, Mar del Plata

Pfeiffer ML (2005) Transgénicos. Un destino tecnológico para América Latina. Suárez, Mar del Plata

6.5.2 *Journal Publication*

Revista de Medicina y Bioética "Quirón" (Director and Founder Prof. José Alberto Mainetti; Fundación Mainetti, Gonnet, La Plata)

Perspectivas Bioéticas (1996) Facultad Latinoamericana de Ciencias Sociales (FLACSO)

Revista Cuadernos de Bioética (Diretora Dra. Dominga Teodora Zamudio, Ad-Hoc, Buenos Aires)

Revista de Filosofía Jurídica y Filosofía Social, Universidad Nacional de Rosario

Vida y Ética, Pontificia Universidad Católica Argentina, Bs. As.

Bioética. Temas y perspectivas (1990) Organización Panamericana de la Salud (OPS) (esp. publicação científica nº 527, Washington)

Yearly Issue of Bioethics (Revista Lexis Nexis-Jurisprudencia Argentina, Edited by Pedro Federico Hooft from 1998 on)

Proceedings of the Yearly Meetings of Asociación Argentina de Bioética (a partir de 1995)

Proceedings of the first Yearly National Meetings on Bioethics and Law (Primeiras Jornadas Nacionais de Bioética e Direito) (I/IV), August 2000, Chair UNESCO, UBA, professor Salvador Darío Bergel (id. www.aaba.com.ar)

6.5.3 *Web sites of Institutions and Organizations*

www.aabioetica.org (Asociación Argentina de Bioética)

www.aghu.org (Asociación Argentina de Genética Humana)

www.elabe.bioetica.org (Escuela Latinoamericana de Bioética, ELABE)

www.uca.edu.ar (Instituto de Bioética, UCA)

www.publicidad-guia.com.ar (Fundación Pedro Goyena)

www.anmat.gov.ar (Administración Nacional de Medicamentos, Alimentación y Tecnología Médica)

http://www.bioetica.uchile.cl (Bioética, Universidad de Chile)

www.cubasolidarity.net/infomed (Sitios web de Instituciones de Salud de Cuba)

www.felaibe.com.ar (Federación Latinoamericana y del Caribe de Bioética)

www.cuidadospaliativos.org (Asociación Latinoamericana de Cuidados Paliativos)

www.paho.org.bioetica (Organización Panamericana de la Salud, Comité de Bioética) 0 utf8.

Chapter 7
Bioethics in Bolivia: Antecedents and Projections

Javier Luna Orosco Eduardo, M.D.

7.1 First Precursors and Antecedents

Although bioethics was born at the beginning of the 1970s with Potter's coining of the term, we do not have records or knowledge of bioethical activity in Bolivia before 1991, when the Jesuit priest Miguel Manzanera proposed to the authorities of the UCB – Universidad Católica Boliviana de Cochabamba (Catholic University in Cochabamba) the creation of a Center of Bioethics.

Around the same time, Drs. Jose Maria Alvarado, Luis Hurtado Gómez, and Javier Luna Orosco, among others, took an interest in the research and development of clinical bioethics to assist in their composition of the first drafts of the Law of the Medical Professional Exercise – a necessary factor to prevent professional malpractice because of its increasing frequency.

In September 1993, another precursor to bioethics involving the State occurred: with the establishment of the PRB (Regional Program of Bioethics) of PAHO/OMS at the University of Chile, a result of the Promotion of Bioethics (HBE-Promoción da Bioética) of PAHO, the Secretariat of Health of the Bolivian Government received pertinent documentation asking for the advice of Dr. Javier Luna Orosco Eduardo. He was asked to consider the program and to express an opinion on its approval. His opinion was presented at the 37th Meeting of the Board of Directors of PAHO/OMS in Washington, September 1993, and during the activities of PRB in 1994. Dr. Luna Orosco declared in writing that:

> Due to the importance that has been attached to the creation of the Regional Program of Bioethics (PRB), an importance that surpasses the merely local aspects and seeks to enable or to spread the potentialities of knowledge and daily handling of Bioethics regarding not only the human resources of health, but rather to extend them to the population as a whole; it is highly recommendable at the level of the country to support the initiative of PAHO/OMS and the University of Chile, to put it in practice, which will result in an

J.L.O. Eduardo, M.D. (✉)
Physician. President of the National Committee of Bioethics, Bolivia.
He is one of the founders of Revista Boliviana de Bioética (Bolivian Bioethics Journal)
e-mail: bioetica@colmedlp.org

L. Pessini et al. (eds.), *Ibero-American Bioethics: History and Perspectives*,
Philosophy and Medicine 106, DOI 10.1007/978-1-4020-9350-0_7,

> enormous benefit for the countries of the region and for Bolivia in particular, where few have any experience in Bioethics (Orosco, 1993).

In addition, he recommended that the newly created PRB establish methods of instruction and evaluation similar to other countries in the region. Such uniform measures would assist in the exchange of experience and technical cooperation. There would be significant benefit from the establishment of a *Dictionary of Bioethics* that could be used for professional reference. This dictionary would standardize the words and definitions of bioethics with all of its implications: technical, biological, legal, social, and philosophical. Finally, the document of Dr. Luna Orosco proposed to require consultation with PRB for: the organization of the Bolivian Institute of Bioethics; qualification of selected human resources in the country that could result from an agreement by the Secretariat of Health, the University of Chile, and the Medical College; the establishment of the Committees of Clinical Ethics and Review of Biomedical Research; and delivering an initial basic overview of bioethics. Unfortunately, none of these recommendations were taken into account until the year 2000, when, coincidentally, the Office of International Relations of the Ministry of Health and Social Security (MSPS) of Bolivia asked Dr. Orosco Luna to interpret the document CD 42/9 of PAHO: "Evaluation of the Regional Program of Bioethics." "This concluded that from the 186 activities that PRB had supported in 6 years (among seminars, workshPAHO, conferences and courses from its establishment), 60% had been conducted in Chile, followed by Mexico, Central America, the Latin Caribbean, and other countries in South America, as well as in North America, Europe, and the English Caribbean – but none in Bolivia. This situation was presented to the representatives of PAHO/OMS in Bolivia and, as a consequence, was the impetus for the organization of a committee composed of representatives from the Ministry of Health and Social Security, the Vice-ministry of Superior Education, Science and Technology, PAHO/OMS in Bolivia, the Bolivian Medicine Academy, the Permanent Assembly of Human Rights, the Medical College of La Paz and the Medical School of Universidad Mayor de San Andrés (UMSA). On September 7, 2000, La Paz signed the "Document of the Establishment of the Committee for the Promotion of Ethics and Bioethics in Bolivia," aiming to establish an institution for advice, promotion, teaching, research, and monitoring of bioethical and ethical principles. Dr. Javier Luna Orosco was the coordinator for the Committee; the goal was to examine and analyze the culture of the medical community with the aim of making recommendations regarding social justice in the medical context for the development of legislation.

7.1.1 Institutional Context of Bioethics in Bolivia

It is worth providing greater detail about the organizations and activities created by the three most recognized institutions, as well as their main goals and objectives. These institutions are the National Committee of Bioethics (CNB), the Institute of

Bioethics of the Bolivian Catholic University of Cochabamba (IB) and the Bolivian Association of Bioethics, Genetic Rights and Biotechnology (ABIODGE).

7.1.2 *National Committee of Bioethics*

7.1.2.1 Foundations

The National Committee of Bioethics (CNB) was first established as the Committee for the Promotion of Ethics and Bioethics in Bolivia (CIEB), September 7, 2000, by means of a document signed by representatives of the Ministry of Health, the Ministry of Education, PAHO/OMS, the Permanent Assembly of Human Rights, the Bolivian Medical Academy, the Medical College, and Universidad Mayor de San Andrés. The CIEB enjoys international recognition from PRB (Regional Program of Bioethics) of PAHO/OMS, as well as from FELAIBE, the Latin American and Caribbean Bioethics Network, and the International Bioethics Committee (IBC) of UNESCO.

7.1.2.2 Initiatives

The initiatives CNB developed were steps towards a human bioethics, or micro-bioethics, and an ecological bioethics or macro-bioethics, through three approaches led by the commissions of Qualification, Research, and Promotion in the Community. In this sense, under the umbrella of the common good, bioethics is the foundation of all who support living and working for a better future for humanity, independent of race, sex, gender, culture, creed, ideology, or social condition. It is a sign of hope, a light that can better illuminate the future paths of the new millennium, especially for those in situations or regions where the appreciation of human dignity and quality of life continue to be marginal.

7.1.2.3 Activities

1. Shortly before constituting CIEB, the founding group organized a bioethics course taught by the Spanish bioethicist Dr. Isolina Riaño Galán, Master in Bioethics. The course was held in Oviedo, Spain, from August 9 to 11, 2000, under the auspices of the Ministry of Health, PAHO/OMS, UMSA, the Medical College of La Paz, the Bolivian Academy of Medicine, the Court Department of Medical Ethics, and the Masters Program in Forensic Medicine and Human Rights.
2. In November 2000, CIEB organized a seminar on Teaching Bioethics, the first activity in Bolivia sponsored by PRB-PAHO/OMS, at the University of Chile and under the auspices of PAHO/OMS in Bolivia, with the hope that a Ministerial Resolution would be issued by the MSPS.

3. In collaboration with the International College of Surgeons, Bolivia Section, PAHO/OMS, and the Bolivian Academy of Medicine, CIEB organized on April 26–27, 2001, the seminar "Medical Bioethics," having the Venezuelan doctor, Gabriel D' Empaire, as the keynote speaker.
4. A year after its creation, CIEB organized the First Bolivian Congress of Bioethics, September 12–14, 2001, in the city of La Paz, under the auspices of the Reformation of Health of MSPS, PAHO/OMS in Bolivia, the Ministry of Education, Culture and Sports, the La Paz Medical School, the UMSA Medical School, the Bolivian Academy of Medicine and the Permanent Assembly of Human Rights. The President of FELAIBE, Dr. Eduardo Sousa Lennox (Panama), bioethicists Volnei Garrafa (Brazil) and Sergio Cechetto (Argentina), Roberto Mancini from PRB-PAHO/OMS (Chile), and the representative of PAHO/OMS in Bolivia, Dr. Jose Antonio Pagés, attended.
5. During the First Bolivian Congress of Bioethics, the Departmental Committees of Bioethics were organized and began functioning with the delivery of documents and basic materials, some of them given by PRB through Dr. Mancini.
6. Again, at the First Bolivian Congress of Bioethics, the "Declaration of La Paz" was created, and the following bioethical topics were assigned to the committees for consideration: ethics in favor of life; bioethics and human rights; justice and the good in social, institutional, scientific, political, and professional performance; medical practice committed to bioethics and human integral well-being; and protection of the environment and bio-diversity.
7. From the end of October through the beginning of November 2001, CIEB organized the lecture "Ethics in Research and Good Clinical Practice," co-sponsored by the La Paz Medical College and delivered by Drs. Jaime Soto and Julia Toledo from Colombia.
8. Under the auspices of the MSPS, the Embassy of France in Bolivia, the Bolivian Institute of the Biology of Height, and the Medical School of UMSA, CIEB organized the seminar: "Ethics in Biomedical Research on Humans." The seminar was held from March 27 to 29, 2003, with the participation of Laura Rueda and Dr. Roberto Mancini of PRB-PAHO/OMS.
9. From August 27 to 30, 2003, the Second Bolivian Congress of Bioethics took place in the city of Cochabamba, organized by CIEB with the support of PAHO/OMS, and together with the Universidad Mayor de San Simón. The director of the IB of the Catholic University of Cochabamba, Dr. Miguel Manzanera, presided over the Congress. Several international guests, such as Drs. José Alberto Mainetti, Pedro F. Hofft, and Sergio Cechetto, along with Patricia Urband (Argentina), Osvaldo Chávez (Venezuela) and Raimundo Rincón (Spain), expert in theology, also participated in the Congress.
10. In 2004, CNB produced an Open Forum of Health Policies via ten seminars with the following themes: Legislation and Sanitary Organization; Frame of Institutional Competencies and Management in Health with Citizen Participation; Levels of Assistance and Urban–Rural Structuring of Service Networks; Regulations for the Construction and Equipment of the Health Area in Search of a Greater Offer of Primary Care; Policies of Human Resources in Health; Financial

Sustainability of the Health Area; Universal Access to Health and Sanitary Justice; Policies of Medicine and Medical Supplies; Preservation and Benefit of the Person in the Process of Research and Techno-Scientific Development; and Basis of a Final Proposal for a New State Policy in the Health Sector.

11. In September 2004, Dr. Susana Vidal, Coordinator of Bioethics for the Ministry of Health in Cordova, Argentina, developed a conference with the workshop: "Clinical Bioethics and the Organization of Hospital Bioethics Committees."
12. November 3–4, 2004, CNB sponsored the course, "Introduction to Bioethics," organized together with Dr. Volga Iñiguez, Director of the Institute of Molecular Biology of UMSA. The course was designed for biologists and students of biology, and had Drs. Martha Pacheco, Ruth Guillén de Maldonado, Beatriz Montoya, and the specialist Emma Aparicio as speakers. Drs. Violet Aragón and Daysi Gutiérrez, all members of CNB, acted as moderators.
13. The same weekend (November 3–5, 2004), the Coordinator of CNB developed the same course, "Introduction to Bioethics," for members of the Institute of Molecular Biology of UMSA.
14. In memoriam of one of the main promoters of bioethics in Bolivia, Dr. Luis Hurtado Gómez, La Paz hosted the Third Bolivian Congress of Bioethics with the theme "Bioethics and Plurality." The event was organized by CNB with the collaboration of UNESCO in Mexico, RED*BIOS* and PAHO/OMS, and was held in Bolivia from October 26 to 28, 2005. At this Congress, participants included the Director of UNESCO in Mexico, Dr. Alya Saada; the President of RED*BIOS*, Dr. Volnei Garrafa (Brazil); Juan Carlos Tealdi (Argentina), Jose Eduardo de Siqueira (Brazil), and Susana Vidal (Argentina).
15. CNB members participated and still participate as guests in courses, conferences, and advanced lectures organized by several institutions. Among them are: the medical course at the Universidad Mayor de San Andrés, University "Nuestra Señora de La Paz" and "Universidad del Valle," the Medical School of La Paz, School of Biochemistry and Pharmacy of Bolivia, Social Pastoral Episcopal Commission (CARITAS), Representation of PAHO/OMS in Bolivia, Federation Department of Professionals of La Paz, Caja Petrolera de Seguridad Social, Seguro Social Universitário, Residency of Hospital Obrero of CNS, Bolivian Society of Urology, Bolivian Internal Medicine Society, Medical Society of Private Consultations (SOMECOP) and ABIODGE.

The Regional Seminar on Bioethics, organized by the Ministry of Justice and Human Rights of Argentina and by the ceaseless efforts of Dr. Juan Carlos Tealdi of *BIOS*UR, was established with support from UNESCO in the city of Buenos Aires, November 4–5, 2004. One focus of the seminar was the analysis of a third draft of the Universal Declaration of Bioethics, prepared by the writing group of CIB-UNESCO. In this seminar, representatives from Bolivia submitted commentary, along with other invited countries, with precise interpretations and revisions to the draft, which more accurately reflected the interests of developed countries in technological and scientific developments, than a desire to solve the conditions of poverty, disease, hunger, and despair that, due to social and economic injustice, affects a high percentage of the population in Latin American countries.

Later, CNB sent to the Ministry of Foreign Affairs and Cult of Bolivia a complete report of the seminar in Argentina, together with all modifications considered advisable to the rough draft of the Declaration of UNESCO. These were sent to the Bolivian diplomat in Paris, to be considered in subsequent meetings together with the proposals of other countries, until the final approval of the Declaration, incorporating pro-social and pro-ecological positions of developing countries, was expressed in the "Letter of Buenos Aires."

Other remarkable meetings of the Latin American RED*BIOS* include the symposium organized in Montevideo in 2004 to consider topics related to the "Epistemological Status of Bioethics," and a subsequent collection of the same title published by UNAM of Mexico and UNESCO, as well as the symposium on "Research in Human Beings and Public Health Policies" that was carried out in Bogota, May 16–17, 2005.

16. June 27–29, 2006, CNB organized a Cycle of Conferences and WorkshPAHO on health policies, ethics in research, and Latin American bioethics, coinciding with the visit of Dr. Daniel Herrera Stone (Cuba) to Bolivia.
17. One of the main activities of CNB's Commission of Research is the ethical review of research sent by diverse institutions, including MSPS, PAHO, research institutions, scientific societies, ONGs, and independent researchers.
18. In 2006, the Commission of Promotion in the Community developed and introduced a radio program promoting a simple approach to bioethics for the general population.
19. Another objective of CNB has been to promote the incorporation of bioethics and medical humanities into the curriculum of social and health professionals' careers. In December 2005, the medical schools of Bolivia's top four State universities and CNB met and reached an agreement for establishing a unit or department within each school that would be responsible for including medical ethics, bioethics, and medical humanities courses in the curriculum of those seeking health service careers and with the respective adjustments to the requirements of the chairs. At present, the Coordinator of CNB is responsible for the only existing chairs of undergraduate courses in the country, namely, history of medicine (University of "Nuestra Señora de La Paz"), and ethics and medical sociology (Franz Tamayo University).

7.1.3 Inter-institutional Relations

Among the most important national relations are those maintained with the Ministries of Health, Education, Justice and Foreign Affairs, as well as with the Caja Nacional de Salud (CNS), Departmental Services of Health (SEDES), public and private universities, professional colleges, the College of Lawyers of La Paz, Caja Petrolera de Seguridad Social, Seguro Social Universitário, medical-scientific societies, the National Academy of Sciences, Bolivian Academy of Medicine,

Institutes of Research (particularly the Bolivian Institute of Biology of Height, and the Bolivian Institute of Genetics), the Social Pastoral Episcopal Commission (Comissão Episcopal Pastoral Social) of the Catholic Church, ONGs in the health area, the media, the Institute of Bioethics of the Catholic University of Cochabamba, and ABIODGE.

At the international level, CNB maintains relations with PRB of PAHO/OMS, FELAIBE, RED*BIOS*, CIB of UNESCO, *BIOS*UR, and the Association of Bioethics of Argentina, with the Brazilian Association of Bioethics, the Foundation "José Maria Mainetti" from La Plata, and mainly with the representation of PAHO/OMS in Bolivia.

7.1.4 Representations

The current coordinator of CNB is a member of the Board of Directors of FELAIBE, RED*BIOS*, and the CIB of UNESCO (for a period of 4 years from 2006 to 2009).

7.1.5 Publications

Although, through the coordinator and its members, CIEB and CNB have several publications in journals and leaflets, it is worth mentioning the contributions made to the international documents: "Ethical and Policy Issues in International Research: Clinical Trials in Developing Countries," National Bioethics Advisory Commission (NBAC) – USA, and "Epistemological Statute of Bioethics," published by UNAM of Mexico and RED*BIOS* in 2005. At the national level, the Bolivian Journal of Bioethics (June 2005) is an important publication, along with the report of the "Open Forum of Health Policies" (2004), both published in collaboration with PAHO/OMS in Bolivia.

From the beginning, Dr. Javier Luna Orosco has been in charge of the general coordination of CIEB and CNB, with the invaluable collaboration of Drs. Luis Hurtado Gómez, Saul Pantoja, Martha Pacheco, Ruth Guillén de Maldonado, Enrique Vargas Pacheco, Beatriz Montoya, Jaime Mollinedo Averanga, and the expert Emma Aparicio.

7.1.6 Motivations and Future Directions of CNB

It is essential to have a clear appreciation of the current state of the world against which one can gauge what needs to be done and what the appropriate actions are to take as a country and as a part of the Latin American continent. Yet, it is a difficult assessment to make because of a number of adverse situations which, beginning with war and violence, have had the consequences of death and desolation as a historical constant that has never been surpassed; it also presents itself as a daily anti-bioethical reality. However, traditional political power has not been able to carry through its schemes, there is an incapacity of global leaders to effect changes, and injustice and corruption continue to increase in a large part of the world; all of these comprise serious events that force us to consider new forms of political behavior with greater commitment and citizen participation.

In many parts of Latin America, political movements do not have clear direction for bringing about a solution to societal structural problems; they respond more to the urgency of immediately vindicating population groups that live in poverty and at the margins of society. This is compounded by economic globalization and market laws that put countries under the hegemony of power groups, which extend the control and sovereignty of States themselves, increasing the gap between the rich and the poor of a progressively increasing world population. This causes forms of aggression among citizens to increase, many times because of a threat to communal property, and expresses the attitude of a "war of all against all" which almost nobody can control.

On the other hand, technological advances provide economic privilege for those who can afford them, preventing social advances, and compounding the attributing factors of submission and dependency in a contemporary society that "reifies" people and "sacralizes" things, with worrisome manifestations of dehumanization, egoism, and hedonism.

In many places, Latin American citizens are uprooted from the earth, causing a loss of respect for nature and "continuity" with it due to an eagerness to obtain material and artificial "goods" from those great human agglomerations that constitute the Western world. Due to this eagerness, people migrate; those societies that feel "invaded" maintain a permanent conflict among the groups that form them, causing xenophobia, racism, marginalization, and eugenic tendencies. In addition, there has been an increase of uncontrolled phenomena of environmental contamination and ecosystem imbalances, along with an unusual frequency of natural disasters that do not seem accidental.

The abandonment and/or substitution of flora and fauna cause the loss of wealth and variety to both man and nature. Many Earth cultures ("deep" cultures or ethnocultures) are disappearing along with many species, due to this "technological revolution" that provides us with a human recreation of the world replacing natural things with modifications or artificial things, putting in jeopardy man's essential, biological, psychological, social, and historical self. However, with this limited diagnosis of the state of the world we must ask: What is our current perception of international bioethics?

The concept of bioethics has been weakened from its original statement by Potter as a global bioethics because it has been delayed and obscured by the utilitarian interests of technological and scientific developments which take advantage of the so-called altruistic rule of "ethics in research" to service hegemonic interests of a diversified character. This is shown by the fact that the benefits of such advancements are limited only to those who can afford to access them, and by the lack of influence bioethics has had in influencing and improving the world – most populations are unaware of its existence.

From the beginning, Western bioethics – linked mainly to scientific development – universalized trends, including in Latin America, where it continues as such, without being sensitive to the need for adjustment in the context of diverse cultural and socio-anthropological realities. This kind of bioethical colonialism is even evident in the guidelines of the first rough drafts of the Universal Declaration on Bioethics and Human Rights (UNESCO), and in the resulting arguments over revisions to accommodate the interests of developing countries.

Bioethics has become more centered around the individual instead of operating at the social or environmental level, maintaining an academic scientific character that adds doctrinal and philosophical analysis but has very little social impact – except for those controversial subjects, such as the amazing possibilities of molecular biology, cloning, and others. Concerning medical-sanitary applications of bioethics, its guidelines are equally individualistic and remarkably influenced by the four paradigm principles established by Tom Beauchamp and James Childress. These principles may be contradictory or inapplicable in terms of sanitary bioethics, which is imperative for many Latin American countries with serious sanitation problems and inequalities in the supply and access of health services for the population.

Latin America is at a point where it is necessary to analyze the effectiveness of the current bioethics and to ask: Has and does bioethics respond to the Latin American reality? The answers to this question may be appropriately diversified, because the different Latin American countries have different realities. Nevertheless, it is also necessary to answer with consideration of the general characteristics and specific advantages that need to be understood and taken into account when establishing a truly Latin American bioethics. Among its advantages, Latin America adds the inheritance of universal culture and its own contributions to world culture. In addition, Latin America, as a continent, has the greatest natural wealth, biodiversity, and ecological diversity, with an ample array of potential and future possibilities, to which scientific and technological development can also be added. In our countries, traditional "values" are also maintained, such as the extended and united family, warm relationships, and community work, all of which are expressions of a population sensitive to the individual and social dimensions.

All of these considerations are necessary components for a Latin American bioethical epistemology (doctrinal and philosophical), grounded on a framework that ranges from the general or Western to the Native American. It is important to make the effort to know ourselves better and to apply a bioethics with a deeply anthropological and social content focusing on the "Earth tracks" or the tracks of identity.

This requires a bioethics of intervention and participation: one that can have an impact at the State level, and promote a pedagogical guideline for educating citizens that make thematic and programmatic adjustments compatible with our own realities and necessities. Furthermore, regarding the relationship of bioethics to human health, it is necessary to go beyond individual clinical bioethics into sanitary bioethics, working on health policies for *a constant improvement of quality services, and a greater non-exclusive user satisfaction.* Finally, we think the perspective of Latin American bioethics must be incorporated into the international shaping of bioethics, not only with an integrative criterion, but also because of the obligation that Latin Americans have to present a very different reality from the prevailing one in the West.

7.2 The History of the Institute of Bioethics of the Bolivian Catholic University in Cochabamba

7.2.1 Antecedents

On November 6, 1992, the Board of Directors of ISET, in the presence of its president, Dr. Hans van der Berg, and UCB's dean, Dr. Luis Antonio Boza, approved the constitution of the Center of Bioethics, the first of its kind in Bolivia, naming as director Dr. Miguel Manzanera, who continues in the position at the present time. In 1995, the Center of Bioethics would be renamed the Institute of Bioethics (IB).

7.2.2 Purposes and Objective

Within the general purposes of UCB, IB has as its specific purpose: To encourage research, teaching, and the spread of bioethics in defense of human life from conception to its natural completion, which includes the care of the social and environmental context, with universal and theological projections, having as reference and direction the teaching of the Roman Catholic Church.

The general mission of the Institute is to promote interdisciplinary dialogue among cultivators of medical, legal, social, cultural, ecological, philosophical, and theological sciences, on the basis of a human- and Christian-guided anthropology respecting the genuine cultural, familial, and religious values effective in the Bolivian population with a special preference for the marginalized and impoverished, who suffer from a high morbidity and mortality rate.

7.2.3 Promoted Activities

One of the most important actions of the first stage was the organization of the First National Meeting of Bioethics (Cochabamba, September 3–4, 1993), dedicated to the study of the Law of Organs and Tissues Transplant, which was blocked for political reasons by the Parliament of Bolivia. The consequence of that meeting was the revision of the legal text that finally was approved in 1996.

As of 1995, the Institute of Bioethics has been dedicated to research, trying to answer the great bioethical questions. Being part of UCB – Universidad Católica Boliviana de Cochabamba (Catholic University in Cochabamba) has provided guidelines for the Institute's work, having as reference the teaching of the Roman Catholic Church, which has contributed to its improvement and development. IB has a library with bibliographical material and documentation. Notably, IB, together with the National Committee of Bioethics, the Universidad Mayor de San Simón, the Universidad Mayor de San Andrés, PAHO/OMS and other institutions, organized the Second Bolivian Congress of Bioethics, "Bioethics and Underdevelopment," August 27–30, 2003.

7.2.4 Inter-institutional Relations

IB has maintained many contacts with several ecclesiastical, governmental, professional, educative, and university institutions that are included in UNESCO's database of bioethics. Among the ecclesiastical institutions of the Vatican, it is worth mentioning the Pontifical Academy for Life, the Pontifical Council for the Pastoral of Health, and the Pontifical Council for the Family. Within Bolivia it collaborates with the Bolivian Episcopal Conference, particularly the Episcopal Commission of Doctrine and Faith, in addition to maintaining close relationships with the local churches of Bolivia and their diverse organizations.

IB is also a charter member of the International Federation of Centers and Institutes of Personalist Bioethics (FIBIP), which was founded on June 10, 2003, in Rome; the ratification of the incorporation of IB took place on October 1, 2005. The Center of Bioethics was a charter member of the Latin American Federation of Institutions of Bioethics (FELAIBE), founded at a meeting in the historical Villa de Leyva (Colombia), November 23–25, 1992.

7.2.5 Publications

One of the aims of the IB has been the diffusion of bioethics by means of books, journals, brochures, and newspapers. The *BIOS* Collection (Colección *BIOS*), beginning in 1996, deserves special mention (for titles, see bibliography).

7.2.6 Motivations and Guidelines of the Institute of Bioethics

Despite the shortage of resources, we have been able to develop a Latin American bioethics with humanist and Christian inspiration, which can enrich the present bioethical debate. The motivations and guidelines of IB are reflected in publications of the *BIOS* Collection, with the following synthesis:

Bioethics of the We-Relationship (*Nostridad*)[1]

One of the contributions of the Institute of Bioethics has been the elaboration of a bioethics within a new Latin American and humanist perspective devoted to establishing a framework of a personal bioethics based on the ethics of solidarity and the philosophy of *nostridad*. Bioethics of *nostridad*, "for one," resists North American bioethics, which is predominantly pragmatic and utilitarian and does not consider the transcendental vision of man.

It also serves as a counterpoint to European bioethics that, although having more depth in its philosophical aspects than North American bioethics, is preferentially oriented towards a consensual dialogue that implies a relativist vision of truth. Bioethics of *nostridad* wants to base its axiological values and its ethical principles on an integral vision of man as a psychosomatic being impelled to transcendence towards the universal anthropological "We." From this perspective, we must reformulate the classic principles of non-maleficence, justice, autonomy, and charity.

Bio-Law

In the context of Bio-Law, it is important to promote the discernment and recognition of authentic human bio-rights based on the natural dignity of man, rejecting abusive exclusions and interpretations. In the present international debate, great importance is attached to the recognition of the objection of conscience and the development of tolerance as an ethical virtue against intolerance and over-tolerance.

Orthogenesis

Regarding initial life, it is important to promote the human bio-right to orthogenesis, that is, the right of all human beings to be generated by the conjugal natural relationship that guarantees to the baby parents identified and united in familial love. Orthogenesis is against not only abortion and eugenesis but also dysgenesis, including extracorporeal fertilization and other techniques that expose human embryos to manipulations contrary to natural human dignity. For that reason, research with adult or umbilical stem cells must be promoted, and cloning and the use of embryonic stem cells must be rejected (be it reproductive or therapeutic).

Further, within orthogenesis, natural family planning as a humanizing alternative acquires importance before the unrestricted invasion of contraceptives, some of them iatrogenic and abortive. Regarding the ontological status of the human embryo, one shows how normal conception corresponds biologically with the penetration of the spermatozoon in the ovum, resulting in a new endogenous entelechical dynamism, which is in metaphysical terms named "soul." From this

[1] "Nostridad" (We-Relationship) is the name of the union of "I" and "Other" for creating an inclusive "we/us". N.T.

stems the support for the theory of the immediate animation of the human embryo, reinterpreting the Thomist–Aristotelian position.

Orthotherapy

Regarding health and disease, it is necessary to defend the right of the patient to orthotherapy, that is, dignified natural treatment and assistance; the humanization of medicine is advocated, and malpractice and other abuses are rejected. Universal medical insurance for all is promoted. Particular bioethical issues that deserve attention are: defending tissue and organ transplants, promoting a greater solidarity in organ donation and transplants, and defending the right of patients to universal insurance.

Orthothanasia

In reference to the final stage of life, we must argue for the right to "orthothanasia" or a dignified natural death, and we must be opposed to euthanasia (i.e., death caused at the request of the patient) as well as to dysthanasia (i.e., the illegal or futile prolongation of life by means of disproportionate or unbalanced procedures).

In the debate on the so-called cerebral or encephalic death, we are convinced of the validity of the neurological diagnosis of death on the basis of parameters regarding the total and irreversible cessation of the encephalon, which was accepted by the teaching of the Catholic Church in 1985.

Ecological Bioethics

With regard to environmental life, we propose an ecological bioethics. This term expresses an understanding of ecology that rejects both the passive attitude before ecological threats and ecologism that does not put man at the center of creation. Thus, for example, before endorsing an extreme position related to genetically modified organisms, it is advisable to hold a position marked by prudence, approval, and evaluation of each specific project, instead of a general rule.

Sexual Pedagogy

Concerning the libertarian and hedonistic sexual education that endorses the pleasurable use of sexuality, it is necessary to transmit an integral pedagogy for the education and understanding of sexuality as an anthropological dimension comprising three fundamental components: the unitive, the procreative, and the recreational. The reasonable control of sexuality, classically the virtue of chastity, allows young people to prepare themselves suitably for true love, marriage, and family. This education is at the same time the best antidote for sexually transmitted diseases and unexpected pregnancies.

7.3 Bolivian Association of Bioethics and Genetic Right

7.3.1 Antecedents

Motivated by an interest in the study of human behavior, as well as its biogenetic relationship and the juridical context that it implies, two law professionals, Alvaro Munguía Becker and Gustavo Sivila Peñaranda, investigated the relationship between bioethics and legislation. Their study included a new biotechnical branch of law compatible with scientific advances, which resulted in the establishment of the Bolivian Association of Bioethics, Genetic Right and Biotechnology (Asociación Boliviana de Bioética, Derecho Genético y Biotecnología – ABIODGE) in 2003, a group whose membership now includes professionals in social, biological, and health sciences.

7.3.2 Purposes and Aims

National seminars with the participation of international speakers, conferences, forums, and the exchange of information with similar organizations in Bolivia and abroad constitute ABIODGE's main purposes. The drafting of laws pertaining to biotechnology, assisted human reproduction, and genetics is one of its legislative tasks. The acceptance of a proposal for the inclusion of matters of bioethics and genetic right in the curriculum of UMSA's law course, as well as the preparation of specialized courses in each, has up until now been its main activities. The effort and dedication of ABIODGE members tending to these tasks is part of the fulfillment of the intention to place Bolivia at the level of world consensus regarding legal scientific research.

7.3.3 Activities

The Seminar on Bioethics and Genetic Right was held July 17–19, 2003, with the co-sponsorship of the Illustrious College of Lawyers (ICALP – Ilustre Colegio de Abogados de La Paz), La Paz, and the Representation of UNESCO in Bolivia. International guest Dr. Enrique Varsi Rospigliosi, Representative of the Republic of Peru before the Intergovernmental Bioethics Committee of UNESCO (IGBC), and Drs. Javier Luna Orosco (from CNB), and Miguel Manzanera (from IB Cochabamba), among other national guests, participated.

From September 17 to 19, 2003, and in the city of El Alto, ABIODGE replicated that same seminar, with the co-sponsorship of the Regional Medical School of El Alto. In addition, the Committee of Bioethics, with the themes of somatic beginning and end of human life, on June 1–3, 2004, developed a third seminar, which concluded with the book *Bioética y derecho* (Bioethics and Rights) of Dr. Gustavo Sivila Peñaranda, Vice-president of the Commission of Bioethics and Genetic Right of ICALP.

From August 2 to 5, 2005, ABIODGE promoted the seminar "Medical Right in Bolivia" with the auspices of ICALP and the Representation of PAHO in Bolivia. On the first day, a film was viewed named "The Verdict" and the seminar included such speakers as the Minister of Health Dr. Alvaro Muñoz Reyes, the Representative of PAHO Dr. Christian Darrás and a special guest Dr. Jose Geraldo de Freitas Drumond, President of the Latin American Society of Medical Right (Sociedad Iberoamericana de Derecho Médico, or SIDEMA).

With the theme "Malpractice Prevention and Medical Responsibility," the Second International Seminar of Medical Right was sponsored with an international guest Dr. Carlos Navari, Professor of Forensic Medicine of Argentina's Pontifical Catholic University, and the participation of the Coordinator of CNB, Dr. Luna Orosco and a representative of PAHO/OMS in Bolivia, Dr. Carlos Yuri Ayala.

7.3.4 International Relations

In 2004, the interest and commitment in the bio-legal context resulted in the establishment of the Commission of Bioethics and Genetic Right of the Illustrious College of Lawyers of La Paz, which is at the moment in complete integration with ABIODGE; these two organizations are making advancements that are able to meet the expectations of professionals interested in biomedicine, biotechnological advances, human behavior, and justice.

7.3.5 Publications

At the time of the first Seminar, "Bioethics and Genetic Right," the book *Derecho genético y procreático* [Procreative and Genetic Right] (edition for Bolivia) of Dr. Enrique Varsi Rospigliosi was published by ABIODGE and ICALP (Rospigliosi 2005). Another publication to emphasize is the book, *Bioética y derecho*, written by Dr. Gustavo Sivila Peñaranda and presented at the end of the Second Seminar of Bioethics and Genetic Right, June 1–3, 2004 (Peñaranda 2004).

7.3.6 Motivations and Directions of ABIODGE

The beginning, development, and biological end of human life depend upon its genetic component and, in turn, on the epigenome. Nevertheless, the techniques of assisted human reproduction, together with the Human Genome Project and the myth of the immortal and perfect human being, are leading to the indiscriminate manipulation of our primigenious material – the essence of humankind. The risks and consequences of such manipulation constitute an attack against biogenetic integrity and individuality, as well as the register and revelation of their structure against genetic privacy. All this continues despite the positive effects of genetic technologies (such as genetic therapy and the possibility of establishing biological identity).

At the present time, it is possible to generate life without fertilization by means of nuclear transference or cloning. For example, in February 2004, in South Korea, it was recorded that human embryos were obtained by means of a technique for deriving stem cells or "mother cells"; similarly, in April of the same year, in a Japanese laboratory, a scientific experiment resulted in obtaining animal life by means of parthenogenesis.

These scientific biomedical and biotechnological accomplishments, and soon quantum and nanotechnology, will be an undeniable benefit for the biological, psychological, and social evolution of humanity, allowing us to extend the limits of knowledge; however, if these accomplishments are not controlled and harmonized within a bioethical and legal frame, they will constitute an attack against the dignity of the human species.

References

Comité Nacional de Bioética de Bolivia (2005) "Breve reseña informativa del Comité Nacional de Bioética." Revista Boliviana de Bioética, 1.1, Enero-Junio, 9–13

Comité Nacional De Bioética De Bolivia (2005) "Carta de Buenos Aires," Revista Boliviana de Bioética, 1.1, Enero-Junio, 15–17

Orosco JL (1993) Interpretación y comentarios en torno al documento 'Establecimiento del Programa Regional de Bioética en Chile, Documento enviado en Agosto 1993 a la Secretaría Nacional en Salud del Ministerio de Desarrollo Humano de Bolivia, para la participación del Secretario General de Salud en la XXXVII Reunión del Consejo Directivo de la PAHO/OMS

Peñaranda GS (2004) Bioética y derecho. Creativa, La Paz-Bolivia

Rospigliosi EV (2005) Derecho Genético y Procreático. Primera Edición para Bolivia, ABIODGE/ Comisión de Bioética y Derecho Genético del Ilustre Colegio de Abogados de La Paz

Bibliography

Bolivia (2000) Acta de Conformación del Comité Impulsor de Etica y Bioética del 7 de Septiembre de 2000

Bolivia (2003) Resolución Ministerial N° 0126 del MSPS, emitida el 27 de Marzo de 2003

Bolivia (2004) Memoria, Foro Abierto de 'Políticas de Salud', Comité Nacional de Bioética/ PAHO-OMS, 294

Bolivia (2005) Ley N° 3131 del Ejercicio Profesional Médico, promulgada el 19 de Julio de 2005 y reglamentada mediante Decreto Supremo N° 28562 de 22 de Diciembre de 2005

Comité Nacional de Bioética de Bolivia (2004). Ponencia del Comité Nacional de Bioética de Bolivia en el Seminario Regional de UNESCO "Hacia una Declaración Universal de Bioética," Buenos Aires-Argentina, 4 y 5 de Noviembre, Revista Boliviana de Bioética, 1.1, Enero-Junio, 13–14

DOCUMENTO CD 42/9 de la PAHO/OMS "Evaluación del Programa Regional de Bioética," con evaluación externa del Dr. James Drane, de la cátedra 'Russell B. Roth de Bioética Clínica, Edinboro University-Pennsylvania, USA

Instituto de Bioética (1998a) BIOS 1: Inicio de la Vida Humana, 2nd edn. Instituto de Bioética de la Universidad Católica Boliviana, Cochabamba

Instituto de Bioética (1997) BIOS 2: Fundamentación de la bioética en la nostridad. Instituto de Bioética de la Universidad Católica Boliviana, Cochabamba

Instituto de Bioética (1998b) BIOS 3: Bioética del trasplante de órganos. Instituto de Bioética de la Universidad Católica Boliviana, Cochabamba

Instituto de Bioética (2004a) BIOS 4: Fundamentación del derecho en la filosofía de la nostridad, 3rd edn. Instituto de Bioética de la Universidad Católica Boliviana, Cochabamba

Instituto de Bioética (2001a) BIOS 5: Bioética de la insuficiencia renal. Instituto de Bioética de la Universidad Católica Boliviana, Cochabamba

Instituto de Bioética (2001b) BIOS 6: Debate bioético contemporáneo: problemas y horizonte. Instituto de Bioética de la Universidad Católica Boliviana, Cochabamba

Instituto de Bioética (2002) BIOS 7: Bioética, ecología y agrobiotecnología. Instituto de Bioética de la Universidad Católica Boliviana, Cochabamba

Instituto de Bioética (2003a) BIOS 8: Ortotanasia: bioética de la muerte natural digna, 2nd edn. Instituto de Bioética de la Universidad Católica Boliviana, Cochabamba

Instituto de Bioética (2003b) BIOS 9: Filosofía de la nostridad antropoteologal. Instituto de Bioética de la Universidad Católica Boliviana, Cochabamba

Instituto de Bioética (2004b) BIOS 10: Manipulaciones lingüísticas en la bioética. Instituto de Bioética de la Universidad Católica Boliviana, Cochabamba

Instituto de Bioética (2005) BIOS 11: Ley marco sobre derechos sexuales y reproductivos: documentación y reflexión crítica. Instituto de Bioética de la Universidad Católica Boliviana, Cochabamba

National Bioethics Advisory Commission (2001) Ethical and policy issues in international research: clinical trials in developing countries, Report and Recommendations of the National Bioethics Advisory Commission, vol 1. Bethesda, Maryland, p 112

Orosco JL (2005) Comentarios a la ponencia de Julio Cabrera, Estatuto epistemológico de la bioética de la UNESCO, 261–266

Orosco JL (2000) Interpretación y comentarios al documento CD 42/9 de la PAHO: Evaluación del Programa Regional de Bioética, Anexo a la nota de 18 de Septiembre de 2000, enviada a la Jefatura de la Oficina de Relaciones Internacionales del MSPS de Bolivia

UNESCO (2005) Estatuto Epistemológico de la Bioética, Universidad Autónoma de México, Red Latinoamericana y del Caribe de Bioética de la UNESCO, México

Vargas Pacheco, Enrique (2005) Investigación en Salud, Adecuada y Probada Éticamente, Revista Boliviana de Bioética, 1.1, Enero-Junio, 24–28

Chapter 8
An X-Ray of Bioethics in Brazil: Pioneering Voices, Institutional and Educational Programs and Perspectives

Leo Pessini and Christian de Paul de Barchifontaine

8.1 Introduction

Bioethics, as an academic and institutionalized discipline, has existed in Brazil for nearly 20 years. It did not come to acquire its academic character until the beginning of the 1990s and, as a result, there have been few historical studies of Brazilian bioethics, or even of Latin American bioethics, which provide a critical appraisal of its development (Anjos 1994, 2000; Pessini 1995a,b,c, 1999; Garrafa 2000; Schramm 2002).

Brazilian bioethics can be considered a young and overdue enterprise, which has been overly anxious to reflect upon, understand, and solve the old and new challenges brought about by technoscience and its implications for human health and biomedical research. It must face the twin challenge of addressing those "persistent problems" that are inherent to a reality marked by social inequality and exclusion, in addition to those "emergent problems" brought about by the biotechnological revolution, which affect human life and health. We consider Brazilian bioethics a young discipline because it emerged almost half a century after the approval of the Nuremberg Code (1946), which established ethical guidelines for research involving human subjects, and nearly two decades after the establishment of bioethics in the United States at the beginning of the 1970s.

Although Brazilian bioethics appeared within a dynamic and globalized context of which the primary bioethical questions had already been determined (e.g., abortion, euthanasia, organ transplants, etc.), we contributed to the agenda by introducing

L. Pessini
Theology/Bioethics. Master Clinical Pastoral Education and Bioethics at St. Luke's Medical Center. Professor of the Master 'Course in Bioethics of Centro Universitário São Camilo, São Paulo. Superintendent of União Social Camiliana
e-mail: pessini@saocamilo-sp.br

C. de Paul de Barchifontaine
Nurse and Master in Hospital administration. Dean of Centro Universitário São Camilo, São Paulo. Professor of the Master Course in Bioethics of Centro Universitário São Paulo. Vice-Superintendent of União Social Camiliana
e-mail: cpb@saocamilo-sp.br

L. Pessini et al. (eds.), *Ibero-American Bioethics: History and Perspectives*, Philosophy and Medicine 106, DOI 10.1007/978-1-4020-9350-0_8,

questions that were original and particular to the social, economic, political, and cultural reality of Latin America and, in particular, Brazil. These issues included questions of public health, social exclusion, and other challenges stemming from unjust circumstances.

We describe Brazilian bioethics as overdue because it emerged after a change in model had already taken place in the global bioethical movement. This paradigmatic transition was characterized by the passing of a markedly individualistic bioethics, one focused on the problems resultant from personal acts (first-generation human rights) to a more collectivist bioethics concerned with the ethical issues related to public health based on social rights (second-generation human rights). The increasing complexity of global circumstances forces bioethics to evolve so that it is capable of addressing those issues relevant to future generations (third-generation rights), as well as environmental and ecological concerns (fourth-generation rights).

In the 1990s, the historical development of Brazilian bioethics began its "infancy stage," which was characterized by a dependence on the North-American principialist paradigm, a foreign model of ethics, which was hegemonic for the initial 25 years of global bioethical history. Subsequently, in the "adolescence stage," a critical attitude developed towards the use of "imported" models, specifically the principialist model, when addressing issues of public health. In reaching its "adulthood," Brazilian bioethics is faced with the complex challenge of addressing bioethical problems of both an individual and public nature in a manner such that they will be distinguished without being disconnected, and united without being confounded. One must be able to distinguish among the relevant types and scopes of problems so that one is better able to integrate them to contribute to a greater understanding. Brazil's sponsorship of the Sixth World Bioethics Congress, held in Brasilia, Brazil (2002), with the theme "Bioethics, Power, and Injustice," may be pinpointed as the inception of its maturity (Garrafa and Pessini 2002).

8.2 The First Congresses of Bioethics and Health in Brazil

It is important to note in the historical record that before the consolidation of the Brazilian Bioethics Society, there were several institutions and study groups in existence that were formed around the discussion and dialogue of bioethical issues in the world of health, with a strong emphasis on humanization. Thus, in São Paulo, under the leadership of the Camillians, a religious order that works in the world of health, and in partnership with several hospitals and universities (both confessional and non-confessional), a series of four annual events on bioethics and health was sponsored during the early 1990s in São Paulo City, State of São Paulo (Pessini and Barchifontaine 1998).

The First Congress of Bioethics and Health (June 11–12, 1993) discussed mainly emergent bioethical questions concerning the beginning of life. The Second Congress (March 9–11, 1994) discussed questions concerning death and dying. The Third Congress (June 15–17, 1995) proposed a profound discussion of its main theme, bioethics and genetics, and the Fourth Congress (August 14–16, 1997) discussed bioethics and globalization.

Another issue of concern for the Camillians was the question of humanization and ministry within the world of health. This is the theme of bioethics, religion, and theology when one thinks about the ethical questions of life from the perspective of Christian values. From 1981 to the present, the Camillian Institute of the Ministry of Health (ICAPS), in partnership with the Ministry of Health of the CNBB (the National Conference of Brazilian Bishops), has organized 26 national congresses dedicated to the issue of humanization and ministry in health (ICAPS 1993–1997).

This Institute advocates for the humanization of health care in the face of the ever-increasing depersonalization and technologization of care, seeking to remedy problems of clinical ethics. We face the emergent ethical dilemmas brought about by science and technology that interfere with human nature (assisted reproduction, transplants, genetic engineering, cloning, etc.). Our reflection stems from a theological, ethical, and dialogical perspective, which encourages dialogue among scientists, theologians, philosophers, and health care professionals.

The humanization and ministry movement persists today in the world of health. A national organization has become part of the Brazilian reality, which serves as a leader of bioethical debate in the country and which has begun to assemble researchers and bioethicists (Barchifontaine and Pessini 1996).

8.3 The Brazilian Bioethics Society (SBB)

Preceding the development of the Brazilian Bioethics Society (SBB), an organization that develops and organizes bioethical initiatives within the country, the Brazilian Association of Medical Ethics (ABRADEM) was responsible for the reflection of not only ethical, but specifically bioethical issues. Within the association, one must acknowledge the leadership of Alfonso Renato Meira.

The Brazilian Bioethics Society began as an informal group, formed August 19, 1992, and was formally established February 18, 1995. Its pluralist and interdisciplinary character is demonstrated by the diversity of its more than 500 members, representative of several disciplines in the life and health sciences, philosophers, theologians, researchers from the human sciences, and others. At current, the SBB is responsible for having organized eight National Bioethics Congresses: in São Paulo (1996); *Bioethics in the Twenty-first Century* (Brasília, 1998); in Porto Alegre (RS), 2000; *Bioethics, Power and Injustice* (Brasília, 2002), held simultaneously with the Sixth World Bioethics Congress; *Bioethics and Citizenship* (Recife [PE], 2004); and *Environment and Human Life* (Iguaçu Estuary [PR], 2005); in 2007, both the First Bioethics Congress of Mercosur and the forum of REDBIOS – UNESCO, *Bioethics and Social Construction Today* (São Paulo [SP]), were held; in 2009, *Rights and Obligations in a Globalized World* (Búzios [RJ]).

In 2005, the SBB began publishing its quarterly scientific journal, the *Brazilian Bioethics Journal*. In addition, several SBB regional divisions both exist with legal recognition and maintain intense educational and publishing activities, including those in: Rio Grande do Sul (Porto Alegre), Paraná (Londrina), São Paulo (SP), Rio de Janeiro (Rio de Janeiro), Brasília (DF), and Pernambuco (Recife).

Brazilian bioethics is receptive to and in continuous dialogue with the global bioethics movement. Beginning in 1997, there were a number of Brazilian bioethicists on the Board of Directors for the International Association of Bioethics (IAB). The Brazilian Bioethics Society also dialogues intensely with the European Bioethics Association whose headquarters, the International Bioethics Society (*Sociedad International de Bioética* – SIBI), is in Gijón, Spain. Under the leadership of Dr. Marcelo Palácios, SIBI has sponsored international bioethics congresses in Spain. In Latin America, Brazil's participation in the Latin American Bioethics Congresses, promoted by FELAIBE, has long been established. We have also developed a relationship with UNESCO's Latin American and Caribbean Bioethics Network, officially established in Cancún, Mexico, in 2003. More recently, the Seventh Brazilian Bioethics Congress (August 29–September 1, 2007) decisively influenced the establishment of the Latin American Bioethics Association (ALBA).

In the domain of scientific development, the Brazilian bioethics community has published important works dealing with diverse themes related to human life. Some of the works of internationally reputed bioethicists have been translated into Portuguese by the Edições Loyola publishing house. The participation of publishers plays an important role in the collection and dissemination of the bioethics literature and its content. One must call attention to *Fundamentos de bioética* (*Foundations of Bioethics*, 1998) and *Fundamentos de Bioética Cristã Ortodoxa* (*The Foundations of Christian Bioethics*, 2000), by H. Tristram Engelhardt, Jr.; *Princípios de Ética Biomédica* (*Principles of Biomedical Ethics*) by Beauchamp & Childress; and *Introdução à bioética* (*Introduction to Bioethics*) by Guy Durand. From the Universidade do Sagrado Coração Press (Bauru – SP), we draw attention to Francisco Bellino, *The Foundations of Bioethics: Anthropological, Ontological, and Moral Aspects* (*Fundamentos de bioética: aspectos antropológicos, ontológicos e morais* – Edusc, Bauru, 1997). An important document from the Council of International Organizations of Medical Sciences (CIOMS), *International Ethical Guidelines for Biomedical Research Involving Human Subjects* (2002), was co-published in Brazil by Loyola Editions (Edições Loyola) and São Camilo University Center (Centro Universitário São Camilo) (cf. Prado 2002).

An initiative of particular international import is the Portuguese-Brazilian Bioethics Meeting. Four meetings have already occurred: the first meeting took place in Lisbon and was focused on the exchange of experiences; the second in Brasília, Brazil (November, 2002), took place during the World Bioethics Congress and focused on the topic of bioethics education; the third (2004) in the Açores Islands, Ponta Delgada, considered the topic and produced a book entitled *One or Several Bioethics in the Evolution of Societies* (Neves and Lima 2005); the fourth meeting, discussing bioethics and vulnerability, occurred in São Paulo (Brazil, 2006).

The Brazilian Bioethics Society seeks to create an integrative and dialogical space for bioethical initiatives within the country. Because of the SBB's work, Brazil had the credibility at the International Bioethics Association to host the Seventh World Bioethics Congress (Brasília, 2002), proposing as its central theme the relationship of *Bioethics, Power and Injustice*. This Congress added to the global bioethics agenda the need to address issues pertaining to exclusion occurring at the periphery of global society in developing or emergent countries (Pessini 2002a). One of the main publications of the Brazilian Society of Bioethics is about the history of Bioethics in Brazil with the publication of the book entitled Bioética no Brasil: tendênciase perspectivas (Bioethics in Brazil; tendencies and perspectives) (Anjos and Siqueira 2007).

8.4 Brazilian Institutional and Educational Initiatives

In Brazil, many bioethics initiatives are evolving, of both confessional and secular character, in both public and private institutions, and including the independent work of bioethicists in various areas of the country, which were more expressly developed in the 1990s.

Among the various initiatives there is a healthy and respectful conviviality that has grown out of a context increasingly secularized and pluralistic, which requires tolerance as indispensable to the dialogical process. Great interest and sensitivity regarding bioethics exist in Brazil. There are innumerable initiatives that demonstrate its vitality, both in the motivation of young researchers and in the significant interest of professionals (primarily from the health field) to contribute to specialized publications, as well as the substantial interest in events, journeys, seminars, and congresses on bioethics. The SBB's regional branches are also appearing with vitality, like Recife's, led by Maria Clara Albuquerque, which organized a Brazilian Bioethics Congress, or the group in Belo Horizonte (MG), which was formed by Geraldo Drumond, Dirceu Greco, and Antonio Mota, or the branch in Bahia at the University of Feira de Santana, where the reputed geneticist Eliane de Azevedo works.

8.4.1 The Federal University of Rio Grande do Sul (UFGRGS) and the Hospital Clinics of Porto Alegre (HCPA)

Between these institutions we have the *Interinstitutional Bioethics Center*, which develops many bioethics activities in the areas of assistance, education, and research. Regarding research, the Commission of Research and Ethics in Health, linked to the Research and Graduate Studies Group of HCPA, was created in 1989 and is responsible for the evaluation and enforcement of ethical guidelines.

The UFRGS Research Ethics Committee (CEP) was established in March 1997 and was coordinated by Jose Robert Goldim. Teaching activities began in 1990, when an intensive bioethics course was provided by the HCPA, with the participation of Robert Veatch of the Kennedy Institute of Ethics (Washington, DC). As of 1994, the Medical Clinic of UFRGS's graduate course in medicine began to include in its curriculum topics linked to bioethics. In the area of clinical ethics, a Program of Attention to Bioethical Problems was established in 1993 under the coordination of Carlos Fernando Francisconi. As of 2006, the program completed its sixth offering of the course "Introduction to Bioethics." The Bioethics Center also maintains a frequently visited web site that is said to be one of Brazil's best.

8.4.2 Pontifical Catholic University of Rio Grande do Sul (PUCRS), Porto Alegre: The Nucleus of Bioethical Studies and the Research Ethics Committee

Since 1988, under the leadership of Dean Joaquin Clotet, the graduate courses in medicine at PUCRS have included topics in bioethics. Among the university's researchers, Délio Kiper, Jussara de Azambuja, and Mariângela Badaloti must be mentioned. It should also be noted that PUCRS was the first Brazilian university with an academic training program for health professionals to incorporate bioethical problems and dilemmas into the curriculum.

The Bioethics Committee for St. Lucas Hospital and the Medical School of PUCRS was founded June 6, 1997, and has relationships with both institutions' administrations. The center has also published several works in bioethics, including those authored and edited by Joaquin Clotet: *Bioethics: An Approach* (*Bioética: uma aproximação* – Clotet 2003); *Bioethics: Environment, Public Health, and New Technologies* (*Bioética: Meio ambiente, saúde pública, novas tecnologias. Deontologia médica, direito, psicologia e material genético humano* – Clotet 2001) and *Bioethics: An Overview* (*Bioética: uma visão panorâmica* – Clotet et al. 2005).

8.4.3 University of São Paulo (USP), São Paulo (SP)

For many years, the *Oscar Freire Institute* has promoted meetings, journeys, and seminars about controversial topics in Brazilian bioethics at the Brazilian public universities. Marco Segre has defended the school of thought known as "autonomous reflection or autonomous bioethics" in collaboration with Claude Cohen, in their work *Bioethics* (*Bioética* – Segre & Cohen 1995). He has also done so more recently in another of his books, *The Ethical Question and Human Health* (*A questão ética e a saúde humana*-Segre 2006). From Segre's perspective, the expression "ethics of autonomous reflection" indicates the personal and individual character of ethical reflection, an ethics in which subjects, by means of introspection, bring to the surface multiple conflicting feelings and seek to think of their own solutions for these conflicts. One refers to a hierarchy of values determined by the individual person with as much freedom as possible. This is a patently libertarian ethic in which the "bioethicist" seeks to choose what he considers to be of greater or lesser value in every situation, either involving another person, the community, or even the planet.

In the College of Public Health, Paulo Fortes leads the reflections on bioethics and public health. He is co-author of the work, *Bioethics and Public Health* (*Bioética e Saúde Pública* – Fortes and Zoboli 2003). In the Nursing School, Elma Zoboli and Cristina Mazzarolo address those concerns related to bioethics and nursing

(Oguisso and Zoboli 2006). And in the Dentistry School, Dalton Ramos, a corresponding member of the Pontifical Academy for Life, has produced pioneering work on dentistry and Brazilian bioethics.

8.4.4 University of Brasília (UB), Center of Advanced Multidisciplinary Studies: Center of Studies and Research in Bioethics (NEPEB), Brasília, DF

Since its foundation in 1994, the center has been under the leadership of Volnei Garrafa. In August 1998, NEPEB launched its first Lato Sensu graduate course in bioethics. It has also published *The Human Market: A Bioethical Study of the Purchase and Sale of Body Parts* (*O mercado humano: estudo bioético da compra e venda de partes do corpo* – Berlinguer and Garrafa 1996); *Bioethics in the 21st Century* (*A Bioética no século XXI* – Garrafa and Costa 2000) and *Daily Bioethics* (*Bioética cotidiana* – Berlinguer 2003).

Beginning in 2000, the Bioethics Center, in partnership with the graduate program in Health Sciences at UB, began offering a Master's degree and doctorate in bioethics. A number of Brazilian Master's and PhD holders have studied in this program. Additionally, the Bioethics Center now holds the Bioethics Chair of UNESCO (Garrafa and Cordón 2006).

Garrafa proposes the concept of an "emergent situations bioethics," which is primarily concerned with historically emergent problems, called "extreme-situation" problems or knowledge "border" problems. "Emergent" refers to situations that have "emerged" only in the last 50 years as a result of technoscientific developments. Among these are included: human organs and tissue transplants; the Human Genome Project and all genomics aspects; new reproductive technologies, including reproductive and therapeutic cloning; transgenic foods; patents; environmental sustainability and biodiversity; and research involving human and non-human subjects. "Persistent situations bioethics" focuses on the historically persistent problems of bioethics, also called "daily problems." "Persistent" refers to situations that insistently "persist" despite the evolution of science and societal mores since the beginning of time. Among these problems we can mention social exclusion; discrimination; racism; labor inequities; vulnerability; violence; the just distribution of health care resources; abortion; and euthanasia (Garrafa et al. 2006).

8.4.5 The Federal Council of Medicine (CFM), Brasília (DF)

The first Brazilian bioethics journal, *Bioethics*, which was titled by Garrafa, first appeared in 1993 and enjoyed broad circulation in the medical community as it predominantly addressed issues of medical ethics. Each volume contains interesting discussions on the current controversial issues within bioethics. Some of the issues addressed have been: AIDS and Bioethics; Terminal Patients, Abortion, Euthanasia, and Medical Errors; Research on Human Beings; Teaching Ethics to Health Professionals; Public Policy; The Ethics of Resource Allocation in Healthcare; Ethics and Genetics; and Ethics and Violence. All issues are made available electronically at www.portalmedico.org.br.

The CFM has also published two noteworthy anthologies: *Ethical Challenges* (*Desafios Éticos*), edited by Jose Eberienos (Assad 1993) and *Introduction to Bioethics* (*Iniciação à Bioética*), which greatly impacted health care (Costa et al. 1998).

8.4.6 The Brazilian Society of Moral Theology

The Brazilian Society of Moral Theology includes among its membership moral theologians whose work in bioethics has gained international repute. The society has also promoted specialized events to address bioethical issues over the last few years. Among the Society's researchers, mention must be made of Márcio Fabri dos Anjos (Alfonsianum, São Paulo, SP) who studies questions of exclusion from the perspective of a theological bioethics, specifically, liberation theology. In the anthology, *Moral Theology in Latin America*, he provides reference material for every Latin American country. He also wrote "Bioethics from a Liberationist Perspective" (Anjos 1994). Another of the Society's scholars, Antonio Moser of the Franciscan Institute of Theology of Petrópolis, published *Biotechnology and Bioethics: Where Do We Go from Here?* (*Biotecnologia e bioética Para onde vamos?* – Moser 2004). Leonard Martin, the Irish Redemptorist theologian, should also be mentioned, because he lived many years in Brazil and published *Medical Ethics and the Terminal Patient: An Ethico-Theological Reading of Brazilian Medical Ethics Codes* (*A Ética Médica e o Paciente Terminal. Leitura ético-teológica dos códigos brasileiros de ética médica* – Martin 1993), which was derived from his doctoral thesis in moral theology. Mention must also be made of Leonardo Boff, who pioneered liberation theology in Latin America and enjoys international repute as a result. A significant part of his corpus consists in reflections on theology and its relationship to ecology and the environment. Boff was also responsible for establishing the group that wrote the famous "Letter of the Land," which UNESCO has consequently used for educational purposes. Additionally, three of his important works should be mentioned: *Scream of the Poor: Scream of the Land* (*Grito dos pobres: grito da terra* – Boff 1998), *Life Ethics* (*Ética da Vida* – Boff 2005a) and *Ethics and Morals: Search for Foundations* (*Ética e Moral: a busca dos fundamentos* – Boff 2005b).

8.4.7 São Camilo University Center, São Paulo (SP)

The São Camilo University Center sponsors the *The World of Health Journal* (O Mundo da Saúde 2007), which has been published uninterruptedly since 1977 and pertains to the specialized scientific work of health professionals. This journal was responsible for the introduction of bioethical questions to Brazil at the end of the 1970s and the beginning of the 1980s. Five specialized volumes in bioethics have been published and include: (1) *Bioethics* (v. 23, n. 5, Sept./Oct. 1999); (2) *Bioethics: A Brazilian Perspective* (v. 26, n. 1, Jan./Mar. 2002); (3) *Bioethics: Caring and Health* (v. 28, n. 3, Jul./Sept. 2004); (4) *Bioethics: Precursors, Foundations and Brazilian Educational Experiences* (v. 29, n. 3, Jul./Sept. 2005); and (5) *Bioethics: Humanization in Health, Vulnerability, Techonoscience and Research Ethics* (v. 29, n. 4, Oct./Dec. 2006).[1] In addition, the São Camilo University Center produced the first Brazilian bioethics manual for health professionals in 1987, originally titled *Bioética e Saúde* and later retitled *Actual Problems of Bioethics* (Problemas atuais de bioética), which was published in its 8th edition in 2006 (Pessini and Barchifontaine 2006). Additionally, in 2008, a special edition of this book (20,000 copies), sponsored by Diagnosticos da América, was published and distributed to doctors throughout the country. The Center also relies on the work of Hubert Lepargneur, author of a great many papers published in *The World of Health Journal* (*O Mundo da Saude*) and books, including *The New Concept of Bioethics: Reaching Consensus* (*Bioética, novo conceito: a caminho do consenso* – Lepargneur 1996), and the internationally recognized theologian Márcio Fabri dos Anjos (Barchifontaine 2005a).

Within this university, research pertaining to end-of-life issues resulted in the publication of a three-volume work by Leo Pessini on bioethics and the limits of life, translated into Spanish in Mexico by Ediciones Dabar. The trilogy was published by Edições Loyola under the titles *Dysthanasia: Extending Life* (*Distanásia: até quando prolongar a vida* – Pessini 2001); *Euthanasia: Why Shorten Life?* (*Eutanasia: por que abreviar a vida*? – Pessini 2004) and *Humanization and Palliative Care* (*Humanização e cuidados paliativos* – 3rd ed., Pessini and Bertachini 2005). Christian de Paul de Barchifontaine addressed problems pertaining to the beginning of life in his works *Bioethics and the Beginning of Life: Some Problems* (*Bioética e início da vida: alguns desafios* – Barchifontaine 2004), *Public Health and Bioethics* (*Saúde Pública é Bioética* – Barchifontaine 2005) and co-authored with Leo Pessini, *Bioethics: Some Challenges* (*Bioética: alguns desafios* – Barchifontaine and Pessini 1998). The university also began publishing the scientific journal Revista Bioethikos, in 2007.

In 2004, the Center created Brazil's first *stricto sensu* Master's course in bioethics. Its research line is ethics in research involving living beings. Regarding international relations, São Camilo University Center has partnerships with the Center for Clinical Bioethics at Georgetown University and the Kennedy Institute of Ethics (both in Washington, DC), the Palliative Care Program of the University of Toronto's College of Medicine, and the Institute of Bioethics at the Portuguese Catholic University (Portugal).

[1]Cf. *O Mundo da Saúde* (v. 30, n.1, 2007).

8.4.8 Unisinos University, São Leopoldo (RS)

Unisinos University maintains the Humanities Institute (IHU), whose main objective is to identify new challenges and solutions to contemporary problems from the Christian social humanist perspective through the integration of the interdisciplinary activities of ethics, work, and public theology.

As a Jesuit university, Unisinos, and therefore the IHU, seeks to realize the mission of the Society of Jesus through faith, work, the promotion of justice, and cultural and interfaith dialogue. Among the other initiatives of the IHU, it publishes *The Humanities Institute*, a weekly online journal, which addresses issues of modern scientific ethics.

Unisinos University was also responsible for publishing the first work on bioethics in Brazil, the translation of *The Main Issues in Bioethics*, by Andrew C. Varga, published in 1980 in the United States, translated by Guido Edgard Wenzel as *Problemas de Bioética* (cf. Varga 2005). Other publications include *Bioethics: Perspectives and Challenges* (*Bioética: Perspectivas e desafios* – Junges 2005) and *Bioethics: Hermeneutics and Casuistry* (*Bioética: Hermenêutica e casuística* – Junges 2006).

In 2003, the IHU translated a well-respected work on ethics and moral philosophy from France, *The Dictionary of Ethics and Moral Philosophy* (*Diccionário de Ética e Filosofia Moral*), in two volumes, edited by Monique Conto-Sperber. Another interesting translation is *Bioethics: From the Approach of Legal Philosophy* (*Bioética: segundo o enfoque da filosofia do direito* – D´Agostinho 2006).

8.4.9 Feminist Bioethics Centers

8.4.9.1 ANIS: The Institute of Bioethics, Human Rights, and Gender

ANIS, under the leadership of Débora Diniz, is the first Latin American non-governmental organization (NGO) devoted to research, technical assistance, and education in bioethics. With its headquarters in Brasilia, ANIS became active in 1999. In 2002, ANIS was officially recognized by Brazil's National Council of Research (CNPQ) as a bioethics research group. Additionally, the ANIS Documentation and Information Center is a bioethics reference center for the Pan-American Health Organization (PAHO).

The Institute promotes research and education in ethics and bioethics as they relate to issues of human rights, feminism, and gender equality. ANIS engages in research and activism geared towards the promotion and protection of women's basic rights, feminist bioethics, and gender equality, in collaboration with other social, educational, and political organizations that also share these ideals.

The initiatives of ANIS are carried out by its four programs. The Advocacy Program coordinates all political actions, including its work as a pressure group in Brazilian Parliament, and assisting and participating in the legislative debate on bioethical themes related to human reproduction. The Education Program seeks to realize the institutional mission of ethics promotion. It offers three qualification workshops on Advocacy, Bioethics, and Tools in all Brazilian states. The Information Program maintains the Documentation and Information Center, which aims to disseminate and democratize bioethical information in Brazil and is coordinated by librarians, specializing in bioethics. The Research Program is the main ANIS program and is responsible for conducting theoretical and ethnographic research in bioethics. The program also has a commitment to promoting the active participation of young researchers in bioethics.

The publishing house Editora LetrasLivres and the independent video producer ImagensLivres are both supported by ANIS. LetrasLivres is committed to stimulating debate on ethics, bioethics, feminism, gender, human rights, justice and social development. ImagensLivres promotes and democratizes themes associated with human rights and bioethics.

The many publications of LetrasLivres include: *Moral Conflicts and Bioethics* (*Conflitos Morais e Bioética* – Diniz 2001); *Who Has Access to Reproductive Technologies? Different Perspectives of the Brazilian Right* (*Quem Pode Ter Acesso às Tecnologias Reprodutivas? Diferentes Perspectivas do Direito Brasileiro)*, edited by Debora Diniz and Samantha Buglione; *Brazilian Bioethics Bibliography: 1990–2002* (*Bibliografia Bioética Brasileira: 1990–2002*), by Kátia Soares Braga; *A Bibliography of Studies on Sexual Violence Against Women: 1984–2003* (*Estudos Sobre Violência Sexual Contra a Mulher: 1984–2003*), by Kátia Soares Braga; *Research Ethics: Learning Experiences in South African Countries* (*Ética na Pesquisa: experiência de treinamento em países sul-africanos*), edited by Debora Diniz, Dirce Guilhem, and Udo Schüklenk/University of Brasília Press (Editora da Universidade de Brasília; *Bioethics and Reproduction in Contemporary Society* (*Bioética, reprodução e gênero na sociedade contemporânea*), edited by Maria Andréa Loyola/Brazilian Society for Populations Studies (Associação Brasileria de Estudos Populacionais); *Admirable New Genetics: Bioethics and Society* (*Admirável Nova Genética: bioética e sociedade* – Diniz 2003); and *Essays in Bioethics* (*Ensaios: Bioética*), by Sergio Costa and Débora Diniz (ANIS/Brazilian Publishing Company). The organization's web site, www.anis.org.br, provides a full list of publications.

8.4.9.2 Bioethics Information Network (RIB): Bioethics and Feminist and Anti-Racist Theory – Belo Horizonte (MG)

This center, under the leadership of Fátima Oliveira, is devoted to studies aimed at the dissemination and popularization of feminist and anti-racist bioethics. Oliveira has authored several books, including: *Genetic Engineering: The Seventh Day of Creation* (*Engenharia genética: o sétimo dia da criação* – Oliveira 2004) and *Bioethics: The Face of the Citizenship* (*Bioética uma face da cidadania* – Oliveira 1997). The RIB works to promote anti-racist theory and is the world's second web site on feminist bioethics, the first one being the *Feminist Approaches to Bioethics* web site, supported by the Kennedy Institute of Ethics.

8.4.10 National School of Public Health/ENSP/FIOCRUZ, Rio de Janeiro (RJ)

The National School of Public Health is where Fermin Roland Schramm and Miguel Kottow established their theory of "protective bioethics." The four tenets for the development of a protective ethics include: (1) the political commitment of all States; (2) a convivial foundation of ethics; (3) limitations on the North-American principlist paradigm of bioethics; and (4) the necessity of an ethics appropriate to Latin America, which reflects the socio-economic reality of developing countries.

From the perspective of Schramm, what is essential to protective bioethics, is the establishment of measures to protect the vulnerable individuals and populations who lack the resources to ensure the basic conditions for a life with dignity and not of mere survival (Schramm et al. 2005).

FIOCRUZ has a long history of making important contributions to issues concerned with bioethics and public health. In addition to conducting important research in public health, it has sponsored bioethics meetings, which were attended by international bioethicists. The institution has also published a special issue (in English) of the *Journal of Public Health* (*Cadernos de Saúde Pública*), which discussed important bioethical questions (Vol. 15, Supplement I 1999). Another noteworthy publication, edited by Fermin Roland Schramm and Marlene Braz in 2005, was titled *Bioethics and Health: Time for Women and Children?* (*Bioética e Saúde: nos tempos para mulheres e crianças*?). The Regional Chapter of SBB has several bioethicists in its membership, including Sergio Rego, Marlene Braz, Olinto Pegoraro, and Marisa Palácios. Pegoraro, a philosopher, has published within the field of ethics, including the titles *Ethics and Justice, An Introduction to Contemporary Ethics* (*Ética é Justiça, Introdução à Ética contemporânea*) and *Ethics of the Great Throughout History* (*Ética dos maiores mestres através da história* – Pegoraro 1999, 2005, 2006).

8.4.11 Center of Bioethics de Londrina (NBL), Paraná

The NBL's membership is comprised of individuals from several disciplines who are interested in considering and discussing ethical questions pertaining to life. The group's web site states: "Bioethics has an all important role in this debate concerning the protection of human dignity and the battle for justice. Reflection and discussion are two key strategies. NBL's aim in gathering professionals is to seriously engage with problems that affect people's daily life and to stimulate the production and diffusion of knowledge in this field."

The NBL is coordinated by José Eduardo de Siqueira. Among other researchers, Leonardo Prota, Nilza Diniz, and Lourenço Zancanaro participate. They offer a *lato sensu* bioethics graduate course, which was established at the end of the 1990s and was responsible for organizing the Sixth Brazilian Bioethics Congress in Foz do

Iguaçu in 2005. The NBL has also published several works, including *Ethics, Science and Responsibility* (*Ética, ciência e responsabilidade* – Siqueira et al. 2005).

Ainda no Paraná, Curitiba, destacamos a obra organizada por Cicero de Andrade Urban, intitulada *Bioética Clínica*, que reúne mais de 20 autores especialistas na área (Revinter, Rio de Janeiro 2003). Na Pontificia Universidade Catolica de Curitiba destaca-se a atuação do teologo Mario Sanchez, autor da obra: *Bioética e transcendência* (Loyola, São Paulo 2003).

The centers presented above are only some of the Brazilian organizations that publish, conduct research, and sponsor events relevant to bioethics. In addition, there are a number of independent initiatives that have been undertaken by Brazilian bioethicists from several Brazilian universities who are working towards integrating bioethics into the humanistic formation of the university, particularly within the health and life sciences.

8.5 Ethics in Research Involving Human Beings (1996–2006)

One of the most important achievements of Brazilian bioethics has been the establishment of a system of social control for research involving human subjects. In October 1996, Brazil developed its own ethical guidelines; they were developed within the purview of bioethics and approved by the Ministry of Health's National Council of Health (CNS). Within the field of research ethics in Brazil, the leadership of William Saad Hossne must be recognized, because in 10 years of work he was able to establish a Brazilian system of social control to govern research involving human subjects, which has consequently served as a model for many countries around the world.

The importance of this system fills the need to provide a historical overview of its development. In 1995, CNS created an interdisciplinary taskforce for the purpose of establishing guidelines. This group, on the basis of data from the Ministry of Health, the Ministry of Education, and the Ministry of Science and Technology, was able to identify about 30,000 relevant personalities or institutions (e.g., scientific societies, associations of individuals with deficiencies, and numerous professional councils), which were then analyzed with the purpose of extracting various norms. After 10 months of activities, a proposal was then presented to the National Council of Health, which formed the basis of Resolution 196/96 (Rules on Research Involving Human Subjects (Res. CNS 196/96 and others) 2000).

The guidelines had an essentially bioethical character and espoused a pluralist perspective. They were not crafted to read like a code, lacking language such as "it is forbidden" or "it is permissible," and they also did not have a mere notary-like or bureaucratic character. In accordance with the norms they had extracted, "nothing was a priori forbidden" but "not everything was allowed;" all depends on the ethical evaluation of a particular research project.

The researcher has full and non-transferable responsibility for having one's research project approved by a research ethics committee (CEP) at the institution where the research will be conducted before the project begins. CEPs have an interdisciplinary composition, and no more than half of its members can be of the same profession; it also must include people from different fields, in particular those of biomedicine, the human sciences, the hard sciences and, always, at least one representative of the institution's clientele. The committee has total autonomy and freedom in acting and, therefore, when a project is approved, it becomes partially responsible for its ethical oversight. The institution also has due responsibilities for the potential circumstances that may arise.

All CEPs must be registered by the National Commission of Research Ethics (CONEP), which is directly linked to the National Council of Health, a legal agency for social control. Thus, CONEP and CEP form an independent system for the social control of research ethics involving human subjects.

At present, Brazil has 475 ethics committees with around 7,000 members, comprised of doctors, nurses, dentists, physiotherapists, sociologists, lawyers, philosophers, engineers, mathematicians, anthropologists, and community representatives (Freitas et al. 2005). Bioethical norms apply to all research involving human subjects, in any field of knowledge (including the human sciences) capable of causing "physical, psychic, moral, intellectual, social, cultural or spiritual damage to human beings, at any stage of the research or resulting from it."

In addition, CONEP, with the interdisciplinary participation of both civil and scientific society, has elaborated seven other specific lines of direction for determined "thematic areas." All texts are available at www.conselho.saude.gov.br. In 2005, about 17,000 research protocols were evaluated (e.g., retrospective studies, phase II and III trial, and stem-cell research), involving about 700,000 subjects, who are, today, duly protected by the CONEP-CEP (Pessini 2002).

8.6 A Prospective Evaluation

Surprisingly, Brazil, in spite of so much vitality in the bioethical movement, has not yet established a National Commission of Bioethics. The SBB has been making consistent efforts to cause this to occur, and has been waiting for the most politically favorable moment to establish an agency to advise the Government, the Parliament, and society at large in matters of bioethical debate. This would prevent "petty politics" from having an advantage in ethical questions fundamental for life, health, and the future of the Brazilian population, which unfortunately did mark the approval of the Biosecurity Law at the beginning of 2005. The same statute regarding the moral status of genetically modified organisms was applied to transgenic food production and embryo (stem cell) research, which served to confuse public opinion.

The theoretical development of bioethics in Brazil is undoubtedly a great challenge. It has surpassed early legalism as a reference for norms creation and now has a place within interdisciplinary dialogue for reaching consensus. A number of lawyers in Brazil have great interest in bioethical issues concerning, to a large extent, the dilemmas caused by new technologies, because they frequently require court intervention. Socio-anthropological, philosophical, and theological arguments and analyses are also well received, in addition to a high degree of scientific seriousness and interdisciplinary dialogue.

The purview of Brazilian bioethics and its themes can be categorized into six different areas. The first is constituted by methodological studies that explain the nature of bioethics, its genesis, importance, methods, principles, and relevant relationship to technoscience, and searches for a philosophical–anthropological foundation. The second group includes mostly humanist health professionals (e.g., doctors, nurses, psychologists, theologians, and philosophers), and has as its main task the analysis and discussion of issues related to questions of professional ethics, medical ethics, and the humanization of health care. The discussion undertaken is interdisciplinary in nature and is concerned with the "macro" or broader social context, without restricting itself to "micro" questions. A third group is constituted of theologians, scholars, and researchers of moral theology who bring to bioethical discussions a religious ethic, a so-called *theological bioethics*, which, in Brazil, has a particular emphasis on the Christian and Afro-Brazilian religions. According to Marcio Fabri dos Anjos, theological reflection can help in the development of a horizon of sense, or a "mystique" for bioethics, that feeds a transforming socio-humanitarian perspective in which all fellow creatures are seen with love, that overcomes inequality by means of justice and solidarity, and helps to promote arguments and proposals aiming at a just and happy future for all. A fourth group espouses feminist bioethics, a group of individuals who champion a bioethical reflection sensible to women's concerns, which is capable of overcoming gender inequalities and eliminating the submission of women in the socio-political context, in addition to addressing racism, etc. Researchers of a social–political bioethics, some of whom champion a "bioethics of intervention," or a "hard bioethics" as Garrafa refers to it, constitute the fifth group. Additionally, this group includes those like Schramm and Kottow who endorse a "protective bioethics," which takes into account an analysis of the social–political structures producing inequalities and exclusions and advocates for changes particular to the defense of society's excluded and vulnerable people. In this same line, there is also the liberation ethics perspective, which was introduced in Brazil through liberation theology. Lastly, the study of bioethics has also awakened an interest on the part of legal professionals, causing a great many publications to appear. The Brazilian Bar Association (OAB), in its various regional branches, has established commissions of bioethics and law. Characteristic of this group is its devotion to the study of the interrelationships of bioethics, law, legislation, and public policies.

Due to the variety of Brazilian sensibilities and bioethical perspectives, we have as a daily challenge the practice of a respectful and tolerant dialogue, an inter-, multi-, and trans-disciplinary dialogue that avoids all forms of dogma, exclusion, and reduction. The greatest challenge for a global bioethics, and a Brazilian one specifically, is to be able to construct one with humility, respect for differences, and an appreciation for diversity and unity. If we are able to guarantee unity and openness as an integral part of each of the different perspectives, Brazilian bioethics will no doubt rapidly evolve and Brazil could be "humbly" proud of itself.

Brazilian bioethics in a short span of time succeeded in forging an identity and character of its own in the context of the global bioethics movement and now enjoys a position of leadership in the Latin American context. We have already produced works of critical analysis in search of a uniquely Latin American approach to bioethics, as is demonstrated in the anthology, *The Conceptual Foundations of Bioethics: A Latin American Approach* (*Bases conceituais da Bioética: enfoque Latino-americano* – Garrafa et al. 2006). To be able to understand bioethics in Brazil from now on, to be able to search for its epistemological structure, it is necessary to read and reflect with pleasure on the content of this work. Additionally, it should be noted that in the mid-1990s, the first critical studies had already begun to appear (e.g., Pessini 1995; Anjos 1996; Drane 1996; Garrafa et al. 2000; Hossne 2006).

In its adulthood, reaching maturity, Brazilian bioethics has an originality and an identity that need to be rescued and appreciated, moving beyond the historical context that was imposed on it due to an incapacity to think for ourselves and to our inferior circumstances as developing countries of the world. This reminds us of a Latin American proverb that states: "journeyer, there is no ready way; we create the way during the journey." We seek to practice a bioethics with reason and heart, with sensitivity and commitment to society's most vulnerable. This is a bioethics that realizes the dream of a better, healthier, and happier future for all.

References

Anjos MF (1994) Bioethics from a liberationist perspective. In: Dubose ER, Hamel RP, O'Connell LJ (eds) A matter of principles: ferment in US bioethics. Trinity Press International, Valley Forge, pp 130–147

Anjos MF (1996) Medical ethics in the developing world: a liberation theology perspective. J Med Philos 21(6):629–637

Anjos MF (2000) Notes on bioethics in Brazil, biomedical ethics. Newsl Eur Netw Biomed Eth 5(1):42–45

Anjos MF, Siqueria JE (eds.) (2007) Bioética to Brasil: tendências e perspectivas. Sociedade Brasileira de Bioética/Idéias e Letras, Aparecida, SP

Assad JE (eds) (1993) Desafios éticos. Conselho Federal de Medicina, Brasília

Barchifontaine CP (2004) Bioética e inicio da vida: alguns desafios. Ideias e Letras, Aparecida

Barchifontaine CP (2005a) Perspectivas da bioética na América Latina e o pioneirismo no ensino de bioética no Centro Universitário São Camilo (SP). O Mundo da Saúde, São Paulo, 29.3, 392–393

Barchifontaine CP (2005b) Saúde pública é bioética?. Editora Paulus, São Paulo

Barchifontaine CP, Pessini L (1996) Bioética a partir de América Latina. In: La vida vale: bioética – nuevos caminos. Centro de Estudos Y Publicaciones, Lima, Peru, pp 33–42

Barchifontaine CP, Pessini L (1998) Bioética: alguns desafios. Loyola, São Paulo

Berlinguer G (2003) Bioética cotidiana. Editora UnB, Brasília

Berlinguer G, Garrafa V (1996) O mercado humano: estudo bioético da compra e venda de partes do corpo. Editora UnB, Brasília

Boff L (1998) Grito dos pobres: grito da terra. Vozes, Petrópolis

Boff L (2005a) Ética da Vida. Sextante, Rio de Janeiro

Boff L (2005b) Ética e moral: a busca dos fundamentos. Vozes, Petrópolis

Clotet J (ed) (2001) Bioética: meio ambiente, saúde pública, novas tecnologias. Deontologia médica, direito, psicologia e material genético humano. Edipucrs, Porto Alegre
Clotet J (2003) Bioética uma aproximação. Edipucrs, Porto Alegre
Clotet J, Feijó A, Oliveira MG (2005) Bioética: uma visão panorâmica. Edipucrs, Porto Alegre
Costa SIF, Garrafa V, Oselka G (1998) Iniciação à bioética. Conselho Federal de Medicina, Brasília
D´Agostinho F (2006) Bioética: segundo o enfoque da filosofia do direito. Unisinos, São Leopoldo
de Freitas CBD, Lobo M, Hossne WS (2005) Oito anos de evolução: um balanço do sistema CEP-Conep. Cadernos de ética em pesquisa 16:20–30
Diniz D (2001) Conflitos morais e bioética. Letras Livres, Brasília
Diniz D (2003) Admirável nova genética: bioética e sociedade. Letras livres & UnB, Brasília
Drane JF (1996) Bioethical perspectives from Ibero-America. J Med Philos 21(6):557–569
Fortes P, Zoboli E (2003) Bioética e saúde pública. Loyola/Centro Universitário São Camilo, São Paulo
Garrafa V (2000) A bioethical radiograph of Brazil. Acta Bioethica VI.1:177–181
Garrafa V, Cordón J (eds) (2006) Pesquisas em bioética no Brasil de hoje. Editora Gaia, São Paulo
Garrafa V, Costa SI (2000) A bioética no século XXI. Editora UnB, Brasília
Garrafa V, Pessini L (eds) (2002) Bioética poder e injustiça. Edições Loyola/Editora do Centro Universitário São Camilo, São Paulo
Garrafa V, Costa SIF, Oselka G (eds) (2000) A bioética no século XXI. Editora UnB, Brasília
Garrafa V, Kottow M, Saada A (eds) (2006) Bases conceituais da bioética. Enfoque Latino-americano. Editora Gaia, São Paulo
Hossne WS (2006) Bioética – princípios ou referenciais. O Mundo da Saúde 30(4):673–676
Instituto Camiliano de Pastoral da Saúde. Boletim ICAPS (1993). Informativo do Instituto Camiliano de Pastoral da Saúde. Specific issues: maio de 1993, n.100, ano XI, p. 1–2; março de 1994, n.109, ano XII, p. 1; maio de 1995, n. 121, ano XIII, p.1; julho/agosto de 1997, n. 123 ano XIII; julho de 1997, ano XIV, n. 143, p.1
Junges JR (2005) Bioética: perspectivas e desafios, 3rd edn. Unisinos, São Leopoldo
Junges JR (2006) Bioética: hermenêutica e casuística. Loyola, São Paulo
Lepargneur H (1996) Bioética, novo conceito: a caminho do consenso. Loyola, São Paulo
Martin L (1993) A ética médica e o paciente terminal. Leitura ético-teológica dos códigos brasileiros de ética medica. Santuário, Aparecida
Moser A (2004) Biotecnologia e bioética: Para onde vamos?. Vozes, Petrópolis
National Health Council (2000). National Commission for Research Ethics–Conep–Brazil. Rules on research involving human subjects (Res. CNS 196/96 and others). Ministério da Saúde, Brasília
Neves MCP, Lima M (eds) (2005) Bioetica ou bioéticas na evolução das sociedades (ed) Gráfica de Coimbra – Editora do Centro Universitário São Camilo, Coimbra/São Paulo
O Mundo da Saúde (2007) Uma marca histórica: 30 anos de publicação ininterrupta. São Paulo, 31.1 (Jan–Feb)
Oguisso T, Zoboli E (eds) (2006) Ética e bioética. Editora Manole, Barueri
Oliveira F (1997) Bioética uma face da cidadania. Editora Moderna, São Paulo
Oliveira F (2004) Engenharia genética: o sétimo dia da criação, 10th ed. Editora Moderna, São Paulo
Pegoraro O (1999) Ética é justiça. Vozes, Petrópolis
Pegoraro O (2005) Introdução à ética contemporânea. Uapê, Rio de Janeiro
Pegoraro O (2006) Ética através dos maiores mestres através da história. Vozes, Petrópolis
Pessini L (1995a) O desenvolvimento da bioética na América Latina. Saúde em Debate 47:57–66
Pessini L (1995b) O desenvolvimento da bioética na América Latina – algumas considerações – parte I. O Mundo da Saúde 19(2):84–91
Pessini L (1995c) O desenvolvimento da bioética na América Latina – algumas considerações – parte II. O Mundo da Saúde 19(3):116–119

Pessini L (1999) Bioetica: Horizonte de esperança para um novo tempo. O Mundo da Saúde 23(5):259–262
Pessini L (2001) Distanásia: até quando prolongar a vida. Edições Loyola/Centro Universitário São Camilo, São Paulo
Pessini L (2002a) Bioethics, power and injustice: some personal thoughts from a Latin American perspective. Iab News 13:9–14
Pessini L (2002b) Building a new culture of ethics in research involving humans in brazil. Notizie di Politéia 67:101–112
Pessini L (2004) Eutanásia: por que abreviar a vida? Edições Loyola/Centro Universitário São CAmilo, São Paulo
Pessini L, Barchifontaine CP (eds) (1998) Bioética: alguns desafios. Edições Loyola/Centro Universitário São Camilo, São Paulo
Pessini L, Barchifontaine CP (2006) Problemas atuais de bioética, 8th rev. (ed) Loyola, São Paulo
Pessini L, Bertachini L (eds) (2005) Humanização e cuidados paliativos. Edições Loyola/Centro Universitário São Camilo, São Paulo
Prado MM (2002) Panorama da bioética no Brasil: um estudo sobre a reflexão bioética desenvolvida no país, Dissertação de Mestrado em Ciências da Saúde. Universidade de Brasília, Brasília
Rules on Research Involving Human Subjects (Rs.CNS 196/96 and others) (2000) National Health Council. National Commission for Research Ethics- CONEP/Brazil. Ministerio da Saúde, Brasilia
Schramm FR (2002) A pesquisa bioética no Brasil entre o antigo e o novo. Cadernos Adenauer, ano III 1:97–101
Schramm FR, Rego S, Braz M, Palácios M (eds) (2005) Bioética, riscos e proteção. Editora UFRJ/ Editora Fiocruz, Rio de Janeiro
Segre M (2006) A questão ética e a saúde humana. Atheneu, São Paulo
Segre M, Cohen C (eds) (1995) Bioética. Edusp, São Paulo
Siqueira JE et al (2005) Ética, ciência e responsabilidade. Loyola/Centro Universitário São Camilo, São Paulo
Varga AC (2005) Problemas de bioética. Unisinos, São Leopoldo

Chapter 9
Bioethics in Chile

Miguel Kottow

9.1 Introduction

For quite some time, Latin American bioethicists have defended the idea that regional particularities require a brand of ethics that is attuned to their own social and cultural idiosyncrasies and respectful of the ethnic diversity of their population. A number of historical and social commonalities allow most of the region's nations to share a bioethical discourse which, in spite of local variations, bears witness to the prevalence of a Latin American brand of what has been called moral acquaintanceship (Wildes 2000). Describing the bioethics scene in one country should help to understand and highlight both their variations and similarities. Applied ethics is especially sensitive to the local circumstances of social practices, and it comes as no surprise that the Sixth World Congress on Bioethics, held in Brasilia in 1999, emphasized "Bioethics, Power and Injustice" as its main theme, considering that social and health care inequities are highly prevalent throughout Latin America.

Chile has been unique in its marked physical isolation, its peculiar geography, a long-held political stability that was violently disrupted in the 1970s, and a pioneering interest in social legislation in contrast to its extreme hesitance to accept any legislation on such issues as divorce, contraceptives, and abortion. On the other hand, the nation shares with its regional neighbors an economic dependence on industrialized countries, a strong commitment to market values, unresolved issues concerning ethnic minorities, and an unfavorable Gini index with simmering social conflicts.

M. Kottow
Department of Philosophy, University of Chile (Universidad de Chile)
e-mail: kottow@hotmail.com

L. Pessini et al. (eds.), *Ibero-American Bioethics: History and Perspectives*,
Philosophy and Medicine 106, DOI 10.1007/978-1-4020-9350-0_9,

9.2 Historical Background

A few historical notes on Chile should serve as ancillary information to illustrate and better understand the present situation. Shortly after Pedro de Valdivia had founded the city of Santiago in the sixteenth century, the first hospital was built by Spanish authorities and run by a religious order. For a long time, publicly provided medical assistance continued to predominate over private medical services. Over the years, public resources became insufficient and for a long time charity was pre-eminent in financing and managing public medical institutions, up until the twentieth century when sanitary and medical affairs became a legally recognized and increasingly comprehensive responsibility of the State, with the creation of a National Health Service in 1952.

Formal medical studies were initiated at the University of Chile in 1842, with a strong European influence. Eventually, medical ethics was taught by professors of legal medicine under the label of deontology, mainly dealing with the profession's code of morality. Issues that nowadays concern bioethics, such as health-related rights, access to medical care, social discrimination, and marginalization, were discussed in the field of public health; this is in continuation of a tradition going back to Rudolf Virchow's student Max Westenhofer, who taught in Chile for many years. Among his pupils was Salvador Allende, a physician who, as Secretary of Health, later a senator, and eventually President of Chile, had a major influence on public health policies in the country (Waitzkin et al. 2001; Porter 2006). Even though bioethics was only slowly incorporated into the graduate curriculum of medical studies, there had been a long-standing tradition of teaching the essentials of medical ethics, as well as taking pains to develop public health policies and a concept of sanitary justice.

The disciplined membership in the Chilean Medical Association with its ethical tuition, and the prevalent commitment to public service in state and university hospitals, were decisive in holding Chilean physicians in high social standing that often led to international prestige. Medical ethics did not seem to be in need of expansion or deliberation, because Chilean culture, medical practice included, had always been paternalistic in an authoritarian way; physicians were by right of profession morally adequate and could self-righteously make decisions in the name of their patients.

The Colegio Médico de Chile – Chilean Medical Association – was created in 1948, with a strong mandate to update a professional code of ethics and oversee the morally adequate practice of medicine. Membership for all physicians was compulsory and constituted a legal requisite to engage in any kind of medical activity. Under the military regime of Pinochet, membership in the Medical Association became voluntary and, although the Code of Ethics was expanded and regularly updated, physicians could easily elude control and sanctions by being non-members. Interestingly, the Medical Association has for many years supported a department of (bio)ethics commissioned to study conceptual and practical moral issues, and to formulate answers to ethical problems of major import, in addition to resolving specific moral conflicts not covered by the Association's ethics committee.

The vast majority of clinicians took up part-time (often full-time) employment in public hospitals which were better equipped and staffed than the private sector, at least up until the 1970s. Over the next decades, private medical services, in the form of private practices and a small number of clinics, began to flourish and increasingly tempted physicians away from hospital service. As a result, most Chilean doctors work exclusively in the rapidly expanding private sector, which takes care of no more than one-fifth of the total population. Furthermore, private medical facilities are over-staffed with physicians and richly endowed with instrumental resources as compared to the public sector. Similarly, private universities outnumber the public ones, so that more physicians graduate from newly created medical schools than from traditional ones that offer training in public hospitals and foster strong social commitments.

Concepts of justice are very much at the center of bioethical concerns, especially in a country like Chile, which has appalling social and income disparities. Nevertheless, distributive justice is handled as a political rather than ethical issue. The Chilean Constitution proclaims a right to health care or, in a variation introduced during the military regime, a right to health protection. Since the 1950s a national health care service has been organized and financed with approximately 3% of the GNP to cover public health needs and medical care to the poor, the unemployed, the labor force, and their families. There were, of course, major gaps and insufficiencies even after the brief period of Allende's presidency (1970–1973), when the budget was increased to 3.7% of the GNP. A major crisis in health care provision was unleashed after the military coup curtailed all social services, including medical assistance, which has slowly regained momentum and benefited from reforms instituted in 1988. Health care coverage has improved for the 70–80% of Chileans who are protected by free or subsidized fiscal medical care, but state-financed programs still compare poorly with privately insured medical services. A two-tiered health care system is now firmly established, where a number of highly sophisticated clinics cater to the affluent, offering access to the latest technologies and the amenities of luxurious in-patient care.

Strong pragmatism has also reached the actual practice of medicine, and continuing education is served to a great extent under the unconcealed patronage of the pharmaceutical industry. Some of the leading private clinics have become HMOs and require their physicians to work in an economically efficient way. Evidence-based medicine is strongly advocated, and ethical concerns regarding randomized clinical trials and the application of scientific knowledge in preference to personal commitment are additional factors that tend to weaken the potential influence of bioethics.

In sum, bioethics makes its appearance in a country that for many decades had experienced a medical profession that was devoted to public service and ethically regulated by a strong Medical Association. Under the military regime of Pinochet, public institutions have been weakened, social services including education and medicine have to a great extent been privatized, and professional associations have lost the power to regularly oversee the ethical conduct of their members. Although these factors do not favor a prompt and strong commitment to bioethical deliberation, there has been a steady growth of interest in the subject.

9.3 Early Bioethics

Historians rarely have the opportunity to record the birth of a discipline, especially if it emerges unconnected to any major scientific breakthrough. The twin birth of bioethics was precisely located and followed by the prompt creation of institutions that were to recruit a number of gifted scholars who rapidly became the founding fathers of bioethics. This fulgent emergence of bioethics in the United States did not repeat itself elsewhere, and in Latin America a much less exciting story must be told, for the discipline entered very hesitantly and quietly into social and academic life.

In the 1980s, Chile did not have any indication of the successful institutionalization of bioethics that had occurred in Argentina, Colombia, and Brazil (León 2004). The need for a new approach to ethical dilemmas – presented by clinical and research practices – was hardly pressing, and problems were discussed in a way that did little more than ratify traditional views. In contrast to other countries, philosophers did not show any early interest in bioethics, the theoretical reflection on medical and biological issues being mainly carried out by our most prominent humanistic physicians, who delved deep into philosophical ethics in order to reflect on medical issues adequately (Vial Correa and de D 1990; Roa 1990). In 1988, a symposium on medical ethics was held under the title "Respect and Promotion of the Human Person in Modern Medicine." The word bioethics was first incorporated in the title of the proceedings, and most Chilean contributors mentioned bioethics only rarely (Lavados et al. 1990).

Schools of medicine taught traditional medical ethics and took little notice of the shift toward bioethics. The first centers for bioethics, alone or combined with humanistic studies, were created at the major medical schools. These were small academic units, mainly concerned with the teaching of optional graduate courses that later became enmeshed in the official curricula (Figueroa and Fuenzalida 1996). These centers have currently expanded their teaching activities, offering post-graduate programs that lead to a Master's degree in bioethics. An Interdisciplinary Center of Bioethics under rectorial supervision was created in 1993 at the University of Chile, where one of the first textbooks on bioethics was conceived (Kottow 1995). University faculties were not familiar enough with the idea of academic bioethics to interact actively with the Center, which consequently stopped functioning for a while. The Center was later revived as the Interdisciplinary Center for Bioethical Studies, dedicated to research activities and post-graduate training programs supported by international funds.

An important milestone in Chilean bioethics was the agreement reached in 1994 between the Pan American Health Organization (PAHO), the Chilean government, and the University of Chile to create the Regional Program of Bioethics, which was aimed at promoting bioethical activities throughout Latin America and the Caribbean. Among its multiple activities, the program published the "Cuadernos del Programa de Bioética" with articles provided by regional scholars, and instituted a 2-year-long course leading to a Master's degree in bioethics. This international post-graduate program was held for two consecutive periods in Santiago, Chile, and is now located at the University of Cuyo, Argentina. The regional program has been reorganized as a bioethics unit, assisted by an International Advisory Board on Bioethics. It continues to publish a biannual journal, now called *Acta Bioética*, and has developed an active and highly productive research and training program of its own (Lolas 2004).

During the 1990s, Chilean scholars began to publish, at first sporadically, in medical journals, in the above-mentioned official publications of PAHO, and, more recently, in the proceedings of meetings held in Chile and other Latin American countries. A small number of authors have also been publishing in international journals or contributing to books published in mainstream bioethics literature, in addition to a few who are members of the editorial boards of prestigious journals in Argentina, Brazil, Colombia, the United States, and Great Britain.

The corporative life of Chilean bioethics is weak. The Chilean Medical Association has created a study group and a Department for Bioethics, which advises the Board of Directors on ethical and bioethical issues. An annual Ethics Prize is given to the best essay presented or published by a collegiate member of the medical profession. The Chilean Society for Bioethics was founded some 10 years ago, and has swelled its membership by resorting to fairly slack admission policies. Meetings were initially scheduled on an annual basis, but have become very irregular. The recent untimely death of its acting president throws a shadow of uncertainty on the Society's future. Membership in regional associations like FELAIBE and FLACEIS has been sporadic, but Chile does have representation in the Directive Council of the UNESCO Network of Bioethics for Latin America and the Caribbean, and in the Council of the Latin American Chapter of the International Society for Bioethics (SIBI). Some Chilean scholars are regularly invited to take part in regional meetings and teaching activities, as well as to participate in international research teams and task forces sponsored by UNESCO, WHO, PAHO, and NIH. Books have appeared on bioethics (Lolas 1998; Escríbar et al. 2004; Kottow 2005), ethics and bioethics (Roa 1998), clinical bioethics (Lavados and Serani 1993), bioethics and medical anthropology (Lolas 2000; Kottow and Bustos 2005), theology and bioethics (Mifsud 1992), bioethics and public health (Kottow 2006a), bioethics and law (Ugarte 2006), and other specific issues (Beca 2002).

9.4 Institutions

The main institutional commitment of bioethics is the creation and proper functioning of hospital ethics committees, which are expected to oversee the ethical aspects of institutional medical care and to protect the rights of patients. The first committees were registered in Chilean hospitals in 1990, but it was not until 1994 that a first ruling was issued, compelling all major hospitals to form a medical ethics committee. Issued by the Ministry of Health, the document was nevertheless hardly heeded: a few committees were formed but never functioned, others allegedly could not find appropriate and willing members, and those that did constitute themselves remained mainly non-operative for lack of experience (Martínez 1995). At present, teaching hospitals have finally formed their committees, often with mixed functions in both medical care and research, and under the widespread impression that medical committees should be formed by a majority of physicians, with the isolated presence of a non-medical health care professional and, eventually, a lay person from the community. Hospital committees have been very conservative, usually abiding by the law, official regulations, or house rules. Respect for life is considered an overruling mandate, preempting any decision concerning life-shortening procedures or treatment rejection by patients (including Jehovah's Witnesses). In extremely exceptional cases, a committee may look favorably at the request to deviate from the strict letter of the law, honoring a petition for the premature delivery of an anencephalic child, or accepting the informed decision of a patient to reject critical treatment.

A law concerning the rights of patients has been under evaluation in parliament for more than 5 years, and is being reformulated in such a way that it will take another 2 to 3 years to reach final agreement. Although favorable to the well-being of in-patients, this law will continue to back up the reluctance of committees to liberalize end-of-life decisions.

The Chilean equivalent of institutional review boards (IRBs) are the Comités de Bioética en Investigación, which are becoming increasingly mandatory, mainly because official funding of research protocols will only consider projects that have been approved by the investigators' institutional research committee. Composition and rulings of these committees are still haphazard, but efforts are being made at different levels to have them certified, and to increase the level of competence of its members (Kottow 2006b, 2007). It has been only very recently that investigations with human subjects and research in animals have received distinct ethical attention by ad hoc committees. Much needs to be done, for many committee members rely on the Declaration of Helsinki and are barely aware of the conflicts that have ensued from the latest version of this document and its modifications. A law requiring the standardization of the regulations of research on human beings has very recently been passed, and possible ways of creating or reinforcing research ethics institutions are now being discussed at different levels.

The year 1968 marks the creation of the National Council for Research and Technology – Consejo Nacional de Investigación y Tecnología (CONICYT) – with the mission of overseeing and funding high-quality research. CONICYT supervises a number of programs, the most important and relevant to bioethics being the FONDECYT: National Fund for Scientific and Technological Development, launched in 1981 and aimed at basic research in the life sciences. Interestingly, ethical consideration first appeared in 1991, when CONICYT "suggested" that research protocols be submitted to an institutional ethics committee; otherwise, CONICYT might consider taking the initiative of requesting an ethics consultation on its own. Between 1993 and 1996, a report from an IRB became increasingly mandatory. One year later, submission of an ethics report was also recommended for animal research, and became mandatory 4 years later. It was not until 1999 that a copy of the informed consent document to be used had to be included in the grant proposal; genetic studies required not only approval but also detailed comments by an ethics committee.

This summarily presented sequence of events suggests that research ethics was quite rapidly incorporated into the fabric of grant protocols; and yet, CONICYT decided to create its own Advisory Committee for Bioethics in 2005. The

Committee has four permanent members whose expertise lies in biomedical and social sciences research, with experience in committee work, and knowledge of theoretical bioethics. After the Committee had reviewed some of the protocols approved and funded in the past, as well as incoming applications, it became painfully clear that most committees (even those in teaching hospitals and universities) were not doing a thorough job of evaluating the ethical aspects of the protocols they reviewed. Many of them issued a *pro forma* approval, or summarily certified compliance with the Declaration of Helsinki. Nevertheless, most approved protocols presented objections that required amendments, a major correction or, more rarely, downright rejection. CONICYT/FONDECYT, being the major research funding institution in the country, can be expected to promote policies and regulations concerning IRBs, such as updating and subjecting them to certification. These endeavors will be supported by the recently passed law that empowers the Ministry of Health, and the about-to-be-created National Commission of Bioethics, to regulate and oversee research with human subjects.

Much discussion about the pros and cons of creating a National Commission for Bioethics has been carried out for quite some time. Those in favor take France as an example of an efficient commission, while opponents point the finger at some poorly functioning commissions in the region. The pro-commission position has finally carried the day, Congress having passed a law creating the commission, but many of the suggestions presented still have not been heeded, and it may well be that Chile will finally have its own less than optimal commission.

9.5 Bioethical Deliberations and Cultural Influences

A history of bioethics is more than the presentation of its actors and their products. More fundamental, perhaps, is the story of its ideas, for bioethics is an applied ethics devoted to social practices of very general concern that are enmeshed with prevailing cultural patterns and moral discourse. Three major forces have influenced the development of bioethical ideas in Chile, as in many other Latin American nations. First, the foundations of Anglo-Saxon bioethics, in particular principlism, were absorbed as the most coherent school of thought available. Second, the Catholic Church developed an early interest in biomedical problems, especially those that were intimately related to doctrine. And finally, market forces have become a major impact on biomedical practices and values.

Although principlism was hailed as a transparent and simple-to-follow normative system, it soon became apparent that the idea of four equivalent principles did not easily fit into a culture where colonialism and class distinctions had played an important part in its history and still remained, to some degree, actively present. As a consequence, autonomy could not be accepted as a universal attribute, for the uneducated, the sick, the young, and, still to a large degree, the female population were seen as limited in their mental competence. Beneficence was also tainted by a long tradition of class and professional hegemony, and the assignation and evaluation of benefits still run under the motto "doctor knows best." In a parallel fashion, nonmaleficence is very often downplayed by the physician, and possible risks are silenced, thus distorting the information passed on to patients or research subjects.

All of these developments occur in absentia of a bioethical debate, and illustrate how bioethics has not been effective in influencing civil society or encouraging public deliberation on some of the most socially relevant issues like abortion, contraception (including the day-after pill), voluntary sterilization, euthanasia, and, of course, justice in health care. All these issues and some laws already in effect – regarding organ transplants and brain death – have hardly been subjected to public debate. Relevant scholarly advice and expertise are rarely sought or heeded, and there is hardly any evidence that law-makers take pains to acquire some sort of bioethics education before legislating in matters of nation-wide concern.

Ever since Catholic missionaries took part in the conquest of Latin America and willingly undertook civil tasks like education, hospital care, and the management of cemeteries, the Catholic Church has enjoyed a position of preeminence in political and cultural affairs. To this day, the Church runs a substantial number of the most outstanding schools and universities in the country. Some of the main political parties are overtly committed to religious doctrine and support conservative views. When bioethics arrived, the Church was already prepared to defend positions and educate the public in terms of not allowing secularity to disrupt religious doctrine. The most controversial topics in bioethics have thus been unable to reach the civil turf, and legislators have been unwilling or unable to even discuss such critical matters as abortion, euthanasia and assisted suicide, the use of embryonic stem-cells, and the production and fate of surplus embryos. Unsettling controversies still rage over access to levonorgestrel as a post-coital contraceptive and the dissemination of free condoms to avoid HIV transmission.

Another major influence on the development of bioethical thought has been the strong neo-liberal brand of economics that dictates public policies and tends to blunt substantial increases in fiscal programs related to many social needs (health care included). Bioethics scholars acknowledge that improvements have been made, but much more needs to be done in a country that still has more than 20% of its population under the poverty line, and where public health care services labor under the burdens of insufficient funds, ill paid and poorly trained personnel, unresolved administrative disorders, and a disturbingly high degree of public distrust. As this article is being written, national statistics inform that the health-gap has increased in recent years between the affluent and educated city dwellers, as compared to the poor, the uneducated, and the geographically more isolated population. Official statistics have also been published that show an increase in medical-care and health-status disparities in accordance with social and educational inequities. The social engagement of bioethics tries to palliate these insufficiencies by training health care professionals to be more aware of social inequities, to take part in hospital and research committees, to assist in the improvement of the ethical quality of pertinent laws, and to expand graduate teaching to create generations of professionals sensitive to the ethical problems of their chosen discipline. Unfortunately, these efforts have not reached public education, while pending tasks and unfulfilled expectations remain prevalent.

In sum, Chile has slowly become aware of the importance of bioethics, developing moderate academic activity, which has yet to gain influence in policy-making instances or in public awareness. Personal achievements, not always devoid of rivalries, have predominated over institutional commitments, and teamwork is only slowly gaining momentum, reproducing conditions and traits that are equally present in other parts of Latin America.

References

Beca JP (2002) El embrión humano. Editorial Mediterráneo, Santiago

Escríbar A, Pérez M, Villarroel R (2004) Bioética. Fundamentos y dimensión práctica. Editorial Mediterráneo, Santiago

Figueroa P, Fuenzalida H (1996) Bioethics in Ibero-America and the Caribbean. J Med Philos 21:611–627

Kottow M (1995) Introducción a la bioética. Editorial Universitaria, Santiago

Kottow M (2005) Introducción a la bioética, 2nd edn. Editorial Mediterráneo, Santiago

Kottow M (2006a) Bioética en salud pública. Editorial Puerto de Palos, Santiago

Kottow M (ed) (2006b) Bioética e investigación con seres humanos y en animales. CONICYT, Santiago

Kottow M (ed) (2007) Marcos normativos de la ética en investigación científica con seres vivos. CONICYT, Santiago

Kottow M, Bustos R (2005) Antropología médica. Editorial Mediterráneo, Santiago

Lavados M, Serani A (1993) Etica clínica. Ediciones Universidad Católica de Chile, Santiago

Lavados M, Monge JI, Quintana C, Serani A (eds) (1990) Problemas contemporáneos en bioética. Ediciones Universidad Católica de Chile, Santiago

León FJ (2004) Diez años de bioética en América Latina: historia reciente y retos actuales. In: Lolas F (ed) Diálogo y cooperación en salud. Diez años de bioética en la OPS. Unidad Bioética OPS-OMS, Santiago, pp 145–152

Lolas F (1998) Bioética. Editorial Universitaria, Santiago

Lolas F (2000) Bioética y antropología médica. Publicaciones Técnicas Mediterráneo Ltd., Santiago

Lolas F (2004) 10 years PAHO Bioethics Unit (1994–2004). Acta Bioethica 10:7–10

Martínez L (1995) Situación de los comités de etica hospitalaria en el sistema de salud pública chileno. In: Kottow M (ed) Temática y funcionamiento de los comités institucionales de ética médica/bioética. Centro Interdisciplinario de Bioética, U. de Chile, Santiago

Tony Mifsud, S.J. (Jesuit Priest) (1992) El respeto por la vida humana (bioética). Moral de discernimiento (tomo II), 3rd edn. Ediciones Paulinas-CIDE, Santiago

Porter D (2006) How did social medicine evolve, and where is it heading? PloS Med 3:1667–1672. (Online) Available: www.plosmedicine.org. Accessed May, 2009

Roa RA (1990) Investigación científica biomédica: fundamentos éticos y antropológicos. In: Lavados M, Monge JI, Quintana C, Serani A (eds) Problemas contemporáneos en bioética. Ediciones Universidad Católica de Chile, Santiago, pp 47–61

Roa RA (1998) Etica y bioética. Editorial Andrés Bello, Santiago

Ugarte JJ (2006) El derecho de la vida. Bioética y derecho. Editorial Jurídica de Chile, Santiago

Vial Correa J, de D (1990) Respeto y promoción de la persona humana. In: Lavados M, Monge JI, Quintana C, Serani A (eds) Problemas contemporáneos en bioética. Ediciones Universidad Católica de Chile, Santiago, pp 23–30

Viel B (1961) La medicina socializada y su aplicación en Gran Bretaña, Unión Soviética y Chile. Ediciones de la Universidad de Chile, Santiago

Waitzkin H, Iriart C, Estrada A, Lamadrid S (2001) Social medicine then and now: lessons from Latin America. Am J Public Health 91:1592–1601

Wildes KW (2000) Moral acquaintances. University of Notre Dame Press, Notre Dame, Ind

Chapter 10
Evolution of Bioethics in Costa Rica: A Recent History

Daniel Bustos-Montero

10.1 Introduction

One of the most important achievements of the small Central American country of Costa Rica is its health care system, considered one of the best in Latin America, making its explanation necessary to understanding Costa Rican bioethics.

The so-called Costa Rican health care sector, constituted by the Health Department, the Costa Rican Social Security Agency, the National Security Institute, the Costa Rican Institute of Aqueducts and Sewerages, the universities, and private health services, has managed to attain levels of health care comparable to those of industrialized countries, which has distinguished Costa Rica from the other Latin American countries.

The Costa Rican Social Security Agency (CCSS–Caja Costarricense de Seguro Social), which was established on November 1, 1941, is a fundamental component of this system. The CCSS functions as an autonomous institution and its philosophy is based on the principles of solidarity, unity, universality, equality, and obligation. Since its creation, the CCSS has been the country's primary health services supplier and has provided coverage for about 87% of the country's population, including both Costa Ricans and foreigners. It also has more than 40,000 employees distributed among 2,695 welfare centers located throughout the country. Its assistance system is divided into three levels, which are shown in Fig. 10.1.

With a basic understanding of the Costa Rican health care system and its function and structure, one can now understand the beginnings of Costa Rican bioethics.

D. Bustos-Montero (✉)
Bioethics, Centro de Desarrolo Estratégico y información en Seguridad Social y Salud (Center for Stragegic Development and Information in Social Insurance and Health), Caja Costarricense de Seguro Social (Costa Rica Insurance Agency)
e-mail: dbustos@ccss.sa.cr

L. Pessini et al. (eds.), *Ibero-American Bioethics: History and Perspectives*, Philosophy and Medicine 106, DOI 10.1007/978-1-4020-9350-0_10,

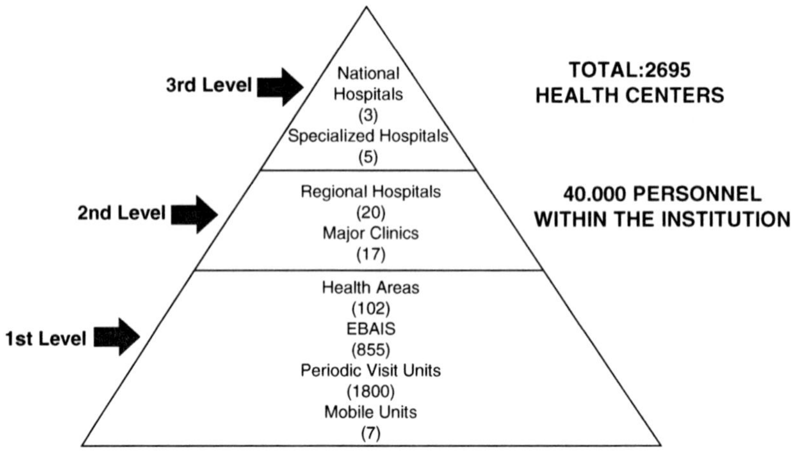

Fig. 10.1 The Costa Rican Social Security Agency's three levels

10.2 The Beginnings of Bioethics in Research

The development of bioethics in Costa Rica in the 1970s is particularly interesting, because its incorporation primarily involved research ethics in the health care sector, which was a welfare system with a very small research culture.

In 1972, long before the Tuskegee study and the Belmont Report were published in the United States, the Costa Rican Health Department set forth the Executive Decree 2393 (Ministerio de la Salud. Centro de Desarrollo Estratégico e Información en Salud y Seguridad Social 2007) providing for the creation of the Committee on Medical Research on Human Beings and the Regulation of New Drug and Medication Assays (Comité de Investigaciones Médicas en Humanos y Reglamenta los ensayos de nuevas drogas y medicamentos). This development presaged a rigorous normative evolution in research ethics that never came to fruition. Additional regulations were put into place, including the General Law of Health (Ley General de Salud) (Imprenta Nacional 1974), which included general regulations for research involving human beings, and the Executive Decree 5463-SPPS1 of the Health Department in 1975 called the Regulation for Research and Experiments in Human Beings (Reglamento para las investigaciones y experimentaciones en seres humanos), which provided for the creation of an inter-institutional scientific committee to evaluate all research projects carried out in the country. A timeline of the development of regulations for biomedical research in Costa Rica is illustrated in Fig. 10.2.

Unfortunately, despite good efforts, these regulations were not adequately implemented and were not recognized by the relevant sectors. It was not until the second half of the twentieth century, with the increased prevalence of clinical research trials, that the importance of regulating research was recognized in Costa Rica. The research trials that took place were primarily drug trials financed by the

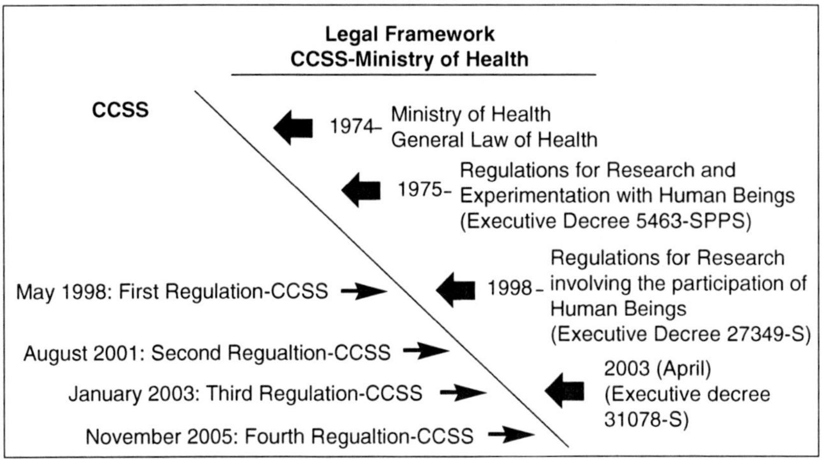

Fig. 10.2 Comparative development of the regulation of biomedical research in Costa Rica. Source: Archivos Área de Bioética – CENDEISSS

pharmaceutical industry in collaboration with paid research organizations, including those trials developed within the CCSS. This increase created a need for regulations that were in accord with international guidelines but were also tailored to the national reality, because many of the previously established regulations had proved to be obsolete. As a result, on May 15, 1998, the CCSS published its first Regulation of Research in the Welfare Services of the Costa Rican Social Security Agency, which established the structure of the Institutional Committee of Bioethics and Research (CIBI) and delegated functions to the research ethics committees located within some of the agency's welfare centers (CCSS-Caja Costarricense de Seguro Social 1998). During the same year, the Health Department implemented the Executive Decree 27349-S4, which included the new regulations for research involving human beings and established the Institutional Scientific Committee (CCI) to govern research at both the public and private levels (Imprenta Nacional 1998).

Once again, due to constant changes and a lack of resources, the regulations were not successfully implemented. In response, the CCSS decreed two new regulations in a 3-year period: the second Regulation of Clinical Research in Welfare Services of the Costa Rican Social Security Agency in 2001 (CCSS-Caja Costarricense de Seguro Social 2001) and the third Regulation of Clinical Research in the Welfare Services of the Costa Rican Social Security Agency in 2003 (CCSS-Caja Costarricense de Seguro Social 2003).

It should be emphasized that the regulations mentioned thus far each proposed a different regulative structure, which produced a period of confusion and a lack of precision in the development of biomedical research in the country, principally affecting the research conducted in CCSS welfare centers. For example, while the

2001 regulation assigned functions to the individual research ethics committees existing in the welfare centers, that of 2003 centralized research decisions to the Institutional Research Ethics Committee (CECI). This type of inconsistency in the required processes gave a political tone to research activities that led to a drastic reduction in the number of CCSS research trials and an increase in those trials conducted in the private sector. One can attribute the growth of biomedical research in the private sector to the creation of private research ethics committees and the consistent decrease of these studies in the CCSS.

Also in 2003, the Health Department enacted a new regulation for research involving human beings, the Executive Decree 31078-S (Imprenta Nacional 2003), which remains the current regulation. The National Council of Research in Health (CONIS), an agency of the Health Department governing research within the country, was established by this decree in addition to the establishment of the so-called Research Ethics Committees (CEC).

In 2005, CCSS presented a new version of this regulation that was not only faithful to the 2003 version but also corrected the errors of previous versions. It proposed a regulative structure for biomedical research inside the Costa Rican social security system that was in accord with international standards and was simultaneously linked to institutional reality to guarantee the protection of the rights of research subjects and the social interests of the CCSS.

10.3 The Beginnings of Clinical Bioethics

As has been noted, the development of clinical bioethics in Costa Rica is relatively new, although for several years there have been discussions related to bioethical topics.

The first point of reference is Act 5560 of 1974, Organ Transplants in Human Beings, which captured the concerns of Costa Rican society regarding issues of organ transplantation, which was beginning to be discussed globally. In the year 1980, the congress of the republic approved Act 6472, the so-called Law Authorizing the Costa Rican Social Security Agency to Donate Organs in Exchange for Medicine (Ley para autorizar a la Caja Costarricense de Seguro Social1 a donar órganos a cambio de medicamentos), which, as is evident in its name, violates all internationally recognized fundamental ethical principles. Both of these laws were revoked in 1994 when the current Act 7409, Authorization to Transplant Organs and Human Tissues (Autorización para trasplantar órganos y tejidos anatómicos humanos), was approved.

Another topic of discussion in Costa Rica, which became relevant in the mid-1990s, was in vitro fertilization (IVF). In 1995, the Health Department published the Executive Decree 24029-S1, In Vitro Fertilization and Embryo Transfer (Fertilización in Vitro y transferencia de embriones). Nevertheless, the same year, the Constitutional Court received a plea against this decree and ultimately ruled that the technique was unconstitutional and the decree was abolished.

In 2002, a major advance for Costa Rican bioethics took place with the approbation of Act 8239, Rights and Duties of Patients of Public and Private Health Services (Derechos y deberes de las personas usuarias de los servicios de salud públicos y privados), in which the rights of patients to information and confidentiality were defined.

In summary, the evolution of the regulation of bioethics in Costa Rica proceeded as follows:

1974 – Act 5560: Organ Transplantation in Human Beings
1980 – Act 6472: Law Authorizing the CCSS to Donate Organs in Exchange for Medicine
1994 – Act 7409: Authorization to Transplant Organs and Human Tissues
1995 – Executive Decree 24029-S: In Vitro Fertilization and Embryo Transference
1995 – Decision by the Constitutional Court FIVET
2002 – Act 8239: Rights and Duties of Patients of Public and Private Health Services
2007 – Renewal of CCSS until 2025
2007 – JD – CCSS Nº. 8123

10.4 Structure and Membership of Bioethics Committees

One can note from the above history that research ethics committees are more advanced than clinical ethics committees and therefore have a more developed structure. For example, in 1975, the first research ethics committee in Costa Rica was created in the National Children's Hospital, impelled by the increasing need to protect the well-being of its vulnerable population. Additionally, in 1977, the Psychiatric National Hospital established the second committee of this kind. At current, both committees are still in existence and functioning in this capacity.

As mentioned, the Executive Decree 31078-S7 established the structure of the National Council of Research in Health (CONIS) and the Research Ethics Committees (CEC). At present, there are seven research ethics committees accredited by CONIS for the review of biomedical research proposals: five in public institutions (CCSS, Costa Rican Institute of Research and Education in Nutrition and Health, University of Costa Rica, National University, Institute of Alcoholism and Pharmacodependence) and two in private institutions (University of Medical Sciences and San Jose CIMA Hospital). In addition, the CCSS has the centralized Institutional Committee of Bioethics in Research (COIBI–Comité Institucional de Bioética en Investigación/CCSS) which oversees 42 local bioethics committees in research (CLOBI–Comités Locales de Bioética): three national hospitals, five in specialized hospitals, twenty in regional and peripheral hospitals, five in general clinics, and nine in health areas.

With the significant development of research ethics committees, the need to promote the development of bioethics within the Costa Rican Social Security

Agency and the country at large became evident. As a result, in 2005, the Bioethics Area was created and assigned to the Center of Strategic Development and Information in Social Security and Health (Centro de Desarrollo Estratégico y Información en Seguridad Social y Salud/CCSS) with the mission of "creating and developing qualified instances of reflection and dialogue for decision making according to bioethical principles with regard to clinical problems or dilemmas of health management and research involving human beings" (Ministerio de la Salud) and to coordinate all activities meant to strengthen the implementation of bioethics in the institutional setting. This area was divided into two subareas: the Subarea of Bioethics in Research and the Subarea of Clinical and Management Bioethics.

In an attempt to fulfill its mission, the Bioethics Area designed and implemented numerous strategies, including:

1. Establishing well-defined and standardized processes for the presentation of biomedical research proposals through the use of standardized forms and guidelines for researchers.
2. Restructuring the Institutional Committee of Bioethics in Research (COIBI-CCSS) as an entity accredited by CONIS for the review of research proposals in the CCSS.
3. The creation of a network of 42 local committees of Bioethics (CLOBI) coordinated by the Advisory Council of CLOBI, which includes the participation of all CLOBI coordinators plus the COIBI-CCSS president.
4. The establishment of a training program to educate CLOBI members to better understand their function.
5. The implementation of an educational program directed towards the institution's staff and the general population to better inform them about different bioethical topics.

In addition to these initiatives, the Bioethics Area also established intra- and extra-institutional contacts as a means to strengthen the growth of the discipline at the national level.

Currently, the Bioethics Area is collaborating with public and private universities to develop an undergraduate curriculum in bioethics to be implemented in the health sciences majors. In reality, there are a number of obstacles to the implementation of this curriculum because there are very few training options available in bioethics within the country. Another institution that has promoted the development of bioethics has been the Costa Rican School of Doctors and Surgeons, which has made efforts to sponsor forums and symposiums within the medical community on relevant issues.

In 2003, with the support of the Pan-American Health Organization (PAHO), the establishment of a Master's program in bioethics in Costa Rica began to be worked out. Aware of the need for the development of national training programs, the National University, the University of Costa Rica, and the CCSS joined this effort and began developing the program. It was implemented in 2006 and the first class of Master's students completed the program in 2008. At present, this is the only program of its kind in Costa Rica.

10.5 Bioethics Legislation in Costa Rica

Currently, Costa Rica has several laws, decrees, and regulations that frame bioethics. The most important of this legislation include:

- Act 8239: Rights and Duties of Patients of Public and Private Health Services
- Act 7409: Organs Health
- Decree 31078-S/2003: Regulation for Research Involving Human Beings
- Legal Guidelines for Biomedical Research in the Welfare Services of the Costa Rican Social Security Agency
- Regulation of Social Security
- Regulation of Health Records Data

10.6 Publications

Since its establishment in 2005, the Bioethics Area of CENDEISSS has understood its function, in part, as a responsibility to publish works that will cultivate the development of bioethics in Costa Rica. Its publications include the anthology, *Bioethics in the Costa Rican Social Security Agency* (*Bioética en la Caja Costarricense de Seguro Social*), which is a compilation of essays written by members of local bioethics committees as part of a basic bioethics course. The anthology provides a realistic picture of the situation in which the CLOBI of CCSS was at that moment.

The Bioethics Area was also responsible for the promotion of the first advertising campaign in this field, entitled *Clinical Researchers: Ask First* (*Investigaciones clínicas: primero pregunte*), for health services users. The campaign consisted of a poster, a brochure, and a video advising people to ask the appropriate questions before agreeing to participate in a clinical research study. The suggested questions included: asking what was involved in the study and what its purpose was, if the research had been approved by a bioethics research committee, what the benefits and risks were of taking part in the study, and whom one could ask for help if one had doubts regarding the research. The campaign was very successful and succeeded in reaching the public as well as many officials regarding these topics.

Later, in 2007, the Operation Manual for Bioethics Committees was published in order to standardize the minimal requisites that CCSS committees must follow to achieve optimization in their work. In December of the same year, the first edition of *Regulations Related to Bioethics in Health* (*Normativa relacionada con la bioética en salud*) was published. This volume was a recompilation of national and international regulations applicable to bioethics for the purpose of continuing to share and exchange knowledge as a means to further implement bioethics in the institutional setting.

10.7 Where Are We Going?

In light of the efforts mentioned in this essay, one is aware of how much work still remains to be done to fully establish bioethics as a discipline in Costa Rica. Nevertheless, the steps for achieving this can be outlined as follows:

1. Emphasize the importance of bioethics in the health sector and society as a whole.
2. Encourage a love for bioethical knowledge among health professionals.
3. Improve intra- and extra-institutional communication to establish strategic alliances for the development of the discipline.
4. Reach a regulative maturity that promotes the appropriate implementation of the respective guidelines.

References

CCSS-Caja Costarricense de Seguro Social (1998) Reglamento para la investigación en los servicios asistenciales de la Caja Costarricense de Seguro Social (March). San José

CCSS-Caja Costarricense de Seguro Social (2001) Available at: www.ccss.sa.cr

CCSS-Caja Costarricense de Seguro Social (2003) Reglamento para la investigación clínica en los servicios asistenciales de la Caja Costarricense de Seguro Social. CCSS, San José

Imprenta Nacional (1974) Ley General de Salud. La Gaceta Jan. 18 (12). San José, Costa Rica

Imprenta Nacional (1998) Decreto Ejecutivo n.27349-S. La Gaceta, Oct. 13 (198). San José

Imprenta Nacional (2003) Decreto Ejecutivo n.31078. La Gaceta, Mar. 27, (61). San José

Ministerio de la Salud. Centro de Desarrollo Estratégico e Información en Salud y Seguridad Social (2007) Available at: www.cendeisss.sa.cr

Chapter 11
Bioethics in Cuba: Responsibility and Solidarity

José Ramón Acosta Sariego

11.1 Introduction

Cuba is a country that represents a unique case in the context of Latin America because, in spite of the political trends of the region, it has persisted in the construction of a social project inspired by the ideas of Marxist socialism and José Martí. The rapid and irreversible diffusion of bioethics throughout Cuba was a surprise for some, due to the individualistic and self-centered nature of a bioethics created in the context of a liberal capitalist economy. For others, who knew about the ideals of justice and equity dreamt of by Potter, the spread of bioethics in Cuba was one of the logical consequences of searching for ways to build a sustainable society based on Cuban traditions and culture.

11.2 A Cuban Perspective of the New Paradigm of the Doctor–Patient Relationship

Since the foundation of the Royal Medical Court of Physicians of Havana in 1711, until the creation of the Cuban Federation of Physicians in 1925 and its later establishment in 1944 of the National College of Physicians, the Cuban model of the doctor–patient relationship has corresponded to the classical paternalistic paradigm, although it maintained a nuance of its own, which distinguished it during the colonial and republican periods.

The proposal for university reform, promoted by Francisco de Arango y Parreño at the beginning of the 19th century, was intended to include the teaching of medical ethics in Cuba. However, a long period of time was required to introduce it fully in practice. Determinants of its definitive acceptance were: the cycle of conferences

J.R.A. Sariego
Physician and Researcher in Public Health, Chair of Bioethics in the Medical University of La Habana, Cuba
e-mail: joseacosta@giron.sld.cu

L. Pessini et al. (eds.), *Ibero-American Bioethics: History and Perspectives*, Philosophy and Medicine 106, DOI 10.1007/978-1-4020-9350-0_11,

about the "Foundations of Morality" directed by Enrique José Varona between 1880 and 1882 at the Royal Academy of Medical, Physical and Natural Sciences of Havana; and the activity of Antonio Jover Puig, Raimundo de Castro y Allo, Raimundo de Castro y Bachiller, and Francisco Lancís y Sánchez in teaching medical ethics and the moral duties of doctors (Delgado 1997, p. 44).

In the 1950s, accessibility to medical services in Cuba was divided: the upper class enjoyed the best technical and human resources, while most of the population was forced to accept political deals in exchange for medical care in an obsolete, insufficient, and Dante-esque public sector. In addition, behind the closed doors of the National College of Physicians, an important issue was being discussed: whether there was an excessive number of physicians. This situation occurred amidst an unstable pre-revolutionary Cuban society. The Moral Code and the Honour Oath of the National College of Physicians, "of incontrovertible validity in its time" (Delgado 1997, p. 45), could not overcome the customs imposed by Thomas Percival of modern medical paternalism.

11.3 Justice as Solidarity

The accession of revolutionary power in 1959 completely reversed the national scene. By promoting the Marxist principle of equality, access to medical services became a human right and the government was held responsible for the adequate provision of health care. This policy resulted in the extension and modernization of services and an exponential increase of human resources in the health services.

The National College of Physicians, in particular, became a battleground for the intensive class struggle that developed throughout Cuba. The climax of the debate ended in ideological and political crisis, as the dissolution of the institution resulted. After the disappearance of the college in 1966, and for almost 20 years after, the management of ethical regulations was assumed directly by the Ministry of Public Health. It was not until the mid-1980s that the Principles of Medical Ethics were promulgated, causing the establishment of medical ethics commissions in all units of the National Health System.

The reinforcement of a unified and public National Health System at the end of the 1960s created the proper conditions for social–democratic criteria to overcome the search for equality among unequal people; to paraphrase John Rawls, it required the unequal treatment of unequal individuals for the purpose of creating an equality of opportunity (Rawls 1999). This revolutionary approach to health care allowed for a moral commitment reminiscent of José Martí's inspiration: "with all, and for the welfare of all," where, rather than donating what is in excess, one shares what one owns.

The task of the Cuban model was not to define and secure a uniform minimum standard of health care, and, therefore, the care of one's health was left a matter of individual interest and economic means; this was the objective of a social democracy following the Kantian principle of universality. For Cuba, the primary objective was to offer the maximal technological and human resources available, while guaranteeing legal, economic, geographical, and cultural accessibility to all citizens. The relevance of the Cuban model is observed in its independence from the Soviet model or any other exemplar of the so-called "Real European Socialism." Instead, it drew from the best international sources of social medicine in order to create its own alternative, which has resisted the loss of ideological references and the consequences of the severe economic crisis in the 1990s (De la Torre et al. 2004, p. 200).

Achieving the sustainability of a health care system with these characteristics in a poor and isolated country such as Cuba has required a wide network of primary health care units along with the population's participation in the maintenance and improvement of their own health. The political will to establish universal coverage, with the most advanced technology possible, has required the deliberation of citizens and the ultimate acceptance of certain sacrifices so that social goals, including full access to employment, education, and health, among others, may be realized.

Sadly, in most parts of the world, artificial limits have been imposed by the market as a result of miserly economic interests and a lack of solidarity, causing the unnecessary suffering and death of millions of people. At present, most health care problems of significant magnitude permeate national borders and therefore require international cooperation and collaboration for their resolution. Facing these realities, Rafael Araujo González proposed an alternative system of ethical principles to those endorsed by the Kennedy Institute of Ethics at Georgetown University: accessibility, equity, and participation, in his opinion, were the most appropriate for Cuba's marginal context (Araujo 1997, p. 30).

This ethical analysis from the underdeveloped countries perspective of the South corresponded with the general principles of Cuban Public Health, where unselfish cooperation plays an important role. Since Cuba's provision of medical assistance to Chile in 1960 and Algeria in 1963, through the emergency aid offered to the victims of natural disasters in Pakistan in 2005 and Indonesia in 2006, a vocation of service has impregnated the historical stamp of Cuban medicine in its contribution to solving local and global health problems. The principle of justice, understood in this way, has found no better expression than solidarity.

11.4 Beneficence as Responsibility

Solving the problem of the just distribution of access to medical care is a basic requirement, although it is not sufficient to resolve the issues inherent in interpersonal relationships within the health care system. The international trends of (1) concern regarding the psychological and social factors in the provision of health care, (2) the new conditions created by the revolution of universal access to health care, and (3) the increased progress of promotion and prevention initiatives in primary health care refocused health management on social medicine. During the 1960s, the teaching of courses called "Medical Humanities" and the "Social Sciences Applied to Medicine" at Cuban University was promoted. Another revolutionary step was the conception of the Integrated Study Plan of Medicine, in which the general unit, entitled "Man and his Environment," acted as a foundation.

During the academic year of 1978–1979, "Medical Ethics and Deontology" was included as an independent subject for the first time in the history of medical education in Cuba. Its textbook, *Medical Ethics and Deontology*, (Alonso et al 1979) can be considered an initial contribution by Cuba within the international context of the new paradigm of medical ethics. Suffice it to remember that the first edition of *Principles of Biomedical Ethics*, authored by Beauchamp and Childress (1979), was published in the same year (1979).

In this way, a particular conception of informed consent was expressed, which required its realization within the context of interpersonal relations characterized by trust. This Cuban perspective begins the move away from classical medical paternalism. Several years later, Edmund Pellegrino and David Thomasma defined this type of doctor–patient relationship as "beneficence with trust" (Pellegrino and Thomasma 1988).

Both the awareness of changes in the health population in Cuba at the beginning of the 1980s and the capabilities of the health care system in responding to emergency situations (successfully tested by the dissemination of hemorrhagic dengue in 1982–1983) revealed certain vulnerabilities in the system and, consequently, the necessity of designing new strategies and policies. Important developments included the publication of "Principles of Medical Ethics" (Anonymous 1983), in addition to the creation of medical ethics commissions for all units and at all levels of the National Health System. Relevant to law, the Public Health Law was passed in 1984. In the field of medical care services, the "Family Doctor and Nurse Plan" was established in 1984 and led to an improvement in the Cuban family medicine system. Finally, in the field of medical education, a new Study Plan of Medicine was created in 1985, based on the identified needs and health problems of the population.

The "Principles of Medical Ethics" constituted the first ethical code written under the new economic and social conditions created by the Cuban Revolution and, if only for this reason, has significant historical value. In spite of its still paternalistic wording, its content was adapted to the particular circumstances and introduced several new precepts, reflecting a change in approach. In fact, the withholding of information from patients and relatives is normally only exercised in those instances of terminal illness. The decision regarding who should receive bad news pertaining to the patient's status is left to the discretion of the medical team; the patient is only included as an option if one's personal beliefs allow for it. Another concept related to autonomy in the "Principles of Medical Ethics" is informed consent. Voluntary consent is also included, but it does not have specific informational standards and is only required for high-risk procedures. However, the inclusion of informed consent in an official document governing the behavior of Cuban doctors was itself very important and should be considered progress.

The increase in biomedical research, together with the introduction and local production of complex medical technologies, induced the moral consideration of related controversial topics typical to bioethics. The work of Ernesto Bravo Matarazzo, promoting a colloquium on "Philosophical Problems of Medicine," was of great value. It began in 1983 and continued for several years. The lectures delivered were published by the Medical University of Havana in several volumes. This colloquium introduced a coherent picture of the bioethical terrain which, at that time, had been treated in a fragmentary manner or was simply unknown, such as the treatment of theoretical and philosophical questions related to the origins of life, genomics, neurosciences, and medical diagnosis based on new technologies. The paper "Ethical Problems of the Development of Contemporary Biology and Medicine," by Abelardo Ramírez Márquez and Raúl Herrera Valdés, is a good sample from this colloquium because it served to introduce the moral conflicts related to scientific research on human beings, genetic therapy, the definition of death, and the donation and transplantation of organs and human tissues (Ramírez and Herrera 1984, pp. 165–179).

The first theoretical consideration of bioethics by a Cuban author was presented by Antonio De Armas during the Third International Science Symposium on Management and Social Planning in the Territory (III Internationales wissenschaftliches Symposium über Leitung und Plannung sozialer Prozesse im Territorium), celebrated in Rostock, East Germany, in 1985. It was published some years later in the *Cuban Journal of Social Sciences* in the January–April 1989 issue under the title "About the Philosophical Orientation of Bioethics."

In 1986, an updated version, including the most current bibliographic support, of the subject "Medical Ethics and Deontology" was published in the textbook *Themes of Medical Ethics*. This book constitutes another step toward the future of Cuban bioethics because it offers a holistic vision of the man–nature relationship and the economic and social factors relevant to the health care system (Borroto et al. 1986, p. 113).

Three years later (1989), the curriculum for the new Undergraduate Studies in Technology of Health program was designed, due to the realization of the Area of Education of the Public Health Ministry (in Cuba medical education is a responsibility of the Ministry of Public Health) that it was necessary to provide resources in this field for the broad coverage of the social sciences and their relevance to health. Three subjects were integrated into a discipline named "Health." The third and last of these subjects, "Health III," was taught in the second year of study and constituted the first educational program in bioethics to be taught at the level of undergraduate medical education in Cuba. This program began in the 1989–1990 academic year and remained through the 2002–2003 academic year. This program was not only one of the first in Cuba, but in Latin America as well. In 40 hours of study, it addressed the traditional content of medical ethics in addition to those special topics considered under bioethics. The results of the first 5 years of the program were published in the records of the Third International Workshop of the Regional Program of Bioethics for Latin America and the Caribbean PAHO/WHO celebrated in Havana in November 1995 (Area of Education of the Ministry of Public Health 1996, p. 22).

Due to limited enrollment during its first 15 years, the "Technology of Health" program had little impact on medical education in Cuba. In 1994, a transformative decision to convert the philosophy program, which had universal application to medical and scientific studies, into a new program called "Philosophy and Health" would focus on the links between theory and practice.

The establishment of the Center for State Quality Control of Medications (1989) and the Center for State Control of Medical Equipments (1992) for the purpose of exerting social control over the applications of techno-scientific advances in medicine was of great importance. Both centers were subordinated to the Regulatory Bureau of Health in 1996. The creation of the Clinical Trials Coordinating Center (1991) promoted the formation of ethics review committees for the evaluation of all clinical trials. In addition, the promulgation of the "Good Clinical Practice Norms" in 1992 (subsequently modified in 1995 and 2000), and the approval of the "Ethical Code for Science Workers" in 1994, stimulated the interest of researchers and officials; there was particular interest in the ethical foundations of scientific research, what the standard procedure for evaluating research projects was, and the emergence of independent organizations to oversee the fulfilment of these standards: the Ethics of Scientific Research Institutional Committees (Institutional Review Boards).

The celebration in Havana of the First International Symposium on Brain Death in 1992 – later renamed International Symposium on Coma and Death – attracted prominent bioethicists from around the world to Cuba. From the symposium exchanges, ideas for the preparation of the first international courses in bioethics emerged: the first course, "The Medical University Facing Current Bioethical Problems" was team-taught by Cuban and American professors (Wikler, Yougner, Charo and Miles) in the former National Center for Medical Improvement in 1993; and the "Introduction to Bioethics" course was held at the Faculty of Public Health (today National School of Public Health) in 1994 and was taught by Juan Carlos Tealdi of the Latin American School of Bioethics, Buenos Aires, Argentina.

During the first half of the 1990s, professorships in bioethics at all medical universities (24 in total) and medical technical colleges (15 in total) were created. Moreover, discussions about the draft of the "Universal Declaration on the Human Genome and Human Rights" also resulted in the foundation of the National Committee of Bioethics in 1996. Under the auspices of Catholic institutions, the first Cuban journal dedicated to bioethics *Ethos*, began to publish in 1996. In 1997, the Juan Pablo II Bioethics Center was founded, which has held nine annual bioethics meetings to date and, since 2000, has published the journal *Annals of the Juan Pablo II Bioethics Center*, which was eventually renamed *Bioethics*.

The rapid diffusion and eagerness with which the first edition of *Bioethics: From a Cuban Perspective* (1997) was received were easily explainable by the precedents leading up to it. This book, co-written by more than 40 Cuban authors, represented the national continuity in thinking about the ethics relevant to life and health. However, at the same time, it demonstrated the break from medical paternalism from the point of view of Cuban cultural traditions, which does not extol individuality, typical of American bioethics. Alternatively, it acknowledges the role of the individual and collective responsibility for the general well-being.

Ricardo González deals with an issue later developed in the text by Núñez de Villavicencio. He specifically addresses the responsibility of the doctor as educator, which emphasizes that the real benefit of the patient or healthy person is only possible to reach, if he is made aware of his own health needs. Far from the coercion typical of the classic paternalistic model and far from the neutral information given in the radical autonomist's model, this Cuban proposal involves the health professional in the education of the client; this approach promotes a deliberation process of deciding together among the best options for a solution. To accept this approach means to overcome the traditional paternalistic paradigm (González 1997, p. 106).

The necessity of additional equality in the interpersonal relations typical of contemporary medical care is dealt with by Varán Von Smith: "... within clinical ethics the respect of the integrity of the individual wins a preponderant place and it must be applied in any clinical environment, and independently of the affectation of the patient" (Von Smith 1997, p. 124). It is very significant that Varán Von Smith uses the term "clinical ethics," created by Mark Siegler, and does not specify a limited set of situations within which the observance of the patient's integrity and, also, respect for the capacity and moral competence of the patient are relevant. The original idea of interpersonal relationships in clinical care being context-dependent, allowing for different models of the doctor–patient relationship to be employed, was presented by Thomas Szasz and Marc Hollender (Szasz and Hollender 1956) and was further developed by Ezequiel and Linda Emanuel (Emanuel and Emanuel 1992). The distinctive features of Varán Von Smith's approach are its recommended application in any clinical environment (for example, primary or secondary health services), in any clinical situation (for example, acute or chronic diseases), and its establishment of a link between the health professional's social role and one's professional responsibility.

Radamés Borroto Cruz and Ramón Aneiros-Riba deepen the questions of respect and dignity through responsible communication, in expressing support for those relations which are of good quality and meet the expectation of participants:

> The essence of medical care is summarized in the satisfaction of the health necessities of the human being. Nobody can be happy in ignorance, and much less, if it is about something related with their own health. The patient will only be satisfied when he knows all desired information about his health or illness. Nobody, except for a doctor, has the possibility to get closer to the most intimate and sensitive aspects of a human being (Borroto and Aneiros-Riba 1997, p. 118).

Developing the skills of effective communication is how one becomes able "to get closer to the most intimate and sensitive aspects of a human being"; this attitude establishes a link between the technical and moral aspects of interpersonal relationships. The social responsibility of the health professional is to act beneficently by satisfying all of the related health necessities of the patient; it is no longer sufficient to satisfy the biological needs of the patient as had been the common trend.

Fernando Núñez de Villavicencio also made an important contribution with his formulation of informed consent as one that must essentially be an educative action in which respect for autonomy is harmonized with the medical needs of the patient or the healthy person:

> We should not limit ourselves to do good or to fight for health; the issue is to warn the physician that, if he prioritizes only the aspects related to biological balance, there will be occasions in which his beneficent actions, in this sense, can produce psychological and social imbalances of greater intensity. To authorize them to impose their charity in these cases would mean to authorize them to perform actions against health.... While analyzing the principle of autonomy, however, we are not in the same situation. The patient's right to

> be informed, consulted, and participate in the actions taken in connection with his own health, which is unquestionable in essence, requires very precise limitations to prevent their inadequate use resulting in a disaster for the patient himself (Núñez de Villavicencio 1997, p. 129).

The analysis of the convergence points of these and other contributions to *Bioethics: From a Cuban Perspective* makes it evident that, even though all the authors move away from classic paternalism, they do not fall into the arms of the autonomist; instead, they propose an alternative model in which the user's well-being is reached by means of the responsible actions of the health professional and the mutual trust engendered with the patient.

At the end of the 1990s, the consolidation of bioethics in Cuba was confirmed by the founding of new institutions that included bioethics in their mission statements, such as the Center for Studies on Bioethics of the Medical Sciences Faculty of Holguín, which has annual international scientific meetings; the Humanistic Studies Center of the Medical University of Havana; and the Bioethics Committee of the University of Havana in coordination with, the Latin American School of Medicine, which has hosted several workshop on Education on Bioethics; in 2002.

Courses on human resources in bioethics and the addition of relevant subjects to the curriculum of traditional introductory courses of the Master's degree program in Medical Genetics and Computer Sciences for Health as well as in courses on the ethics of scientific research (sponsored by the Finlay Institute for Vaccines and Serums in 1996) were established. Specialized development in bioethics began at the postgraduate diploma level at the same time, in the 1998–1999 academic year, as those academic courses at the Victoria de Girón Institute of Basic and Pre-clinic Sciences and the Medical Sciences Faculty of Holguín, and later at the Medical Sciences Faculty of Sancti Spiritus. In addition, one must note the intense editorial activity in bioethics at the Félix Varela Center (a non-governmental organization), which has been imperative for the diffusion of work by Cuban authors.

Cuban bioethics does not forsake the contribution made by the system of principles created by Beauchamp and Childress in clinical ethics, but it has not been blindly adopted. The characteristic of responsibility, with which beneficence should be exercised, highlights solidarity as the maximum expression of justice and signifies a unique component of the Cuban approach. However, the period between 1997 and the current day has witnessed debate over the validity of bioethical discourse, in addition to the discipline's evolution from a restrictive biomedical focus toward a more comprehensive environmentalist vision.

11.5 Cuban Contributions to Sustainable Global Bioethics

The book, *Bioethics: From a Cuban Perspective*, primed the search for a necessary balance between medical bioethics and global bioethics. Already in 1997, awareness of the importance of Van Rensselaer Potter's conception of global bioethics as a theoretical and methodological development within the discipline was growing. The scientific editor of the book intended to incorporate these ideas into the project modestly. To a certain extent, this objective was achieved, as enough material was gathered to be able to dedicate a chapter to it, entitled "Civilization, Environment and Health."

The chapter, "The Postmodern Scenario of Bioethics," addressed the intersection of the notion of progress stemming from the material development typical of modernity, which has been apparent in moments of neo-liberal capitalism, and the necessity of a bioethics of intervention:

> If there is a real will to save mankind from an ecological holocaust, and to undertake the way to sustainable development, a new mentality is necessary, an effective commitment with Man and with Life, a new planetary culture "with all and for the welfare of all"... It is required to create consciousness in the spiritual field, and to claim changes in the social and economic fields, this is the great challenge of such current thinking trends as bioethics, ecosophy, and political ecology, but furthermore, it is the great contemporary challenge of mankind, if it doesn't want to cease to be (Acosta and González 1997, p. 21).

Another of the flashes of a sustainable global bioethics included in the first two editions of *Bioethics: From a Cuban Perspective* is expressed by Ubaldo González Pérez, Jorge Grau Avalo and María Antonia Amarillo Mendoza, when they criticize the emphasis of medical bioethics on an individual-centered approach to the quality of life, which includes those clinical events related to the beginning and end of human life:

> ... If medical bioethics acknowledges and works eulogistically in relation to the quality of life in the moment of death.... The polemic about all the global, social, group and individual problems that affect life; the ecosystem and the quality of human life should be prioritized and it also must focus on what socio-economic conditions of life, what juridical guarantees, and what moral education a man needs so that his decisions don't constitute a violation of the moral principles of the universal culture (González et al. 1997, p. 285).

In 1999, two books were published, *Ecology and Society: Studies* (with a scientific edition by Carlos Jesús Delgado Díaz and Thalía M. Fung Riverón) and *Green Cuba: In Search of a Model for Sustainability* (also with a scientific edition by Carlos Jesús Delgado), which marked the confluence of environmentalist and bioethical perspectives in contributing to a characteristically Cuban vision of sustainable global bioethics. In the contributions of José Ramón Acosta Sariego to both books, he points out the need for medical bioethics to concentrate on questions of interpersonal relations pertaining to medical care and biomedical research and the necessity of enlarging the horizon of bioethics (Acosta 1999a, pp. 77, 78).

Also in 1999, the editorial house of the Genetic Engineering and Biotechnology Center convened the First National Workshop on Genetically Modified Organisms in Havana, sponsored by ELFOS. The reports presented were published in the journal, *Applied Biotechnology*. The following ideas of Acosta Sariego were an attempt to offer another perspective when considering the appropriate ethical foundations for the analysis of the environmental impact of artificially designed living organisms:

> The observance of the principle of responsibility promotes the preservation of the general welfare, contributes to creating an appropriate material and social context for the balance between man and nature, where the individual values and rights can find true realization… The principle of justice will be effective regarding the investigation and use of GMO and biotechnologies in general, if the necessary equity is reached when: sharing benefits, assessing and facing potential risks, and guaranteeing access to the accumulated genetic information and transference of technologies. This purpose will only be attainable if the necessary North–South cooperation is reached, which would mean to overcome the unjust neo-liberal conception of justice…. Responsibility and justice constitute the ethical imperatives for the investigation and ulterior use of the GMO. The observance of both principles is consubstantial so that this achievement of culture results in the benefit of society in general and does not become another instrument for the exercise of hegemonic power (Acosta 1999b, pp. E29–E31).

A global focus of bioethics cannot ignore the economic and social problems resultant of technological developments, for which the theoretical and methodological framework of medical bioethics is not sufficient. Although Araujo had already outlined a reference system as an alternative to individualism, which can be applied to the analysis and solution of the problems characteristic of a medical macro-bioethics (accessibility, equity, and participation) (Araujo 1997), it is necessary to specify that just utilization should also be a requirement, since the processes involved reach beyond human health to the stability of ecosystems and the survival of life in general.

In the *Glossary of Bioethics*, by Rafael Torres Acosta, the terms "environmental bioethics," "global bioethics," and "deep bioethics" all appear (Torres 2001, p. 14), providing another indication that Cuban bioethics employs a holistic view.

Bioethics for Sustainability, published in 2002, represents the true establishment of sustainable global bioethics in Cuba, not only because the entire book floats an homage aura to Potter, but also, independently of the dissimilarities of the collective work, for its contributions to the consolidation of the environmentalist perspective in bioethics. Jesus Armando Martínez Gómez, in his article, "Projects for a Global Bioethics," has refined the necessary criteria for defining a holistic interpretation of bioethics:

> Medical bioethics has insisted more on group solidarity, based in the 'ethics of having', rather than in global solidarity based on the way of being…. The bridge conceived of by Potter was the development of a global ethics, but the beams and pillars of this bridge cannot be other than global solidarity and responsibility (Martínez 2002, pp. 228–231).

The unique perspective that was previously attributed to Cuban medical bioethics, for defining "beneficence" as responsibility and "justice" as solidarity, is worth considering within the context of sustainable global bioethics. For example, the excerpt above suggests that the principles of responsibility and solidarity are the appropriate foundation from which the deliberation process and search for valid solutions to moral conflicts should begin.

The global conception of bioethics and its interrelation with the sustainability of development lead, inevitably, to biopolitics, defined as civic action taken to awaken responsible solidarity and the establishment of policies for the inclusion of all: civil society, the State, and international organizations (governmental or non-governmental in character). To achieve organization and coherence in these efforts, substantial changes to the manner in which values are taught are necessary. In teaching values, one should not isolate scientific knowledge from the relevant moral issues; instead, they should be presented as intrinsic parts of each other. Bioethics, interpreted in this way, becomes a challenge for society as a whole, and not just a topic of academic discussion meant to be decided on by the initiated elite.

Bioethics, as formulated by Potter, indicates a deep cultural fissure. Man is required to reconcile morality and knowledge in the creation of a unique entity. The moral issue, as it is incorporated into knowledge, becomes an important consideration of the objectivity and legitimacy of knowledge. It also provides a proposal for developing responsible agents in an environment of cultural change. Bioethics has been called upon to produce a revolution in human knowledge, and it has been defined by its creator in terms that emphasize this claim (Delgado 2002, p. 153).

The problem outlined by Carlos Delgado regarding the responsibility of every member of society in defining knowledge is also dealt with by Luis López Bombino in *Ethical Knowledge from Yesterday to Today* (Bombino 2004). Bombino recaptures the topic of the moral legitimacy of scientific work and its unavoidable social commitments. As a specialist in values education, he expresses the mission of the scientist's ethical development in the following way:

> To think about science and technology is also to consider the responsibility of those who make and apply it, because what would scientific creativity be if one did not think of its social and moral consequences? It is not for its own sake that the cult of novelty, for the original thing, cannot neglect its axiological meaning, because the longing for new things has led scientists to extreme anguish. Science cannot remain distant from social and human conflicts; for that reason the function of the scientist is not just to produce neutral objective knowledge, without their work being influenced by the society where they live, work, and create (Bombino 2004, p. 81).

All of these factors indicate that the cultural revolution (toward responsible solidarity in the use of knowledge) ultimately implies a restatement of the social role of science and technology. In a time when biological and technological knowledge dominate scientific progress, it is unacceptable for their discoveries to be controlled by private and corporate interests, allowing for the exclusion and limited access of less fortunate segments of the population. Freyre defends a common and recurrent position in Latin American bioethics, which addresses the illegitimacy of an unequal distribution of the fruits of knowledge:

> … although bioethics was promoted under the conscience of establishing moral barriers to new forms of intervention in the biological processes which carried serious bio-risks. It should not be forgotten that in the present-day connotation of bioethics, other factors intervene, for example, an interest in the existence of a more just international distribution of the benefits of science and technology (Freyre 2004, p. 277).

Carlos Delgado in "Social Heterogeneity in Cuba Today," indicates three rupture points of bioethics which have methodological value for the analysis of social inequalities. These are (1) a consideration of nature and its resulting knowledge as a source of morality; (2) the demand of considering all perspectives (social, collective, and individual) as integrated; and (3) the evaluative approach to reaching a sustainable social state that can overcome political agendas and capitalist ethics (Delgado 2004, pp. 325, 326). Sustainable global bioethics represents the synthesis of these ideas, and it connects bioethics to political ecology in an attempt to discover sustainable models for social organization as an alternative to neo-liberal capitalism.

The twenty-first century, as Potter stated, should be the century for global bioethics; otherwise, we will witness the holocaust of the sixth extinction. Pedro Luís Sotolongo is optimistic:

> … And maybe going along that road of this time we will arrive at the promised land of a holistic vision of life (human and other), with a comprehensive and global focus concerning life whose basic metaphor is not that of fight and competition (survival of the fittest), but fraternity and cooperation among human beings for the sake of global preservation. For that purpose a global bioethics will also be necessary (Sotolongo 2002, pp. 84, 85).

The search for a model of sustainable society is one of the primary aims of Cuban thinking in global bioethics. The achievement of this ideal is only possible in an environment of responsible solidarity. To be successful, this principle must be jointly exercised by the whole of society, inside and outside national borders; modifying the maxim of José Martí: "homeland is mankind," so that "homeland is biosphere," for which, and in which, Man exists.

11.6 Bioethics as a New Type of Knowledge: Applied or Meta-Ethics?

The introduction of novel issues to bioethics initiated the first round of national debate pertaining to the validity of this ideological discourse for the objective and subjective conditions of a country which was, at the time, immersed in deep economic and social change as it struggled to preserve the revolutionary project (Pérez et al. 2000, pp. 157 – 158). A trend in Cuban authors recognized the characteristics inherent in bioethics which could motivate and accommodate change in the right direction, in spite of its origins in a liberal capitalist society, which had conferred certain particular characteristics, which would need to be revised to reconcile with Cuban culture and identity.

Recognition of the validity of bioethics in Cuba was evident in the television series "Ethics and Society" which was aired in 2006 national channels. Additional support from the tabloids was elaborated under the direction of Nancy L. Chacón Arteaga, and was circulated widely throughout the country. The following ideas were presented:

> Bioethics is becoming a universal language of remarkable ethical dimensions. In its effort to emphasize the beneficent role that science must play for the welfare of mankind, bioethics offers interdisciplinary solutions and is opposed to disrespect, corruption, and any discriminatory intent that affect both the human being's dignity and have disastrous impact on the environment. From this perspective, bioethics constitutes a responsibility that should reach all citizens as new knowledge. For this reason, it is indispensable to educate the

> population about the fundamental principles of bioethics in the sphere of education and their rights as potential research subjects in all fields of knowledge (Chacón 2006, p. 9).

Despite the advances in recognizing the legitimacy of bioethics as a discipline in the Cuban context, the national theoretical discussion about its place within the structure of ethics has not yet reached a conclusion. Well-known ethicists, such as Luís López Bombino, consider bioethics to be an application of ethics to the problems and conflicts of moral values created by the technological uses of scientific knowledge and their impact on the culture of contemporary society. On the other hand, Thalía Fung argues:

> ... bioethical knowledge is still in construction... one of the characteristic elements of this knowledge is studying the link between conception and instrumentation, regarding which it differs from a great part of contemporary philosophy. Its global and local character engages it closely with "environment" and suffers the same operational difficulties that affect it. Bioethics as the environment conjugates the theoretical thing and the empirical thing, the absolute thing and the thing contaminated with diverse sciences, the circularity of its concepts and its mediating role, both horizontally and vertically. This type of knowledge includes not only the specific phenomena of life, but also its interrelationships with non-organic components. ... In this, bioethics differs from philosophical generalization as such, but compromises subjectivity and nature, without giving priority to either of them, because both constitute one, with a diverse predominance identified by happenings (Fung 2002, p. 48).

In one of his most recent works, *Toward a New Knowledge: Bioethics in the Contemporary Revolution of Knowledge*, Carlos Delgado carries out a careful historical analysis of the development of bioethics as a discipline since its division and reinterpretation as both medical bioethics and global bioethics. His analysis determines that the distinctive characteristic of bioethics as both a theoretical and ethical application is that it has constituted itself as a new type of knowledge, which goes beyond modern rationality:

> Global bioethics completes the integration of new knowledge and the rupture with classical rationality altogether expressed in the epistemology of the second order, complex thinking, and holistic environmentalism... in summary, the overcoming of the traditional notions of human superiority based on scientific knowledge, the rescue of Man as a person and the integration of his social and natural worlds (Delgado 2007, pp 187, 188).

This debate over the place of bioethics in the structure of ethics is one of paramount theoretical value, and its performance constitutes a contribution to the development of the discipline in Cuba.

11.7 Conclusion

Bioethics in Cuba was initially understood as a biomedical ethics and, in its development as such, has established a model of the doctor–patient relationship based on responsibility, trust, and solidarity, with concrete contributions to the theory of informed consent, the definition of human death, and the quality of life.

During the last decade, the reinterpretation of the discipline as a sustainable global bioethics has been addressed with such fervor that it compares in impact with technological and biomedical advances. A consequence of this intellectual effort has been the understanding of bioethics as a new type of knowledge that transcends modern rationality and reconciles Man with Nature. The integration of global environmental problems into the context of bioethics has reinforced responsibility and solidarity as its ruling principles. The dual role of bioethics (medical and environmental) has determined guidelines for a Cuban global bioethics committed to biopolitical action addressed to the rational and equal use of the common products of knowledge, which frame a sustainable society and a just world order.

References

Acosta JR (1999a) Bioética, civilización y desarrollo sostenible. In: Delgado CJ (ed) Cuba verde. En busca de un modelo para la sustentabilidad. José Martí Publishing House, Havana, pp 74–80

Acosta JR (1999b) Los organismos modificados genéticamente. El poder blando del Tercer Milenio. Revista Biotecnología Aplicada 16(Special issue):E25–E31

Acosta JR, González MC (1997) El escenario postmoderno de la bioética. In: Acosta JR (ed) Bioética. Desde una Perspectiva Cubana. Acuario Publishing House, Félix Varela Center, Havana, pp 17–24

Alonso D, Von Smith V, Ramírez A, Ortega A (1979) Etica y deontología médica, Provisionalth edn. Collection of the Students of Medicine. Ministry of Public Health, Havana

Anonymous (1983) Principios de la etica médica. Editora Política, Havana

Araujo R (1997) Hacia una bioética latinoamericana. In: Acosta JR (ed) Bioética. Desde una perspectiva cubana. Acuario Publishing House, Félix Varela Center, Havana, pp 25–31

Area of Education of the Ministry of Public Health (1996) Memoirs of the third international workshop of the regional program of bioethics for Latin America and the Caribbean PAHO/WHO. In: Beca JP (ed) Etica de la investigación científica. Regional Program on Bioethics PAHO/WHO Editions, Santiago de Chile, pp 18–34

Beauchamp T, Childress J (eds) (1979) Principles of biomedical ethics. Oxford University Press, Oxford and New York

Bombino LR (2004) Ética, ciencia y responsabilidad. In López Bombino LR (ed) El saber ético de ayer a hoy, vols 2. Félix Varela Publishing House, Havana, pp 78–86

Borroto R, Núñez de Villavicencio F, Martínez H (1986) Repercusión de la revolución científico-técnica sobre el proceso salud-enfermedad y la organización de la salud pública. In: Lancís F et al (eds) Temas de etica médica. Department of Psychology, Institute of Basic and Preclinic Sciences "Victoria de Girón," and Ministry of Public Health, Havana, pp 105–146

Borroto R, Aneiros-Riba R (1997) La comunicación humana y la calidad de la atención médica. In: Acosta JR (ed) Bioética. Desde una perspectiva cubana. Acuario Publishing House, Félix Varela Center, Havana, pp 112–123

Chacón NL (2006) Etica y sociedad. In: Rebelde J (ed) Tabloid of the course. Ethics and Society of University for all, Havana

De la Torre E, López C, Márquez M, Gutiérrez J, Rojas F (2004) Salud para todos sí es possible. Cuban Society of Public Health, Section of Social Medicine, Havana

Delgado G (1997) Raíces históricas del pensamiento bioético y de la investigación médica en sujetos humanos en Cuba. In: Acosta JR (ed) Bioética. Desde una perspectiva cubana. Acuario Publishing House, Félix Varela Center, Havana, pp 43–52

Delgado CJ (2002) Cognición, problema ambiental y bioética. In: Acosta JR (ed) Bioética para la sustentabilidad. Acuario Publishing House, Félix Varela Center, Havana, pp 135–156
Delgado CJ (2004) Bioética, desigualdad y política. In: Iñiguez L, Pérez OE (eds) Heterogeneidad social en la Cuba actual. Center of Studies on Health and Human Well Being, University of Havana, Havana, pp 324–344
Delgado CJ (2007) Hacia un nuevo saber. La bioética en la revolución contemporánea del saber. Acuario Publishing House, Félix Varela Center, Havana, pp 187–188
Emanuel EJ, Emanuel LL (1992) Four models of the physician–patient relationship. JAMA 267(16):2221–6
Freyre E (2004) La bioética: enfoque imprescindible. In: López Bombino LR, De Armas A, Porto ME (eds) Por una nueva ética. Félix Varela Publishing House, Havana, pp 267–279
Fung T (2002) La bioética: un nuevo saber? In: Acosta JR (ed) Bioética para la sustentabilidad. Acuario Publishing House, Félix Varela Center, Havana, pp 45–54
González R (1997) La nueva dimensión de la relación médico-paciente en nuestros días. In: Acosta JR (ed) Bioética. Desde una perspectiva cubana. Acuario Publishing House, Félix Varela Center, Havana, pp 105–111
González U, Grau J, Amarillo MA (1997) La calidad de vida como un problema de la bioética. In: Acosta JR (ed) Bioética. Desde una perspectiva cubana. Acuario Publishing House, Félix Varela Center, Havana, pp 279–285
Martínez A (2002) Proyectos para una bioética global. In: Acosta JR (ed) Bioética para la sustentabilidad. Acuario Publishing House, Félix Varela Center, Havana, pp 211–238
Núñez de Villavicencio F (1997) Bioética: el médico un Educador. In: Acosta JR (ed) Bioética. Desde una perspectiva cubana. Acuario Publishing House, Félix Varela Center, Havana, pp 128–134
Pellegrino E, Thomasma D (1988) For the patient's own good – The restoration of beneficence in health care. Oxford University Press, Oxford and New York
Pérez M, Flores JL, Singh C, Paredes G (2000) Ética médica y bioética. In: Colectivo de autores. Lecturas de filosofía, salud y sociedad. Editorial of Medical Sciences, Havana, pp 140–164
Ramírez A, Herrera R (1984) Problemas éticos en el desarrollo de la biología y la medicina contemporáneas. In: Varios autores, Problemas filosóficos de la medicina. Coloquio, vol 1. Medical University of Havana, Havana, pp 157–181
Rawls J (1999) A theory of justice, Revth edn. Harvard University Press, Cambridge, MA
Sotolongo PL (2002) La bioética como una disciplina crítica. In: Acosta JR (ed) Bioética para la sustentabilidad. Acuario Publishing House, Félix Varela Center, Havana, pp 69–96
Szasz TS, Hollender MH (1956) A contribution to the philosophy of medicine: The basic models of the doctor–patient relationship. AMA Arch Internal Med 97(5):585–592
Torres R (2001) Glosario de bioética. Acuario Publishing House, Félix Varela Center, Havana
Von Smith V (1997) La ética clínica. In: Acosta JR (ed) Bioética. Desde una perspectiva cubana. Acuario Publishing House, Félix Varela Center, Havana, pp 124–127

Chapter 12
The History of Bioethics in the Dominican Republic

Miguel Angel Suazo

12.1 Antecedents: The Birth

The year 1990 can be considered the beginning of bioethics in the Dominican Republic. In that year, the Pan-American Health Organization (PAHO) in the Dominican Republic extended an invitation to the academic and medical communities to attend an important meeting. At this meeting, a very special guest was welcomed who spoke of a new and foreign subject called "bioethics."

The guest was Dr. Eduardo del Caño from Argentina, who came to the country for several reasons, including the delivery of this talk. The invitation was taken very seriously in academic circles. We from the universities were among the first to show interest, accompanied by those from the Ministry of Health, other government officials, and those within religious circles.

The full magnitude of the proposal was not immediately appreciated; nevertheless, it can be said that it was well received. Argentinians already had much experience with bioethics, and bioethicists such as Mainetti were already part of the history of bioethics. Dominicans, on the other hand, were still only trying to conceive what the landscape of bioethics would look like. The institutes and bioethics centers of Argentina were a reality separate and distant from us.

This meeting can be considered the spark that started the fire, so to speak, and during the following years the battle was long. Meetings, seminars, symposia, and so forth culminated in the establishment of the *National Commission of Bioethics* (*Comisión Nacional de Bioética* – CNB). It began with a managing committee in charge of electing interested individuals from the participating institutions into formal offices. The first president was Dr. Milciades Albert, who, at that time, was

M.A. Suazo
Physician. Universidad Autonomous Santo Domingo, Dominican Republic. Specialized in sexual education. MA, sexology. MA, Bioethics - University of Chile/Pan-American Health Organization. Dean, The Technological Institute of Santo Domingo,
Director of Intec Bioethics Center and coordinator of the Specialization course in Bioethics
e-mail: msuazo@mail.intec.edu.do

L. Pessini et al. (eds.), *Ibero-American Bioethics: History and Perspectives*,
Philosophy and Medicine 106, DOI 10.1007/978-1-4020-9350-0_12,

the executive director of the APEC Institute of Sexual Education; Dr. Andrés Peralta from Madre y Maestra was vice-president.

After only a few months, the resignation of the president caused vice-president Peralta to take charge. He began a process of consolidation and held a series of meetings in universities and public ministries that led up to the First Dominican Congress of Bioethics.

These events led to the establishment of rules, legal incorporation by the executive authority, work commissions, foreign guests, and national congresses; this was followed by the qualification of the commission itself, which had already established a formal structure and division of responsibilities by area: committees of welfare, environment, research, teaching, religion, and philosophy of bioethics, to name a few.

These beginnings were brought about by individual research and efforts by members, as well as by contact with international organizations like Chile's Bioethical Unit of Pan American Health Organization (PAHO) and its directives.

With a certain sense of humor, we remarked that we established a National Commission of Bioethics that was not a Commission – since the number of people that constituted it overflowed those limits – was not national, because most representatives were from the capital city, and, regarding bioethics, we knew very little about it. A providential hand acted in the shadows for a long time while we tried to discover exactly what it was in which we had agreed to participate.

12.2 Stage of Formalization (1998–2001): Development

At the time of the establishment of the CNB, important events in the life of Dominican bioethics had already begun to transpire. One event brought about the specialization of different sectors, as well as to make international contacts with FELAIBE, the Regional Program of Bioethics of the PAHO in Chile, and other global institutions. Two national congresses had been promoted and partnerships among Caribbean Bioethics commissions had been formed, leading to the establishment of the Caribbean Commission of Bioethics, which included Cuba and Puerto Rico.

In that year, Miguel Suazo was the Intec candidate in the Master's of Bioethics program at the University of Chile under the auspices of PRB, while our president, Dr. Andrés Peralta, participated in international bioethics courses with esteemed professors of bioethics in Puerto Rico with the support of the PAHO Chilean program.

With the knowledge we acquired from orienting ourselves in the academic setting, we began to gain clarity in our understanding of what "bioethics" was. Two years of participation in the Master's program before receiving a degree, the conclusion of the courses in Puerto Rico, and many events at the local level began to give a sense to what would be the guiding principles of bioethics in the Dominican Republic.

Some of the participant universities gave (and continue to give) important support to this process of development. They have not only given us support, but have served as officials and sponsors to our organization as well.

12.3 Internalization

In 2000, the Academic Council of the Technological Institute of Santo Domingo welcomed a request from the Health Area for Dr. Miguel Suazo, once Chair of Health at the Institute, to be a member of the *Intec Center of Bioethics* (*Ceninbio*), which requested the participation of several professionals in the field of bioethics. Its objective was to support, to advise, and to serve as a resource in the Dominican setting for the propagation of bioethics, as well as to start a process of sensitization and awareness in the country.

At the end of the second Master's program in Bioethics at the University of Chile, Intec of the Dominican Republic, with PAHO, and under the direction of Professor Diego Grácia and his team from Complutense University, as well as other Latin American countries, was asked to host the first Master's program outside of Chilean territory, a request that Intec promptly accepted.

The Center of Bioethics was expecting this opportunity with its attendant responsibility and took charge of the technical coordination of the new course. The course coordination commenced immediately, and the participation of students from Colombia, Chile, Peru, Ecuador, Argentina, El Salvador, Mexico, Cuba, and the Dominican Republic was obtained.

The *National Commission of Bioethics*, whose president then was Dr. Andrés Peralta, played a primary role in the negotiations and guarantees for executing the Master's program in the Dominican Republic, since it was a private university and the PAHO was accustomed to working with public universities.

12.4 Growth: Broadening and Development

The Center was given support by the dean of Intec at that time, Dr. Altagracia Lopez, who organized the Master's course and charged the Center with its academic management as a counterpart to PAHO'S educational and technical body.

Some of its accomplishments include:

1. The coordination of the International Master's course in bioethics with the Regional Program of Chile during the years 2000–2001
2. The qualification of Hospital Committees of Bioethics
3. Formation of the Intec Forum of Bioethics (at the undergraduate level in the medicine program of Intec)
4. Conferences hosted in the Dominican Republic
5. Curricular implementation of bioethics in the transversal axis of the medicine program of Intec
6. Partnerships with the Regional Program of Bioethics of Chile
7. Support to the National Commission of Bioethics

From then on, the Center took charge of these processes and became a national resource in addition to promoting the aforementioned activities.

While these academic processes were being developed, the National Commission of Bioethics continued its own development through assemblies and the election of new directors. After two consecutive mandates of Dr. Peralta, Monsignor Ramon Alonso, the director of Santo Domingo Catholic University, a prestigious academy, who gave a seat to the Commission, was elected president.

In this period, the most important event was the decree of the Dominican government recognizing CNB as an advisory organization to the executive authority in bioethical matters and asking for its regulation. Dr. Miguel Suazo was later elected its president.

12.4.1 The Academic Setting

Intec University, with the support of CNB, took up the challenge of establishing continuity in the academic process. Intec began and created its own Master's program in bioethics, and with its establishment the second class of students arrived from several related disciplines. As these processes developed, the graduates of the Master's program began to participate in the National Commission of Bioethics; in the recent elections a group of them, presided over by Dr. Togarma Rodriguez, presented as candidates.

12.4.2 Representation

Because CNB is already recognized at the national and international level, its relationship with the PAHO at the international and local levels has been so limited that the PAHO is an advisor and seat of the commission.

At United Nations Education, Scientific, and Cultural Organizations (UNESCO), the CNB has been represented at multiple international events where proposals relevant to bioethics and human rights have been discussed, and also at the local level within the headquarters of the country.

At the governmental level, CNB has made many contributions, including serving as an advisory body to the Secretariat of Health and the National Council of Research in Health.

12.4.3 Caribbean Commission of Bioethics

At the regional level, the Caribbean Commission of Bioethics was established with the partnering of Venezuela, Puerto Rico, Cuba, and the Dominican Republic.

12.5 Legal Aspects

The National Commission of Bioethics established its legal framework with the approval of the necessary statutes during the assembly of October 4, 1995, and its recognition by the executive authority by means of a decree by President Leonel Fernandez.

With its legal recognition, the mission and reach of the CNB was broadened to allow for the inclusion of any individuals involved in or interested in bioethics. As such, bioethics was born and found that modern legislation pertaining to issues of respect for life, abortion, research on human beings, or assisted reproduction was limited.

In 2001, the general law of health was approved. Its articles referred to general subjects that appeared to endorse the rights of patients and imply – without referring to it by name – the concept of "informed consent," establishing the right of the patients to be informed; however, when addressing "bioethics" properly, the concept of informed consent is narrowed in an interesting way to research on human beings, indicating in a vague reference that research must be based in international codes of ethics like those of Nuremberg and Helsinki.

Subjects pertaining to sexual and reproductive life, including abortion, were the topics of heated debates, and pressure, mainly of a religious kind, was used to prevent the explicit treatment of these topics in legislation. Abortion, for example, is still punishable under the penal code of the time which calls for the imprisonment of all involved persons, considered accomplices, and thereby criminalizes and prohibits the possibility of a therapeutic abortion.

The great paradox of the text is that just one hospital in the capital reported more than 100,000 abortions in a year, which the law neither considered nor sanctioned, allowing for the conclusion that abortions are acceptable when the intention is to save the mother's life. This meant that medical assistance and shelter from the law could be obtained by many pregnant women interested in terminating pregnancy. Furthermore, regarding organ donation, in 1981 the organ donation act (Act 391) was passed, followed by the cornea donation and transplant act (Act 60–88) in 1988. However, the general population has not seen the intended benefits of these laws, and the anticipated results have not been actualized. This process will take time, because the attitudes surrounding organ donation need to be modified, since they tend to be rooted in myths, religious beliefs, and personal beliefs that regard the practice negatively.

CNB has been distanced from these subjects since its inception, because the Commission has no reputation in society, not to mention that bioethics lacks an autonomous statute to be its Letter of Presentation. The process of incorporation into civil life for CNB is slow because of its lack of recognition by the general public.

The Health Area and the Secretariat of State of Public Health and Social Assistance (Sespas) are the settings where bioethics has grown and become recognized. We have already indicated that the establishment of an official bioethical evaluation of research protocols by the National Council of Bioethics in Health (*Consejo Nacional de Bioética en Salud – Conabios*) – wherein paragraphs explicitly place bioethics in the general law of health, in the clinical context in the case of informed consent, in the respect of human dignity and values, and in the research context – legitimizes bioethics.

Conabios' legal identity credits it with a statute requiring that all research on human beings be evaluated from a bioethical perspective. For a credible evaluation to take place, an official in the field must be present, as well as a balanced staff of professionals in the areas of research, policy, and bioethics. Master's students and professors of bioethics at Intec University have produced for *Conabios* national and international members able to evaluate these protocols, or to cooperate in the technical formation of its members. The minister of Health has delegated to CNB the development of a proposal to address the use of drugs and treatment in addressing cases of undesired multiple pregnancies.

Given the strong religious roots of the population and the power of religious spheres, there are subjects that are not openly addressed in the legal context. This is evident in the adoption of a new penal code addressing abortion which fails to make a concession for therapeutic abortion and instead makes a blanket prohibition on all types of abortion. The case is similar regarding euthanasia: a request has been made of congress to debate and discuss this issue for the purpose of exposing the problems surrounding it, but this has only been met with silence and disregard.

CNB has proposed to open the debate in its context, serving as a platform for a generation of secular thought, but it has not been possible to go beyond this intention, given the plurality of its membership.

12.6 The Present Situation of Bioethics in the Dominican Republic

At this point, we have considered the founding of bioethics and its recognition as a discipline in the Dominican context. The CNB has a number of subcommittees in such areas as the environment, ethics and bioethics, and education, giving an interdisciplinary character to the discipline.

In terms of academics, unlike in the beginning, there are now at least six medical programs at six different universities that have incorporated bioethics into the curriculum and employ innovative pedagogical modalities and methodologies. The State University (Universidad Autónoma de Santo Domingo) has created short courses in bioethics for their instructors. The specialized medical societies of the Dominican Medical School have included the subject in their congresses, as well as other instances in the academic world and the civil society. Both the Intec Center of Bioethics and the National Commission of Bioethics are mandatory references in the national context. Furthermore: a group of Master's students are even now studying at Intec; advisory work is being done for the Dominican government on the Humanization of Health Services; CNB is promoting elections, and its board of directors is composed of Master's students coming from the said Master's program, something that increases the quality of its service.

The support of international organizations has been beneficial, and with it we have developed specialized consultants and formation workshops for ethics committees to assist in the hinterland, as well as international workshops supported by PAHO Chile and its Ethics Unit on the Didactics of Bioethics Teaching in the Dominican Republic.

Our members and Master's students educated at Intec have contributed to the bioethics literature. The following are worth mentioning: *Bioética para Nuevos* (*Bioethics for the Young*) (Míguelo Suazo); a co-authored book, *Bioética para la Sustentabilidad* (*Bioethics for Sustenance*) (Andrés Peralta and Miguel Suazo); *Bioética y Gestión de los Servicios de Salud* (*Bioethics and Health Services Management*) (Rafael Montero, Miguel Suazo and Francia Reynoso); and *Adolesceré, un Nuevo Marco Axiológico* (*I Will be A Teenager: A New Axiological Framework*) (Miguel Suazo).

Although bioethics does not have a significant presence in the legislative world, there is no doubt that this revolution in the last 15 years has brought to life a critical mass, a group of specialists in the subject, and a potential impetus for developing the subject in the professional and social contexts. We know with certainty that bioethics is an instrument not restricted to the health arena but pertains as well to the professional world. In addition, its interaction with the world of values has been developing in the last few years.

The present account of bioethics in the Dominican Republic must recognize that its bigger accomplishments are: first, the development of the academic context and the development of professionals to take part in this social process; and second, its contributions at the State level, because it was nominated adviser of the executive authority in matters of bioethics immediately following its legal incorporation in the last government, that is, three consecutive governments have provided legal space for it (since its expertise has not been directly sought by the Secretary of Health).

Our history has developed in a logical way and we can say that, starting from a distant and uncertain initiative, we have been able to successfully establish a discipline that the country already recognizes.

References

Asociación de Bioética Fundamental y Clínica (eds) (1999) La educación en bioética de los profesionales sanitarios en España. Asociación de Bioética Fundamental y Clínica, Madrid

Comisión Nacional de Bioética (2000) Estatutos. Republica Dominicana, Santo Domingo

Cuceiro A (1999) Bioética para clínicos. Editorial Triacastela, Madrid

Facultad de Educación Universidad El Bosque (1999) Bioética, origen y tendencias. Universidad a Distancia, Programa de Bioética, Bogotá, Colombia

Gracia D (1998) Profesión médica, investigación y justicia sanitaria. El Buho, Bogotá

Pichardo A (1997) Responsabilidad civil y penal del médico. Impretur S.A, Santo Domingo

Presidencia de la República Dominicana (2005) Reglamentos de la Ley General de Salud (42–01), vols 2. CERSS, Santo Domingo

Reboredo J (2004) Inserción de los comités de ética en los hospitales públicos. Buenos Aires

Secretaría de Estado de Salud Pública (2001) Ley General de Salud de la República Dominicana

Secretaría de Estado de Salud Pública. Reglamento Hospitalario de la República Dominicana

Suazo MA (2002) Bioética para nuevos. Instituto Tecnológico de Santo Domingo, Santo Domingo

Suazo MA (2004) Adolesceré, un nuevo marco axiológico. Instituto Tecnológico de Santo Domingo, Santo Domingo

Chapter 13
Historical Aspects of the Development of Bioethics in Ecuador

Katya Rodríguez

13.1 Introduction

In 1971, Van Rensselaer Potter's book, *Bioethics: A Bridge to the Future*, introduced the term "bioethics" to the world's scientific literature. In recent years, the term has remained in common usage, although its meaning has continued to evolve beyond what Potter had originally envisioned (Lolas Stepke 1998).

In the last four decades, ethical concerns have gained significance due to the rapid development of extraordinary scientific technologies. These developments have had direct consequences for life and health, making them appropriate issues of bioethical consideration (Lolas Stepke 1997). This requires that one ethically reflect on one's own responsibility for the impact human development may have had on the biosphere, biology, social and population policies, and more. One must reflect on all dimensions of life, including those considerations relevant to future moral agents, the environment, and, more broadly, the future of humanity.

Since the 1970s, the concept of "bioethics" has been adapted by countries all over the world and has caused the emergence of various speakers who have taken its language as part of their functional structure. The adoption of bioethics in Latin America began in the 1980s in the countries of Argentina, Chile, and Brazil (Mainetti 1989). The reception of bioethics was found primarily in medical schools, causing a reorientation of their thinking about medical ethics, and eventually reached the universities and those professions related to the social and human sciences. Interest in bioethics grew, although often without a local identity. However, according to historical record, Ecuador did not become involved in the dialogue or social process of bioethics until the early 1990s (Rigail 2003).

K. Rodríguez
Research and Professor in the Universidad Central del Ecuador Quito, Ecuador
e-mail: katyarodriguez@hotmail.com

L. Pessini et al. (eds.), *Ibero-American Bioethics: History and Perspectives*, Philosophy and Medicine 106, DOI 10.1007/978-1-4020-9350-0_13,

13.2 Legal Framework

One of the advancements of Ecuadorian bioethics was the promulgation of the Code of Medical Ethics, published in the official Gazette in 1992. The Code came to occupy an important role for the development of guidelines pertaining to health and health care in Ecuador. However, in 1993, flaws in the Code led the Court of Constitutional Rights to defer its application. Later that year, an appeal was made to the Supreme Court to declare its nullity, thereby creating a legal "knot" without a definitive resolution.

In 1995, the Law of Patient Rights and Protection served to guarantee that the principles of bioethics would be respected. The same type of guarantee appeared in other texts within the Constitutional Legal Framework, stating that one must "observe," "follow," or "adhere" to the principles of bioethics.

Specific mention of bioethics also appeared in the health section of article 44 of the 1998 Constitution. Considered as an aim "to guarantee health to the population," it is also mentioned in articles 42, 45, and 46.

While mention of particular bioethical issues within the law is uncommon, the National Law of Transplants does exist. However, issues concerning topics such as abortion and euthanasia are often insufficiently addressed. Unfortunately, the influence of law is substantial in Ecuador; there are very few laws pertaining to topics in bioethics, and those that do exist do not effectively deal with the subject matter.

13.3 The Sowing of Bioethics

The acceptance of bioethics as a discipline with a particular set of values and field of knowledge allows one to respond to the academic, scientific, and professional activities of the biological and human sciences. Bioethics advocates taking a reflective position, which allows one to question, for example, scientific rationality and its sometimes pernicious consequences. It has the ability to challenge preconceived ideas, like the common conception of science as being morally neutral. Bioethics has refuted this claim by demonstrating that science, in its conception, development, and application, always implies an agent with intention, necessarily making them moral agents and their actions classifiable as morally good or bad.

In Ecuador, some advances towards adopting a bioethical attitude have been accomplished. However, for the most part, things remain unchanged. We wait expectantly, almost in a state of inertia, believing ingenuously, for example, that scientific and technological developments will solve our serious social problems without the help of an ethical framework or an administrative and political restructuring. There is no single way to reach a national consensus about the extensive debates induced by the bioethical approach. Due to this, the soil in which the real "sowing" of the development of bioethics needs to take place is still in its beginning stages.

Topics such as cloning, transgenic food, and genomic medicine cannot even be raised within a context having no legal guidelines and, even worse, no rules for deliberation. However, in Ecuador, a topic receiving some attention has been the establishment of ethics committees and a national research ethics. Some advances have already been made, but the topic is still far removed from substantial debate.

13.4 Bioethics in Professional Training

Bioethics, within the context of professional training, is meant to serve as a tool for changing one's perspective based on a specific set of values. The infusion of bioethics at all levels of education (undergraduate and graduate) within the health professions and the human and biological sciences has been considered essential by many authors (Fierro 1998). In spite of these recommendations, the universities that have integrated bioethics into the curricula of their human and biological science programs remain isolated, even in 2008. The situation has improved from years past, but it still remains unsatisfactory.

In our case, for example, as doctors trained at the Central University of Ecuador's medical school during the period of 1976–1983, we completed 7 years of formal undergraduate study without encountering bioethics as a discipline or subject in the curriculum. There may have been "moments of reflection," "an evolution of conscience," a certain "sensitization" that took place or, ofttimes, a sort of "challenging attitude" in confronting death, pain, and injustice, but it was in a non-formal and almost personal way that our professional training introduced us to bioethics. We all experienced it with differing intensity, but, undoubtedly, it has had effects on all of us during the last 25 years of our professional achievement.

The closest we came to an ethical dialogue during the training process was when we collectively heard the reading of the Hippocratic Oath at the University Theater on August 5, 1983, the day of our graduation as doctors of medicine and surgery. We swore to uphold this code of ethics promulgated more than 2000 years ago. Without question, this activity was probably, in most cases, performed in an unconscious manner. However, the action can be considered an engagement with a component of bioethics, an ethical obligation, that is, a professional ethic, which we were bound to respect and uphold in our professional conduct and development.

In asking some of our colleagues who graduated before and after 1983 in various parts of the country, whether they remembered being formally introduced to bioethics and its deliberative dialogue during their professional training, they all responded in the negative. Although there appears to be record of a "Seminar of National Medicine," which all doctors graduating in 1983 were required to take, we have no recollection of this seminar, nor of there being a requirement to take it. Supposedly, the Directive Council approved the seminar in an attempt to introduce an analysis of the national medical practice into the educational process as a means of relating it to bioethics. It was also recorded that the seminar was a negative experience and was consequently cancelled.

The perspective in medical schools today is different and has been ever since the 1990s, when the late Dr. Eduardo Estrella Aguirre, as chair of the faculty of medical sciences at the Central University of Ecuador, introduced bioethics into the curriculum as a branch of the medical humanities. As a result, some activities in bioethics were developed, focusing primarily on the Ecuadorian actors in bioethics, instead of on the global movement, which helped pave the way for the founding of a national bioethics.

Additionally, undergraduate chairs of bioethics in the medical schools of some of the most important universities in the country were established. However, their bioethical approach has focused primarily on health problems and not necessarily on ethical conflicts in a strict philosophical sense. It must be realized, however, that the bioethical approach goes much further than academic formalism. Bioethics has more to offer than that which can be learnt in a university classroom and applied to practical matters. It is undoubtedly a continuous process of learning how to act; a process in which reason, passion, conscience, and action are united. This is evidenced in the way those who truly study bioethics are encouraged by it and, at least from our perspective, deepen its reflections by legitimating its practice and contributing to the training of new professionals.

Thus, we are grateful for the introduction of bioethics into graduate and undergraduate courses by visionaries. An example is the graduate medical specialties course at the University of San Francisco, Quito, as in the capital of Ecuador, (USFQ), which has introduced bioethics as an essential way to induce dialogue and deliberation for reaching a consensus, a context for moral decision making, and as a means for giving science a conscience. The course has realized bioethics as a necessary practice in medical training, and in doing so it has encouraged a value-based education, which the medical profession demands. As a result, the course has become a pioneering effort in the clinical and medical specialties. Graduate medical students have been doing their residence at the Carlos Andrade Marin Hospital, under an agreement with the University of San Francisco of Quito, as in the capital of Ecuador, for several years now.

13.5 Bioethics and Institutions

Since the establishment of the Intergovernmental Commission of UNESCO's International Committee of Bioethics in 1998 and Ecuador's subsequent membership for a year, a series of inter-institutional activities meant to encourage the dissemination of bioethics in Ecuador has taken place (Comité Internacional 1998).

One of the institutions, the National Academy of Medicine, sponsored several activities during Dr. Rodrigo Fierro Benítez's presidency of the Latin-American Association of National Academies of Medicine (ALANAM) with the sponsorship of the PAHO/WHO (Pan-American Health Organization/World Health Organization) of Ecuador and the House of Ecuadorian Culture. In 1998 the book, *Dehumanization of Medicine and Bioethics*, was published as a collection of the letters and presentations of ALANAM's meeting of the Managing Council in

Madrid on November 23, 1997. The content of the book approaches bioethics from the perspective of its being a discipline restricted to professional establishment.

The precursor to such substantial bioethical movements in Ecuador was the meeting of the 37th managing committee of PAHO/WHO to create the Regional Bioethics Program in 1994 (PAHO/WHO 2007). The program's head office is in Chile and is now called the Bioethics Unit. Its director and coordinator, Dr. Fernando Lolas Stepke, has given momentum to the consolidation and development of a regional bioethics and has also developed a national bioethics course. This program has been responsible for the bioethics training of a limited number of Ecuadorian professionals, most of whom were doctors. Among the first to attend the program during the period of 1998–2000 were Dr. Antonio Crespo, Dr. Domínguez, Dr. Tenorio, and Dr. Hermida. During 2003–2004, Dr. Katya Rodríguez attended the graduate course in Chile with the assistance of a Fogarty Scholarship from the NIH-USA and the support of the PAHO/WHO. In addition, there are other professionals who have received an education in bioethics at other schools. Including those previously named, the number of professionals in Ecuador who have received academic titles in bioethics is less than 15. However, those professionals who have studied or engaged in bioethics in some capacity remain unknown.

13.6 The National Commission of Bioethics

Since the establishment of the National Commission of Bioethics in 2001 as a technical advisory committee for the Department of Public Health (MSP), regular meetings have been held with the assistance of the National Council of Health (CONASA).

The Commission is comprised of representatives from the Association of Medical Faculties and Schools, a non-governmental organization (not necessarily specializing in bioethics), the National Agency of Health of the Joint Command of FF the Armed Forces (AA) (two representatives), The Charity Board of Guayaquil, the Ecuadorian Institute of Social Security, the MSP Institute of Science and Technology, the Nurses' Federation of Ecuador, the Ecuadorian Red Cross, the National Agency of Health of the National Police, the PAHO/WHO – Ecuador, the Ecuadorian Medical Federation, the Ecuadorian Bioethics Society, the Department of Public Health, the Dentists' Federation, the Consortium of Provincial Councils of Ecuador, and the Technical Coordinating Committee of CONASA. As a technical commission, its membership appears inflated with a number of members and institutions not involved in bioethics.

The various functions of the National Commission of Bioethics were established in article 50, which states:

The commission will fulfill the following functions:

1. To guide and promote the essentials of bioethics in the country, especially in defense of and respect for life
2. To propose initiatives incorporating the ethical aspects of research, professional training, and health, and to establish relevant guidelines

3. To propose the incorporation of bioethical principles into the national public health policies
4. To design strategies and to establish mechanisms and procedures for the inclusion of bioethical principles in official health programs and plans
5. To advise the National Council of Health and other entities and to assist in the production of technical guidelines for the fulfillment of bioethical principles and other related aspects
6. To promote the deliberation of current ethical dilemmas in health research and practice
7. To create spaces for the discussion and solution of ethical problems and dilemmas related to health by means of publications, events, and the creation of study groups, centers, or specific entities for this purpose
8. To perform other functions in its field of competence, which are assigned to it by the Council, its board of directors, or the President

13.7 Institutionalization of Bioethics

Since 2000, the expansion of educational activities related to bioethics in Ecuador has primarily occurred in non-academic settings. The primary focus has been on professional organizations and the inclusion of bioethics in their training modules at different courses or congresses run by various associations. For instance, at the National Congress of Internal Medicine in 2002, space was made for bioethics in their scientific and academic programs. In that year, Dr. Katya Rodríguez was president of the bioethics module and was responsible for developing it. She was also in charge of the first meeting of the Latin-American Congress of Internal Medicine, held in Quito (the capital of Ecuador), in June 2005, where she created an outstanding module for Latin American bioethics. Since then, forums, roundtables, symposiums, courses, and congresses have all incorporated bioethics into their programs.

It is often times the case that indicators of the development of bioethics within a country do not necessarily guarantee any *real* development in terms of its principles being put into practice. A good measure of the development of bioethics is reflected by the number of institutional bioethics committees (both assistance committees and research ethics committees) a country has, which operate in accordance with international bioethics guidelines. In this vein, the bioethics committees in Ecuador and their guiding principles were the focus of a study conducted as part of the graduate course at the University of Chile, in alliance with its Interdisciplinary Center for Studies in Bioethics, the Regional Bioethics Program (PAHO/WHO), and the American National Institutes of Health (NIH) (Rodríguez 2004a). The published results of the study indicated the existence of 19 institutional committees, which were regrettably constituted and working in irregular ways and, in most cases, were operating on good will and not within any established codes or guidelines.

In 2004, when Alfredo Palacio was vice-president of the Republic, Dr. Katya Rodriguez submitted a plan for establishing bioethics and creating hospital committees as components of a Universal Insurance Project, but the project failed to gain the necessary support.

These facts, taken in addition to the lack of a formal position or institutionalization of bioethics, lead one to conclude that it remains an underdeveloped field in Ecuador, due in large part to the absence of any real formulation or implementation of relevant governmental policies.

Despite the efforts of the past few years specifically related to the education and training of professionals to become members of Institutional Ethics Committees (IECs), with strong support from the PAHO/WHO in Ecuador (especially the national bioethics representative, Dr. Granda, and the regional representative, Dr. F. Lolas Stepke), the situation is still far from ideal. Nevertheless, bioethics workshops have been developed by the College of Exact and Natural Sciences at the Pontifical Catholic University of Ecuador (PUCE), including a workshop meant to train hospital managers about bioethics committees, supported by MSP, CONASA, PAHO/WHO-Ecuador, the Medical College of PUCE, and CEPAR.

In May 2005, an international seminar took place at the PUCE, Quito, sponsored by TDR, PAHO, WHO, Ohio University, and FLACEIS, which focused on the establishment of an IEC, the preparation of its official statute document, the creation of an operational guide in accordance with the International Bioethical Guidelines, and, also, the training of the members of bioethics committees at the national level. Dr. Katya Rodríguez, appointed by Ohio University, directed the seminar and was responsible for the development of the course and workshop for potential members of IECs, which was attended by several representatives from institutions around the country and many of the professors from PUCE. Other course topics included the "CIOMS Guidelines" presented by Dr. Peralta; "International Recommendations for Organizing IEC" presented by Dr. Robert Mancini (consultant for the PAHO/WHO of Chile); "The Ethics of Ethics Committees," a roundtable discussion moderated by Dr. Katya Rodríguez and participated by Dr. Mancini, Dr. Francisco León (Spanish bioethicist working for several universities in Spain and Chile), Dr. Andrés Peralta (bioethicist from the Dominican Republic and vice-president of FLACEIS), and Dr. Santacruz; "The Ethics of Research" presented by Dr. Fernando Lolas Stepke (Director of the Regional Program of Bioethics); and "The What, How, What For and Why of ICEs" presented by Dr. Katya Rodríguez.

13.8 Activities in Bioethics

In 2002, at the PUCE, due to the initiative of Dr. Pablo Maldonado Schullo, a lawyer specializing in bio-law, a course was developed primarily concerning the relationship between law and bioethics, which was taught by Dr. Ricardo Rabinovich from Argentina.

In 2005, there were a number of academic and scientific activities taking place in the field of bioethics, including the international congress, "The Human Face of Medicine: Advances in Palliative Care," directed by Father Alberto Readelli, on

February 22–25, with the support of the Ecuadorian Foundation of Palliative Care (FECUPAL), the Ecuadorian Episcopal Conference, and the Camillian Center of Humanization and Pastoral Health. The Brazilian bioethicist, Father Leo Pessini, was in attendance and made outstanding contributions to the conference.

The Ecuadorian Foundation of Palliative Care, managed by the Camillian Religious Community, offers integral care to patients in terminal stages of disease and seeks solidarity with those who suffer. The Foundation's work is an important part of bioethics because it functions in accordance with the message, "a life with dignity is more than just existing," and seeks to sensitize the community to this important aspect of bioethics. Their actions consolidate a fruitful 10 years of bioethical activity in Ecuador.

In May 2005, the Fourth National Forum of Health Research took place in the city of Cuenca and with the support of Fundacyt, the MSP's Institute of Science and Technology, CONASA, CONESUP, and PAHO/WHO. The focus of the forum was not bioethics, but its debate program included the topic of bioethics and scientific research with a conscience. Also in 2005, the Fifth Latin-American Congress of Bioethics (FELAIBE) occurred in Quito, as in the capital of Ecuador, and again in Panama, due to temporary disputes between the presidencies of FELAIBE and the Ecuadorian Bioethics Society (EBS).

13.9 The Ecuadorian Bioethics Society

In an effort to try to institutionalize bioethics, the Ecuadorian Society of Bioethics was established in 2003 as a result of an initiative of the members of the National Commission of Bioethics of CONASA (Dr. Antonio Crespo, Dr. Patricia Moncayo, Dr. Katya Rodríguez, Dr. Dimitri Barreto, Dr. Edmundo Granda, Dr. Luis Sarrazin, Lic. Jacqueline Bonilla, Dr. Gladis Baldeón, Dr. Enrique Hermida). The founding members of the Society included Dr. Domínguez, Dr. Oswaldo Chávez (the founding president), Dr. Agustin García, and others, (the SEB is currently chaired by Dr. Agustin Garcia (2008)).

13.10 Publications on Bioethics

Ecuador has also produced a number of publications in bioethics, including: *La equidad en la mira: La salud pública en Ecuador durante las últimas décadas* (Equity in Focus: Public Health in Ecuador During the Last Decades), PAHO/WHO 2007, in which the chapter, "Apuntes de Bioética en América Latina" ("Notes on Bioethics in Latin America"), written by Dr. Fernando Lolas Stepke, stands out; as well as *El cóndor, la serpiente y el colibrí: la PAHO/WHO y la salud pública en el Ecuador del siglo XXI* (The Condor, The Snake and the Hummingbird: The PAHO/WHO and Public Health in Ecuador in the 21st Century, 2002), which addresses bioethics in Chapter 61; *Memoria del Museo Nacional de Medicina Eduardo Estrella* (Memory of the Eduardo Estrella National Museum of Medicine, 2003), which mentions bioethics in Chapter 26.

In 2007, the document *Políticas para la normativa y aplicación de la ética y bioética en investigación y tecnología en salud* (Policies for the Regulation and Application of Ethics and Bioethics in Health Research and Technology) was developed by the Department of Public Health's National Institute of Science and Technology and will be accessible soon at http://www.conasa.gov.ec.

13.11 Final Considerations

We find that state policies in bioethics should go beyond national health politics and biomedical research by extending its borders to include other areas of the biological, human, and social sciences. Even though the application of ethics is not mandatory, we hope that the previously mentioned document prepared by CONASA-MSP will eventually make possible the institutionalization of a national bioethics, allowing for a reflective conscience inclusive of all involved. In this way, all citizens, even those incapable of participating in action, would see their rights defended, whether they were research subjects or users of the health system. Ethical codes would govern research, the health care system would be equitable, the basic bioethical principles of non-maleficence and beneficence would be respected, and persons would be treated with dignity. When this has become the national reality, we will finally be satisfied that bioethics has taken roots in Ecuador. Bioethics will then be a concrete reality for Ecuador instead of just a theoretical construct. The interdisciplinary potential of bioethics is also still unknown in our country, because bioethics tends to be intricately related to medicine instead of public health. Therefore, the inherent possibilities are yet to be realized. The course of action is just as much determined by human will as it is by any natural or man-made law. Thus, it appears that efficient intervention relies on our comprehension of bioethics, because there are no clear limits as to what practices can be established.

Therefore, the construction of Ecuadorian bioethics still remains to be completed. There is a long journey ahead, which will depend on the attitudes and actions of future agents to bring about dignified social practices related to health and human life, to ensure technological and scientific advances that will promote the well-being of all, and to base their decisions on principles and values that will allow for one to consciously take responsibility for future generations. We must also take responsibility for the current trend threatening the human species with extinction by establishing a critical, deliberative, ethical conscience to limit development and reorientation.[1]

[1] We especially recommend reading the chapter "Apuntes sobre Bioética en América Latina", written by Dr. Fernando Lolas Stepke, in La equidad en la mira: la salud pública en Ecuador durante las últimas décadas (Quito 2007), which adequately addresses the Ecuadorian reality of bioethics.

References

Fierro R (1998) Deshumanización de la Medicina y Bioética. ALANAM, CCE

Lolas Stepke F (1998) Bioética. Editorial Universitaria, Santiago de Chile

Lolas Stepke, F (1997) Mas allá del cuerpo. Ed. Andrés Bello, Santiago

Mainetti JA (1989) Ética médica. Editorial Quirón, La Plata

PAHO/WHO (2007) La equidad en la mira: la salud pública en Ecuador durante las últimas décadas. Quito. Available at: http://www.uchile.cl/bioetica/doc/perspectivas.pdf

Rigail F (2003) Memorias del Museo Nacional de Medicina "Eduardo Estrella". Quito

Rodríguez K (2004a) Línea de base sobre funcionalidad y constitución de Comités de Ética de la Investigación en Quito. Available at: http://www.uchile.cl/bioetica/doc/linea.pdfhttp

Rodríguez K (2004b) Plan para desarrollar una estrategia de vinculamiento del Proyecto de Aseguramiento Universal (a cargo de la Vicepresidencia), FUNDACYT (Fundación para la Ciencia y la Tecnología) y LA BIOETICA. Quito. Available at: www.uchile.cl/bioetica/doc

Chapter 14
A Survey of the Development of Mexican Bioethics: Genomic Medicine as One of Its Greatest Challenges

Gerardo Jiménez-Sánchez, Cesar Francisco Lara-Álvarez, and Alberto Arellano-Méndez

14.1 Posing the Problem

Bioethics brings forth the conscience of both a right and a duty of justice and also of responsibility linked to science and the ethics of behavior before life.

Manuel Velasco-Suárez

Before one considers significant scientific advances, the development and proliferation of new medical technologies, or the relationship of man and the environment, one must first reflect on the close connections between ethics and other areas of knowledge. Thus, *bioethics* is born as a "new interdisciplinary method of study and debate about the new problems created by the development of science" (Santos y Vargas 2002, pp. 58–59), which tries to produce consistent answers to meet the current demands of society.

Although more than three decades have passed since the founding of bioethics as a new discipline, the concept is not univocal. In Latin America there is a consensus, more or less generalized, that bioethics is: "the study of human values and their relation to science and technology as applied to the different contexts of life"

G. Jiménez-Sánchez (✉)
PhD, Medicine – Johns Hopkins University, General Director of Instituto Nacional de Medicina Genômica do México (National Institute of Genomic Medicin), Professor of Genomics of Uma, is resident researcher of Funsalud – Fundação Mexicana de Saúde (Mexican Health Foundation)
e-mail: cflara@inmegen.gob.mx

C.F. Lara-Álvarez
MA, Ethics of Biomedical Research – University of Chile, Director of Educational Programs, National Institute of Genomic Medicine, Mexico. Coordinator of Ethical, Legal and Social Issues of the research Center of Genomic Medicine
e-mail: cflara@inmegen.gob.mx

A. Arellano-Méndez
Graduated by the Law School of National Autonomous University of Mexico (UNAM) and researcher of Health and Law Studies of the Law Research Institute (IIJ-UNAM)
e-mail: cflara@inmegen.gob.mx

L. Pessini et al. (eds.), *Ibero-American Bioethics: History and Perspectives*, Philosophy and Medicine 106, DOI 10.1007/978-1-4020-9350-0_14,

(Kuthy Porter 1999, p. 17). In a sense, bioethics is understood as an attempt to humanize scientific development by establishing dynamic relationships between science and the humanities and by striking a balance between the developmental path of science and the ethical boundaries that restrict it.

14.2 The Construction of Bioethics in Mexico

14.2.1 The Origins of Bioethics in Mexico: Manuel Velasco-Suárez

Dr. Manuel Velasco-Suárez is recognized as the father of bioethics in Mexico; he was a man of science and letters and the author of six books in addition to 200 journal articles published both nationally and internationally. During his lifetime, he attended more than 1,200 conferences in Mexico and around the world and was a member of more than 25 medical societies and academies (Carrasco-Rojas 2001, pp. 316–320). He received a great many honors and distinctions from associations, universities, and both private and public organizations from around the world, in addition to having been awarded several honorary titles by the governments of different countries. Dr. Velasco-Suárez was a visionary and a man ahead of his time. In March 1992, he established the National Commission of Bioethics (CNB – Comisión Nacional de Bioética) with Dr. Jesus Kumate Rodriguez who was the Secretary of Health at the time. Later, in 1995, he was a charter member and the first president of the Mexican National Academy of Bioethics (ANMB – Academia Nacional Mexicana de Bioética) (Mateos 2002, pp. 387–388). This renowned and enthusiastic promoter of Mexican bioethics once said:

> Bioethics is an interaction between the biological systems, which obey physical laws, and ethical–moral conscience. Without having relation with physical laws, it weighs the conduct of those who intervene or interfere with life. It is not "the ethics of life," but of the systematic study and reflection of behavior towards life, health, and human rights, in light of the advances of biological sciences and the necessary philosophical reflections of ethics (Velasco-Suárez 2002, p. 195).

It is pertinent to emphasize the magnitude of the contributions that this illustrious bioethicist made. In 2002, the Manuel Velasco-Suárez Scholarship in Bioethics (Beca Manuel Velasco-Suárez en Bioética) was created by the Pan-American Foundation of Health and Education, in cooperation with the PAHO, to stimulate – between young teachers and researchers – the development of one's capacities for bioethical analysis.

14.2.2 The National Commission of Bioethics

It was not until 2003 that the CNB was granted a permanent statute. On November 8, 2001, the Secretary of Health officially designated Dr. Manuel Velasco-Suárez as the Executive Secretary of the CNB. In September 2005, the CNB became a decentralized organ of the Secretary of Health (SSA), with technical and operational autonomy. With its new status, the CNB was charged with defining Mexican policy as it was proposed within bioethics, with the aims of (a) establishing bioethics-related public health policies; (b) acting as a national advisory agency for pertinent issues in bioethics; and (c) encouraging participation in bioethical debates among the various sectors of society, among other aims.

After the death of the first executive president of the CNB, Dr. Fernando Cano-Valle was left in charge of its direction, creating the *Summa Bioética* journal, the official publication of the CNB. Later, Dr. Juan Garza-Ramos was the Interim Executive Secretary until 2004 when the illustrious Dr. Guillermo Soberón-Acevedo permanently undertook the position, which he still holds.

Among the most important accomplishments of the CNB was the organization of seven conferences which were well attended by both national and international participants. The first six conferences had their respective proceedings published. Conference themes included: (a) "Bioethics, Health, Human Rights and Scientific Responsibility" (the First National Congress of Bioethics 1997); (b) "Bioethical Culture for Human Development" (the Second National Congress of Bioethics 1998); (c) "Bioethics at the End of the Century and for the New Millennium" (the Third National Latin American and Caribbean Congress of Bioethics 1999);[1] (d) "Bioethics for the Development of the Human Conscience in the Sciences" (the Fourth National Latin American and Caribbean Congress of Bioethics and Second International Congress of Bioethics 2000); (e) "Bioethics of Human Life Events: From the Dawn to the Eclipse of Life" (the Fifth National Latin American and Caribbean Congress of Bioethics 2001); (f) "Bioethics of the Quality of Medical Assistance" (the Sixth National Latin American and Caribbean Congress of Bioethics 2002); and (g) "Bioethics in Science and Society" (the Seventh National Latin American and Caribbean Congress of Bioethics and Third International Congress of Bioethics 2003).

The various conference events attracted the participation of several Mexican and foreign universities, in addition to an endless number of national organizations, including the SSA, the Mexican Institute of Social Security (IMSS – Instituto Mexicano del Seguro Social), the Institute of Security and Social Services of State Workers (ISSSTE – Instituto de Seguridad y Servicios Sociales de los Trabajadores del Estado), the National System for the Integral Development of the Family (DIF – Sistema Nacional para el Desarrollo Integral de la Familia), the Secretaries of Health from Chiapas, Federal District, Jalisco, and Nuevo León, and the Center for the Study and Research of Bioethics of Guadalajara (CEIB – Centro de Estudios y Investigaciones de Bioética de Guadalajara). At the international level, the promotion of the meetings was supported by WHO, PAHO, UNICEF, FELAIBE, International Physicians for the Prevention of Nuclear War (IPPNW), and the Universal Movement of Scientific Responsibility (MURS, México – Movimiento Universal de la Responsabilidad Científica).

[1] From this congress forward, the expression "Latin American and Caribbean" was added to "National Congress," as a result of an agreement made a year prior between the CNB and the Latin American and Caribbean Federation of Bioethics Institutions (Federación Latinoamericana y del Caribe de Instituciones de Bioética – FELAIBE).

The conference proceedings make apparent the emphasis of participants on points of connection between bioethics and scientific responsibility, as well as the characteristic conflicts and controversies that arise between researchers and society in the context of modern techno-science. Of further concern was the modified relationship between society and the new techno-scientific power, which evolved from society's simple and passive acceptance with total confidence to a preoccupation with controlling its possible negative effects. However, among the different events, it was emphasized that this framework of social controversies is not entirely new and has been significant in approaching biotechnology, as well as the debates over the security of the nuclear and pharmaceutical industries. As a result, it is clear that the relationship between techno-science and society has become one of conflict and controversy because of an increased social interest in the reduction of risks to the environment and human health caused by techno-scientific advances.

Another interesting fact worth mentioning is that the seven conferences involved the participation of more than 500 lecturers from around the world, including Argentina, Belgium, Brazil, Canada, Chile, Colombia, Costa Rica, Cuba, the United States, England, France, Germany, Guatemala, India, Japan, Mexico, New Zealand, Panama, Peru, Portugal, Puerto Rico, the Dominican Republic, Spain, Uruguay, and Venezuela, all of them academic professionals and world renowned experts in the different fields of human knowledge.

The Mexican CNB, under the direction of Dr. Guillermo Soberón-Acevedo, has taken on a number of important international roles. For example, it was the Mexican representative who participated in the elaboration of the Universal Declaration of Bioethics and Human Rights, along with the Intergovernmental Bioethics Committee (IGBC) and UNESCO.

More recently, the CNB participated in the Latin American and European Ethical Regulation Systems of Biomedical Research: Comparative Analysis of their Pertinence and Application for Human Subjects Protection Project (EULABOR), which arose from the interest of diverse European and Latin American countries to study their systems of research ethics thoroughly, to share experiences, and to design new frameworks for solving the ethical dilemmas raised by biomedical research.

From all of the available data, it appears that the greatest bioethical challenge in Mexico is the stimulation of research and scientific education rooted in ethical principles. Therefore, supporting efforts to improve understanding of scientific progress in the context of novel scientific fields, such as human genetics, is imperative. In this respect, the participation of educational institutions is important, mainly in developing countries like Mexico, for the promotion and modernization of education in science and bioethics.

14.2.3 Educational Offerings in Bioethics

Bioethics is a discipline that has acquired vital importance in different professional contexts and from diverse philosophical perspectives. In Mexico, there are three undergraduate, eight Master's, and one doctoral program in bioethics. In addition to these programs, there are also a number of others in different disciplines that include bioethics in their curriculum. The authors of this essay were able to identify 235 programs and/or disciplines related to bioethics existing at different levels of education, including the baccalaureate, the Master's degree, the doctorate, *lato sensu* graduate courses, seminars, advanced training courses, and online courses. Four of the identified programs are distance-learning courses, and the others are distributed among 28 of the 32 states of the Mexican Republic.

Regarding the distribution by discipline, more than 70% of the relevant courses are in medicine, nursing, odontology, social work, and psychology, while 30% occur in other areas. The National Institute of Genomic Medicine (INMEGEN) has implemented two highly specialized courses (the Introduction to Genomic Medicine and Genomic Applications in Internal Medicine), in addition to another class for the graduate program in Medical, Odontologic and Health Sciences of UNAM (Genomic Applications in Pediatric Medicine), with the purpose of promoting the knowledge of the basic principles of genomic sciences and their applications for the improvement of health care. The curriculum of UNAM's graduate program includes work in the areas of ethics, law, and the social sciences, focusing on their applications for genomic medicine for the purpose of demonstrating the limits imposed on genomic medicine.

14.2.4 Bioethics Organizations

Besides the CNB, other groups exist that make outstanding contributions to the development of bioethics in Mexico. Not all of the groups to be mentioned are primarily focused on bioethics, but, by the types of questions they address and/or the tasks they undertake, one can see that they can be categorized as groups contributing to the study of bioethics.

(1) *National Commission on the Human Genome* (*Comisión Nacional sobre el Genoma Humano*) This commission was founded on October 23, 2000, with the primary aim of advising the Secretary of Health regarding policies and initiatives for research and educational efforts pertaining to the human genome. The commission was comprised of six committees, one of which was dedicated to the study of ethical, legal, and social issues, and whose members included researchers Rubén L. Yourkowitzky, Marcia M. Alba Medrano, Marco Antonio A. Castillo, Alessandra C. Cantoni, and Víctor M. Martínez Bullé-Goyri. The Commission was dissolved on August 2, 2004, by a presidential decree for the creation of the National Institute of Genomic Medicine (INEMEGEN).
(2) *Mexican Foundation for Health* (*Fundación Mexicana para la Salud A.C.* – FUNSALUD) This foundation is a civil non-profit association servicing the community and is included in the RENIECYT registry of the National Council of Science and Technology (CONACYT). It is not formally a bioethics research

group, but its mission is related to the tasks of bioethics, such as contributing to scientific and technological knowledge, the analysis of health policies as a means of encouraging research, and the formation of high-level human resources and technological advancements.

FUNSALUD has conducted 14 studies, each examining a "state-of-the art" medical treatment for different health problems. The studies have primarily included projects in the area of nutrition, health education, and t-genomic medicine. Regarding this last topic, under the direction of Dr. Guillermo Soberón, FUNSALUD participated in the creation of INMEGEN along with Dr. Julio Frenk Mora, the director of SSA (2005–2006), and Dr. Gerald Jiménez-Sánchez, the President of the Promoting Partnership of Genomic Medicine (Consorcio Promotor de la Medicina Genómica) in Mexico.

(3) *The Group of the University Project for the Human Genome* (*Grupo del Proyecto Universitario del Genoma Humano – PUGH*) at UNAM This project takes a multidisciplinary approach to research relative to the human genome. It directs and reports efforts made by UNAM relevant to this and other related subjects. PUGH includes multidisciplinary research projects relating to technological support and also promotes the establishment of activities, trainings, and the qualifications of human resources. Lastly, PUGH is responsible for the dissemination of bioethics in the university community.

(4) *The Intersecretary Commission of Biosecurity of Genetically Modified Organisms* (*Comisión Intersecretarial de Bioseguridad de los Organismos Genéticamente Modificados* – CIBIOGEM) This group is responsible for collecting specialized information on the security of biotechnology within the system of the Agreement of Biological Diversity. The members of CIBIOGEM include scientists and experts in modern biotechnology and biosecurity, representatives for civilians and entrepreneurs, and Chambers of Commerce.

(5) *Nucleus of Studies of Health and Law* (*Núcleo de Estudios de Salud y Derecho* (*NESD*) – NESD) of the Institute of Legal Research at UNAM (*Instituto de Investigaciones Jurídicas*) This group was founded in 1991 by Dr. Fernando Cano Valle. Through the application of bioethics, NESD has been able to integrate diverse professional methodologies and discourses for the purpose of determining their relationship to the law. Over the past 15 years NESD has held seven international events in addition to a great number of seminars, academic colloquia, courses, conferences, and meetings, which have drawn the attendance of specialists from around the world. The center also has a prestigious publishing house specializing in materials related to the connection between law and bioethics.

(6) *Interdisciplinary Group of Bioethics of the Autonomous Metropolitan University – Xochimilco Campus* (*Grupo Interdisciplinar de Bioética de la Universidad Autónoma Metropolitana Campus Xochimilco* – UAM-X) Since January 2002, this group of outstanding researchers has sponsored more than 20 conferences pertaining to particular aspects of genomic science, their social impact, and bioethics.

(7) *The Autonomous Group of the Technological Institute of Mexico* (*Grupo del Instituto Tecnológico Autónomo de México* – ITAM) This group is recognized

as a layperson's organization and is the first center of legal studies to implement a course specifically designed to educate lawyers in topics of bioethics. The group has also published on specialized topics in bioethics.

(8) *Bioethical Studies of the Pan-American University* (*Grupo de Estudios Bioéticos de la Universidad Panamericana* – UP) This Christian university has assembled experts in the areas of medicine, philosophy, and law for the purpose of studying bioethics from a personal perspective.

(9) *Study Group of Anáhuac University* (*Grupo de Estudios de la Universidad Anáhuac*) This group is responsible for founding the second college of bioethics in the world, at Anáhuac University (the first being at the Ateneo Regina Apostolorum in Rome), and has been a pioneering institution for the dissemination of bioethics in Mexico. The group has a conservative philosophy and oversees the university's bioethics programs at all levels (baccalaureate, Master's degree and doctorate).

(10) *National Polytechnic Institute* (*Instituto Politécnico Nacional – IPN*) Along with UNAM, IPN is a leading lay non-profit educational institution for the generation, application, diffusion, and transference of scientific and technological knowledge. It was created with the aim of contributing to the economic, social, and political development of Mexico with a commitment to quality, responsibility, ethics, tolerance, and social responsibility. The Institute offers internships at the pre-graduate, undergraduate, and graduate levels and conducts research projects whose findings are made publicly available. Although this institution does not have a specialized bioethics group, it has recently established a Master's of Sciences program in Bioethics.

(11) *Department of Studies and Research of Bioethics* (*CEIB – Centro de Estudios y Investigaciones de Bioética de Guadalajara*) at the Institute for Technological and Advanced Studies of the West (ITESO – Instituto Tecnológico y de Estudios Superiores de Occidente) This department offers a specialization in bioethics during the course of their 3-year Master's program.

(12) *Ethical, Legal and Social Study Center* (ELSI-INMEGEN – Centro de Estudios Éticos, Legales y Sociales del Instituto Nacional de Medicina Genómica) at the National Institute of Genomic Medicine. This center is still in the process of identifying and selecting individuals qualified to perform highly specialized research. ELSI is meant to be a support tool for INMEGEN for approaching the ethical, legal, and social aspects of genomic medicine in both practice and theory. Its aim is to increase public awareness regarding the procedures and products involved in teaching and researching genomic medicine and other related areas.

Among the most important accomplishments of ELSI was the consolidation of a strategic alliance with the Program of Law Studies at the medical school of Vanderbilt University, directed by Dr. Ellen Wright Clayton, an international leader in the field of law and genetics and an advisor to the United States' government. In addition, alliances have been forged with Dr. Fernando Lolas Stepke, an outstanding author and researcher in bioethics and the director of the Unit of Bioethics of PAHO/OMS and the Interdisciplinary Center of Studies in

Bioethics at the University of Chile and, from Canada, Dr. Bartha Maria Knoppers, who coordinates the Public Population Project in Genomics (P3G).

The above list of organizations is by no means comprehensive, and the omission of some groups is inevitable. The choice of organizations presented was based on their solid foundations and publishing records. What should be evident from this diverse list is the necessity of raising awareness of the need for interdisciplinary dialogue among scholars and professionals to facilitate the development of bioethics in Mexico.

14.2.5 Bioethics and Research Centers in Mexico

The exact number of biomedical research centers currently operating with an ethics commission in Mexico is unknown. However, within UNAM and IPN, there are several groups of scientific research that maintain a communication network with professionals of different areas and promote bioethics forums.

Of the Mexican National Institutes of Health, all of which are part of the SSA, the Institutes of Oncology, Respiratory Diseases, Medical Sciences and Nutrition "Salvador Zubiran", Public Health, and Genomic Medicine are the only institutes that currently have ethics committees with a minimum of 6 and a maximum of 12 members.

Outside the scope of the National Institutes of Health and according to information provided by the Federal Commission for the Protection Against Sanitary Risks (Comisión Federal para la Protección Contra Riesgos Sanitarios – COFEPRIS), there are approximately 50 institutions, both public and private, that have registered their respective ethics commissions, which sometimes address issues of bioethics, with COFEPRIS. Despite evidence of a fair number of ethics committees in the country, it is important to recognize that this number is still insufficient as a greater number of hospitals and institutions perform research on human beings.

14.2.6 Bioethics in the Legal System

In Mexico, innumerable laws related to diverse issues have been catalogued by specialists as having relevance for issues of bioethics. In the following paragraphs, the most important of these laws are presented:

In the Mexican Constitution (Constitución Política de los Estados Unidos Mexicanos –CPEUM) there are diverse propositions related to bioethical subjects, such as the right to scientific development, which can be linked to scientific and ethical principles and translated into an obligation to promote and support scientific and technological research (Art. 3°, Sec. V). The Law of Science and Technology (LCyT) establishes rules for section V of article 3 of the CPEUM and aims to establish the support of researchers by the federal government to promote, strengthen, and develop scientific and technological research in Mexico.

One of the principles established by LCyT is that the federal government must guarantee the freedom of scientific and technological research, except in those cases where regulations or limitations are determined by law for the preservation of health, ethical reasons, or any other cause of public interest (Art. 12, Sect. X).

The General Law of Health (Ley General de la Salud – LGS) also indicates that the development of education and medical research relating to scientific and technological advancements is important for the nation (Art. 2°, Sect. VII). The LGS contains a special title dedicated to medical research which is divided into eight articles. This title establishes that medical research includes the development of actions that contribute to the knowledge of biological and psychological processes in human beings; knowledge of the causes of diseases; medical practice and social structure; the prevention and control of health problems considered a high priority for the population; the knowledge and control of damaging effects of the environment on health; the study of the techniques and methods recommended or used for the benefit of health services; and the national production of medical materials (Art. 96).

The Law of the Mexican National Institutes of Health (Ley de los Institutos Nacionales de Salud – LINS) advocates for the stimulation of medical research and education as one of the fundamental objectives of Mexico. In addition, other objectives include the description and explanation of the origins of disease, its prevention, diagnosis and treatment, the rehabilitation of people affected by deficiencies, and the maintenance and protection of human health (Art. 2°, Sect. II). In support of these objectives, Mexico has created an effective and functional network of the National Institutes of Health. This network is a decentralized organization of the federal government with an autonomous legal personality. It is identified as a part of the health sector and its main objective is to perform high-level medical research.

Another issue of bioethics that appears at the constitutional level is the right of all persons to the protection of health (Art. 4°). This establishes the social security system and, for people without other means of access, includes the popular insurance system and the national institutes of health. LGS is a regulation of Art. 4° of the Constitution and establishes the cooperation of the federal government and the States regarding issues of health. It establishes general areas related to health among which emphasis can be given to those areas which are high-priority bioethical subjects, including the organization, control, and monitoring of health services and institutions, the social protection of health (distributive justice), family planning, mental health, the coordination of medical research, the regulation of research involving human beings, and the control of the sanitary disposal of human cadavers, cells, organs, tissues, and other biological matter.

LINS emphasizes the rehabilitation, maintenance, and protection of health for all people. One of the greatest accomplishments of the Institute is the provision of external consultations, medical care, and emergency services to the extent of its capacities while serving a population requiring treatment in its areas of specialization.

At the constitutional level, the right to a suitable environment is also recognized (Art. 4°, CPEUM). This article of the Law of Biosecurity of Genetically Modified Organisms (Ley de Bioseguridad de Organismos Genéticamente Modificados – LBOGM) aims to maximally reduce the possible risks of genetic manipulation as a safeguard for human health, biological diversity, the environment, and the preservation of the health of animals, water, and vegetation.

In the area of criminal law, there are scattered dispositions, including the prohibition of euthanasia in all states of the republic. On the issue of abortion, it is legal in 13 states for eugenic reasons and allowed in 10 states if an artificial reproductive technique was utilized without the consent of the affected women.

Another interesting example is in the Penal Code of the Federal District, which, in its Book II, has dispositions on sanctions against biotechnological crimes, including the prohibition of conduct involving the non-authorized disposition of gametes, failing to gain consent for assisted reproduction, genetic manipulation with eugenic aims, and human reproductive cloning. Both the states of Veracruz and Chiapas have established in their respective penal codes the same sanctions.

The civil law established that biological tests for paternity research are allowed; also, in almost all civil dispositions of the country the legal consequences of methods of assisted fertilization are mentioned.

It should be noted that many of the regulations derived from the mentioned dispositions have not been included. For example, the Regulation of Sanitary Control for the Disposal of Organs, Tissues, and Human Cadavers applies to the Mexican Republic as a whole and regulates scientific advances in the area of human organ and tissue transplants as therapeutic procedures.

The other regulation of extreme importance is the General Law of Health regarding Research for Health. It provides for the fulfillment of the LGS in the administrative sphere with respect to health research in the public, social, and private sectors (Art. 1°). In addition, it establishes ethical guidelines for research protocols involving human subjects: the criterion of respect for human dignity, the protection of human rights, and the well-being of the subject (Art. 13). Other principles include respect for privacy (Art. 16), the protection of research subjects (Art. 18), the responsibility of researchers (Art. 19), and the freedom to choose to participate in research (Art. 19). This last principle, based on international declarations, translates into the well-known concept of informed consent, which is defined in Mexican legislation as an agreement in writing by means of which the research subject, or his legal representative, authorizes participation in research with total knowledge of the nature of the procedures and risks to which one will be subjected, with the capacity of free choice and without coercion (Art. 20).

Finally, the federal system of Mexico allows for each state to determine its own legislation and, as a result, could generate endless legal dispositions that may not be recognized as bioethical but would have an impact on relevant issues anyway.

14.2.7 Bioethics in Jurisprudence

Only a few bioethical questions have been addressed by the courts. Their resolutions have included issues of abortion, genetic privacy, diagnostic and paternity-determination tests, organ transplantation, and euthanasia.

Regarding abortion, 71 resolutions exist, among which the criteria for allowing eugenic abortion should be emphasized. The resolution dictates that no criminal responsibility is assigned when two specialist physicians find sufficient evidence of genetic or congenital alterations to the fetus which may cause physical or mental damages leading to an increased risk in its ability to survive. In all cases it is mandatory for the assessment to be based on medical findings that contain objective, truthful, sufficient, and opportune information and that the free, informed, and responsible consent of the pregnant woman must be obtained (*Semanario Judicial de la Federación y su Gaceta; Tomo: XV; Febrero de 2002, Tesis: P./J. 10/2002; Página: 416*).

Regarding genetics, there are 20 resolutions that refer to various aspects of genetic privacy, including the establishment of some measure of respect for privacy being taken from the moment a genetic test is offered to determine a question of paternity. These measures include referring the individual for tests at a laboratory that has been previously accredited (*Semanario Judicial de la Federación y su Gaceta; Tomo: XXIV; Agosto de 2006. Tesis: VI.1o.C.88 C, Página: 2317*). In addition, the limitations of accessing genetic information may include any criterion considered relevant by a judge to assure that procedures are carried out with discretion, reserve, and sanitary measures that safeguard the health of the parents and the child. It is also established that information obtained from this scientific procedure must be concrete and objective and used only to solve the specific question at issue (*Semanario Judicial de la Federación y su Gaceta; Tomo: XXII; Noviembre de 2005; Tesis: II.2o.C.501 C, Página: 911*).

Given these restrictions, genetic paternity tests cannot be forcibly imposed on the accused person and the donor of the biological sample has the right to refuse donation, but in such a case paternity would be assumed (*Semanario Judicial de la Federación y su Gaceta; Tomo: XXIII; Enero de 2006; Tesis: 1a. CCXVII/2005; Página: 736*). Another court interpretation establishes a child's right to have an identity and a genetic origin (*Semanario Judicial de la Federación y su Gaceta; Tomo: XXIII; Enero de 2006; Tesis: 1a. CCXVIII/2005; Página: 737*).

Another widely debated bioethical question that went before the courts relates to organ transplantation. Previously, the LGS indicated as a criterion for organ transplantation involving living donors the necessary relation of kinship by consanguinity, affinity, or marriage between donor and receiver. The Supreme Court of Justice determined that this disposition violated the right to the protection of health already mentioned. For a sector of legal and bioethical doctrine, this resolution prevents the illegal commerce of organs (*Semanario Judicial de la Federación y su Gaceta; Tomo: XVIII; Agosto de 2003; Tesis: P. IX/2003; Página: 54*).

Finally, there are two resolutions related to euthanasia. In summary, it is recognized that from the perspective of morality this practice has abundant justification and endorsement because of its human content, but nevertheless it is prohibited due to the damage done to the concept of human inviolability in society (*Quinta Época; Instancia: Primera Sala; Apéndice 2000; Tomo II; Tesis: 1232; Página: 578*).

14.2.8 Bioethics in Legislative Projects

In general terms, there are proposals for including in the CPEUM the prohibition of genetic discrimination. Some want to address the objection of conscience in the LGS and to create a special chapter to bolster basic and clinical research on the stem cells of adults and newborns. Another interesting initiative is one that would force transgenic food producers to affix a clear and visible label to their products.

In other initiatives, the creation of new laws is considered. For example, the creation of the Law of the Rights of Terminal Patients (which surely will be approved due to the news about the Italian citizen Piergiorgio Welby, who was disconnected from life support), constituted by 53 articles, would make it possible for terminal patients to establish a living will and would also establish their right to ask for the voluntary termination of life by means of active or passive euthanasia.

It is worth emphasizing that bioethical issues generate controversy within the different political groups represented in Parliament. As a clear example, we have three initiatives of law to regulate Techniques of Assisted Reproduction. The first was proposed by a member of Partido Verde Ecologico Mexicano and contains 53 articles. Among the most interesting aspects of this proposal is the introduction to the legal system of terms like "human genetic material," "subrogated maternity," "embryo transference," and "pre-embryos." It would allow research with supernumerary embryos of in vitro fertilization techniques, the creation of chimeras with the aim of research in human infertility (the hamster test), and the application of prenatal genetic diagnoses.

The law project proposed by PAN – Partido Acción Nacional–would consist of 14 articles, including a special chapter of the LGS. This law would prohibit positive eugenics and choosing the sex of embryos, except when the possibility exists of inheriting a genetic disease bound to sex. It would also allow for research into genetic identity in cases of risk to the life of a child. It would prohibit the manipulation of human genetic material and the commercialization of germ cells or embryos, and would not allow for the creation of supernumerary embryos.

Finally, the legal initiative of the PRD – Partido de la Revolución Democratica – consists of 35 articles to be added to the LGS. It would allow for pre-implantation genetic diagnosis in order to prevent hereditary diseases and would introduce the terms "pre-implantation embryo" and "post-implantation embryo." It would also allow research with supernumerary embryos, although it indicates a limit of the 14th day of development for use in research. This law would also prohibit the rent of uteri and the modification of the genetic patrimony with eugenic aims. On the other hand, it would create banks of semen and embryos and, like the two laws mentioned above, it would allow prenatal genetic diagnoses to detect congenital defects.

14.3 Bioethics and the Platform of Genomic Medicine in Mexico

It is not the aim of this section to analyze all the general aspects of the development of genomic science, which in recent years has generated abundant information both in scientific papers and in the mass media. A brief account of what is considered the immediate bioethical challenges to be faced by the ELSI Center will be presented.

14.3.1 General Aspects of Genomic Medicine

The Human Genome Project (HGP) has come to be one of the greatest scientific challenges faced by humanity, while providing greater knowledge about our species. It is now known that human beings share 99.9% of the sequence of the human genome; this sequence is constituted by 320 billion nucleotides or letters (A, G, T, C) forming the almost 30,000 genes that constitute the genome. The 0.1% of the sequence that varies from individual to individual typically involves a variation where only one letter changes, that is to say, the single nucleotide polymorphisms (SNPs). The number of possible combinations resulting from genetic variation implies that each member of our species has unique genomic characteristics.

At the end of the HGP, important challenges were identified, and five main areas were defined in which efforts and resources would be invested during the next 10 years. These areas would be dedicated to turning genetic information into tangible realities for the general population by means of the study of the structure and function of genes and proteins. The Haplotype Map (HapMap), a project whose purpose is to accelerate discoveries about genes related to common diseases like asthma, cancer, diabetes, cardiovascular diseases, and others, should be mentioned as an area that must interest more governments.

At the moment, INMEGEN is developing the HapMap of the Mexican "mestizos" that will allow for the identification of the positions in which variations within the human genome of Mexicans exist, that is to say, the variations that confer individuality to each member of our population. There will be a special interest for those variations related to the susceptibility to common diseases. For this reason, it is important for us to integrate the development of a scientific platform to create a solid ground on which to transform genomic medicine so that it is understood as a more preventive, predictive, and individualized medicine that contributes to the improvement of the quality of life of individuals and reduces, in the long term, the expenses of health care, allowing for a more just distribution of resources.

14.4 Final Reflections

The implications of bioethics and genomic medicine go beyond scientific valuations, including important ethical, legal, and social challenges. Because of this, INMEGEN has created an Ethical, Legal and Social Study Center on Genomic Medicine to analyze the best methods for facing challenges in these areas. In addition, it has established a clear separation from other important areas of scientific research with which it has no relations. Thus, genomic medicine, as developed by INMEGEN, does not relate to human cloning, the manipulation of stem-cells, or the procedures of assisted reproduction, and has much less to do with the manipulation of human embryos.

Genomic medicine in Mexico, in its first stage, is devoted to the study of born individuals and seeks to identify genetic predispositions to common diseases in order to formulate lifestyle recommendations with an aim of delaying or avoiding the manifestation of these diseases. The relationship between bioethics and genomic medicine will create landmarks in advancing the knowledge of life, the prevention of diseases, and the promotion of health as a part of preventive medicine, a fundamental concept in use since Hippocrates' epoch in the sixth century B.C.

The development of genomic medicine undoubtedly evokes many bioethical questions that will have to be solved after significant interdisciplinary debate, which must be framed under the aegis of fundamental rights, including the right to scientific and technological progress, as well as the right to health. A progressive bioethical framework will be, for scientists, the reference for their mandatory rights and obligations in the exercise of their functions and will also recognize the protection of scientific projects, expectations, and efforts.

Among the subjects that are presently undefined and require deeper elaboration is the principle of presenting all necessary information to research subjects participating in a research project, which must include the purpose and consequences of the experiment. In addition, it will be mandatory to obtain the voluntary acceptance of participation, that is, informed consent, of participants.

Another controversial subject is genetic engineering, which is widely considered to be ethically acceptable for treating hereditary diseases but not for modifying the genetic code for eugenic purposes or for changing the physical or intellectual characteristics of individuals.

A third subject, among the many we have glimpsed, concerns genetic information. The principle of autonomy must be respected, so that each individual is capable of accepting or rejecting the study of her or his genome and cannot, in any way, be forced to participate in any such study. Additionally, all information must be confidential so as not to cause damage (non-maleficence) before the impossibility to produce a benefit (beneficence); also, the diffusion of the information must be fair, that is to say, must employ statistical aspects. In general, this information can influence the labor market, hiring for work, the right to medical assistance, and life or health insurance, as well as the cost of insurance premiums.

A fourth subject is one of genetic determinism. All research must take into account not only predisposing genetic factors but also environmental factors.

A fifth subject is the rights of patients in the area of genomic medicine, which has many implications for biomedical research and the industry. In the first case, it is very useful in diagnosing and treating genetic diseases, whereas in the second it is used to obtain useful substances in the pharmaceutical industry; this is the reason why so many companies have appeared with anti-hemophilic A and B globulin, the growth hormone, human insulin, interferon, tumor necrosis factor, and vaccines against hepatitis B and C and influenza, among others. A revision of legal dispositions for the promotion of intellectual property rights through the protection of creativity, development, and other accomplishments surely will arise in the future. Due to this, it is vital that multidisciplinary organizations create and apply local and ethical regulations.

It is obvious that science must not freely control itself, even though it has technical means for this task. To this, the decision and commitment imposed by the society to which scientific progress is directed must be added. The intervention of society involves not only an ethical and social responsibility, but also mainly a legal one. Science, like the arts, philosophy, and literature, is a human construction and therefore depends on its creative forces, that is to say, human beings.

If its mission is to be developed thoroughly, bioethics must take into account and duly adjust to the requirements of the members of the current society, be they scientists or not. It must acknowledge the answers created by science and regulate them in terms of ethical permissibility. For this, bioethics must take advantage of the contributions of human self-understanding and reserve its place as the discipline that provides the elements with this self-understanding that science has no conditions to grant.

Bioethics is not against the development of techno-science, but is against such developments outside of a framework of legal, social, and ethical values. Mexico has already secured a special place in the world of bioethics, thanks to Dr. Manuel Velasco Suárez and Dr. Guillermo Soberón; because of this, it is certain that in the next years this new discipline will play an important role in the fight for applying ethics to the new discoveries of genomic medicine. Only then will a science that is able to respect the just requirements of a social conscience and a society developed by scientific knowledge exist.

References

Carrasco-Rojas JA (2001) Distinción Dr. Clemente Robles Castillo al Dr. Manuel Velasco Suárez Humanista Universal, Cirugía y Cirujanos, 69, 6 (Octubre–Diciembre), 3–4

Kuthy Porter J (1999) Deontología, ética y bioética en la medicina. In: Kuthy Porter J (ed) Temas Actuales de Bioética. Porrúa, México

Martínez Bullé Goyri VM (1997) Bioética y derecho. In: García Ramírez S (ed) Los valores en el derecho mexicano. Una aproximación. UNAM y FCE, México

Mateos JH (2002) Manuel Velasco-Suárez, médico y maestro. In Memoriam, Gaceta Médica de México, 69.4 (Julio–Agosto), 375–382

Santos y Vargas L (2002) La bioética como una disciplina crítica. In: Acosta Sariego JR (ed) Bioética para la sustentabilidad. Acuario, Havana

Velasco-Suárez M (2002) Derecho y salud, su protección y fomento. Bioética para el respeto al derecho a la vida y la promoción de la salud. In: Muñoz de Alba Medrano M (ed) Temas selectos de salud y derecho. UNAM, México

Legal References

México. Constitución política de los estados unidos mexicanos

México. Ley de bioseguridad de organismos genéticamente modificados

México. Ley de ciencia y tecnología

México. Ley de los institutos nacionales de salud

México. Ley general de salud

México. Reglamento de la ley general de salud en materia de control sanitario de la disposición de reglamento de la ley general de salud en materia de investigación para la salud

México. Código penal del distrito federal

Chapter 15
The History of Bioethics in Panama

Claude Vergès

15.1 Introduction

Panama has subscribed to all of the international protocols relevant to the founding of a Panamanian bioethics and has afforded them significant legal force. Included among these protocols are: *The Universal Declaration on Human Rights*, *The Declaration of the Rights of Children*, *The Declaration of San Jose about Human Rights in Latin America*, and the *Convention for the Elimination of all Forms of Discrimination against Women*, along with the *National Constitution of Panama*, which, as a whole, constitutes the legal basis of any health policy and dictates the appropriate ethical guidelines.

However, until 1992, academic research dedicated to issues of medical practices and protocols, along with matters concerning ecology and a global bioethics, was severely lacking in Panama. The authority of science in matters of development and technological advances was widely accepted, and the problems this approach encountered were treated as mere accidents without importance. From 1972 on, the state adopted a benevolent and paternalistic system of health services that impacted the relations between physicians and patients. The political crisis between 1987 and 1992 affected these relations, and different segments of the population began to criticize the health sector.

In 1992, Panamanian and American investigators failed to obtain informed consent from individuals and their tribes when gathering tissue samples for genetic testing in the United States for the assessment of the incidence of malaria in an indigenous region of Panama. Informed of this occurrence, Panamanian physicians contacted the Indigenous Congress and its advocates to oppose the continuation of this research; however, it could not be challenged in Panama. It was a California Court that condemned the US investigators and terminated the investigation

C. Vergès
Pediatric pulmonologist. President of the Ethics Committee at the Hospital Del Nino, Panama; Teacher Medical Ethics and Bioethics, Medical School, Panama University, Panama
e-mail: cverges2004@yahoo.es

L. Pessini et al. (eds.), *Ibero-American Bioethics: History and Perspectives*,
Philosophy and Medicine 106, DOI 10.1007/978-1-4020-9350-0_15,

(Gabe, 1995). This incident elicited preliminary discussions among physicians, advocates, and representatives of society about the ethics of research in indigenous populations and the necessity of informed consent in Panama. Up until this point, bioethical discussions occurred primarily among human rights advocates due to its lack of development in the country and its status as a group of issues relevant only to developed countries. After 1992, discussions began to occur pertaining to medical problems and poor treatments from physicians, but they still remained primarily as issues of discussion for the media.

In 1998, Dr. Aida Libya Moreno de Rivera, Minister of Health, accepted the invitation of the Pan-American Health Organization (PAHO) to send Doctor Picard Ami (specialist in psychiatry, Chief of the Cathedra of Deontology and History of Medicine of the University of Panama) to a bioethics course in Havana, Cuba. When he returned to Panama, Dr. Picard Ami assembled physicians and philosophers to discuss bioethics, organize bioethics committees in the public hospitals, and promote the formation of the National Association of Bioethics Studies (Picard Ami et al. 2003).

The word bioethics has Greek origins: *bios* meaning human life and *ethicae* meaning human thinking, character, and customs. In 1970, Van Rensselaer Potter defined bioethics as a "science of survival" and "a bridge to the future" meant to respond to the ecological problems of modern technology. During that same period, André Hellegers at the Kennedy Institute of Ethics advocated for the application of humanistic thinking to medical practice as a way of dealing with medical technology. This ecological movement was poorly developed in Panama and, given its origins in the medical field, has been greatly influenced by Hellegers' definition and the four principles articulated by Beauchamp and Childress (2001).

15.2 Bioethics in Public Services

15.2.1 The National Level

In 1998, the Ministry of Health issued a decree, the *Ministerial Resolution Number 0573* (October 21), which "created a bioethics committee in every public hospital under the administration of the Ministry of Health," later published in the *Official Gazette* Nº 23,663 (October 30, 1998). The Resolution used the recommendations of the PAHO to define the composition of the committee, its resources, and its functions (education, consultation, and normalization) (Álvarez et al. 2006); (Lolas Stepke 2006). Only one hospital, the National Institute of Oncology, applied the Resolution in 1999. The committee went through three reorganizations before 2007.

Another Ministerial Resolution on Bioethics was signed on January 19, 1999, with the number 00496, but it was not published in the Official Gazette.[1] This second resolution established that:

[1] To be legally effective, laws, decrees, and resolutions have to be published in the Official Gazette. We researched all the Gazettes from 1998 to 2006 and did not find it. We present a copy of the original from Dr. Picard Ami, ABIOPAN.

- Panama approved the creation of the Regional Program of Bioethics during the 37th meeting of the Directory Council of PAHO/WHO, September 29, 1993, (Lolas Stepke, 2006) and considered it a necessity to create a ministerial group of coordination to promote the development of a national and international discussion about health and bioethics.
- Panama approved the creation of a *National Bioethics Commission* (CONABIO) dependent on the Minister of Health for designating its members: the chairman of Ethics of the Faculty of Medicine of the Panama University, five national directors of the Ministry of Health, the director of Gorgas Institute of Health Studies, and a representative of public hospitals.
- The functions of CONABIO were: the education and promotion of bioethics, the establishment of bioethics committees, and providing consultations for defining public health policies.

The members of CONABIO were designated in February 1999, but the commission never officially acted, due to the election of a new government.

The Ministry of Agriculture and Development published the Executive Decree Nº 137 on May 29, 2001, with the signature of the President, in the Official Gazette Nº 24,317 (June 6, 2001), which "created the *National Commission on Biosecurity and Bioethics*." This Commission's goal was to promote the "Project of Law which established the national regulations for the development of the activities of genetic engineering and the applications of the corresponding measures of biosecurity" and the "Project of Law which established the National Code of Biosecurity and Bioethics." The members of the commission were from the Ministries of Health, Agriculture, and Commerce, research institutions, universities, non-governmental ecological organizations, and medical associations. Both projects were considerably complex and put limits on the development of science, which elicited objections from researchers and scientists in the health and agricultural sectors. As a result, the law was not adopted and the Commission is now working on the issue of biosecurity in agriculture and farming.

In November 2003, the Ministry of Health, through Resolution 390, promoted the "Operational Guidelines for Research Ethics," which adopted the guidelines of the International Commission of Bioethics of the World Health Organization (ICBWHO) on this topic. In December 2003, Law 78 created the National Bioethics Research Committee located in the Gorgas Institute of Health Studies (NBRC - GIHS) to guarantee the rights and the quality of life of human research subjects in Panama. To guarantee compliance with these guidelines, the NBRC-GIHS evaluated the scientific design of the study, the competency of investigators, the process of obtaining informed consent, the selection process of human subjects, the risks and benefits to subjects, and the provision of compensation for any negative effects from the study. The committee included physicians, pharmacists, and nurses nominated by the Minister of Health. In 2004, the regulations of the committee were published, which included a provision for its auto-financing through the payment of a document management fee by sponsors. In addition, Family Health International provided a course for the members of bioethics committees at the request of the Ministry of Health. In 2005, a commission of representatives of WHO, Family

Health International, and the Latin-American Forum of Bioethics Research Committees (FLACEIS in spanish) evaluated the national bioethics committee and presented its conclusions to the committee. In 2007 the committee nominated new members.

During this same year, the Ministry of Health started to integrate a "social audit of health services" as part of the evaluation of the private services of non-governmental organizations paid for by the Ministry. This social audit evaluates 5% of the annual contract and its report is necessary in order to pay for the private service. Starting in 2007, the social audit will be progressively extended to all health services.

In 2004, the Ministry of Health created the Office of Ethics and Security for Health Attention, which depended on the Department of Vigilance and Regulation in Health in the General Direction of Health (www.minsa.gob). This office has three objectives:

1. Promotion and enforcement of guidelines for the application of bioethical principles in research and health services
2. Promotion and enforcement of guidelines for the application of ethical principles in the administration and work of health professionals
3. Enforcement and regulation of guidelines for biosecurity in health installations

The department had only one employee and a small budget. The first objective replicated the functions of the National Committee of Research Bioethics of the Gorgas Institute defined in Law 78; the second objective replicated the functions of the Technical and Health Council defined in the Code of Health (1946); and the third objective replicated the functions of the Departments of Biosecurity and Ambient Health. The signature of a Convention of Cooperation with Japan for the development of the quality of service committees redirected the focus of this department to the implementation of a new program with its own budget.

Since 2004, the National Secretary for Science and Technology (SENACYT in spanish) has been developing a financial program for national research evaluated by external academics, both domestic and international, using the criteria of ICBWHO. The evaluators were nominated by SENACYT based on academic criteria for each investigation (www.senacyt.gob.pa). SENACYT nominated six national commissions to design a strategic research plan for the next 5 years; one of the commissions was the National Bioethics Commission with Dr. Picard Ami and Dr. Sousa Lennox as representatives. In 2007, the commissions were meant to present their proposals; however, the proposals of the bioethics commission were not achieved.

Beginning in 2006, under the promotion of the Ministry of Health and Japan, the public hospitals have nominated a Quality Commission for the evaluation of their services. This commission is composed of doctors, nurses, pharmacists, a lawyer, and representatives from the administration and the clinical laboratories. The Hospital del Niño's quality commission included a representative of the Institutional Bioethics Commission, in accordance with the 68 Laws of Patient Rights and the mission of the Joint Commission on Accreditation of Healthcare

Organizations to provide a patient-centered approach. These laws include: patient rights, the ethics of the organization, evaluation of patients, assistance to patients, education, and continuity of assistance. Patient rights require that the values and preferences of patients and their families (including the decision to stop treatment) are considered, along with the realization that it is the legal responsibility of the hospital to inform patients of their responsibilities in the care process, and to ensure that the relationship between the hospital and its patients is ethical. The incorporation of a member of the Bioethics Commission remained a local initiative, independent of the Joint Commission on Accreditation of Healthcare Organizations (which has no representative in Panama) and the national Quality Commission. Until 2007, it has been unique to the public sector. For the Ministry of Health and for the other public installations, the Quality Commissions only evaluate functional and financial efficiency.

15.2.2 The Local Level

At the Hospital del Niño (the national children's hospital), the director, Dr. Jose Renan Esquivel, prohibited any medication research trials involving children as subjects in 1979 because he thought it was unfair to experiment on Panamanian children for money. In 1989 a new director took over and allowed funded research trials and established a committee to evaluate the protocols. From 1992 to 2003, the members of the committee were exclusively physicians; three of them were professors of medicine and one was a specialist in epidemiology. In 1998, the research commission changed its name to the *Committee of Research Ethics*. In September 2002, the hospital came under new administration, and in March 2003, the committee was restructured, retaining three of its initial members, and adding to it the chief of pharmacies, a social worker, a nurse, a community member, and a representative from the Commission of Bioethics (www.hden.sld.pa). Its new name was the Committee of Bioethical Research in Health of the Hospital del Niño (2004). The patronage approved its regulations in 2005, and it was published in the Official Gazette in 2007. The purpose of the committee is to evaluate all research protocols that take place in the hospital.

In 2000, health care workers of the hospital were preoccupied with bioethics and its relationship to the issue of the vulnerability of children; they proposed the creation of a new committee, the "Bioethics Commission of the Hospital del Niño." One member with post-graduate training in bioethics was nominated Coordinator and the hospital administration recognized its autonomy, but refused to allocate hospital funds for it. The composition and role of the commission were defined on the basis of the recommendations of PAHO/WHO for institutional committees (Tealdi and Mainetti 1990). During the first 3 years of the commission's existence, its members dedicated themselves to self-education, and eventually began promoting bioethics among the physicians and nurses of the hospital by offering conferences and seminars. In 2004, the commission began discussing clinical cases, and members of the commission participated in local courses and online education. The commission has become known for its strong moral reputation, and, in 2007, the administration of the hospital approved its regulation and published it in the Official Gazette.

In 2004, the Institute of Mental Health created a bioethics committee with roles in both the clinical and research settings. The committee is autonomous under the authority of the director of the institute and still functions today with its founding members.

Another important provincial public hospital, Mother and Child Hospital in Chiriqui, created two committees: the Bioethics Research Committee, which adopted the regulations of the National Bioethics Research Committee, and the Committee on Ethics and Evaluation. Both committees were under the authority of the director of the hospital; although a number of the committee's members have changed over the year, it is still active at present. The research committee of the hospital of the National Security Cash Desk adopted the guidelines of CIOMS and Good Clinical Practice, and changed its name to the Bioethics Research Committee in Health. The committee is under the administrative order of the Sub-direction of Education and Investigation.

In 2005, the research committee of the National Adult Santo Thomas Hospital adopted the CIOMS guidelines. Despite numerous administrative changes of the members of this committee, it is still functioning and evaluating local research protocols.

In 2006, the authorities of the General Sub-Direction of Education and Research crafted a proposal for the creation of a national committee of bioethical research, through a convention with the National Committee of Bioethical Research of the Gorgas Institute, and it nominated a consultant to work on a plan for its structuring. The governmental decision for a unique health system in Panama will dictate the future of this committee.

15.3 Bioethics and Bioethics Committees

The history of bioethics in Panama is intimately bound to the history of bioethics committees. The Panamanian Bioethics Research Committees (CBIs), as in other countries, are commissioned by national and international institutions to maintain ethical standards of research:

- Respecting the autonomy of research subjects through the process of providing adequate information about the research trial and gaining each subject's informed consent
- Protecting research subjects from harm during and after the completion of the research trial
- The promotion of the comfort of the subjects
- Equity in the selection and treatment of the subjects

The references of the bioethics research committees are: the *Declaration of Helsinki* (1964 and its modifications to 2002), the *Guidelines of the International Committee of WHO* (1991, 2005), the *Good Clinical Practice* guidelines established by the Federal Food and Drug Administration of the United States, and national research laws (Resolution 390 and Law 78). The committees have authority over the approval, postponement or rejection of research protocols, and their decisions have remained unchallenged. Beginning in 2007, the national bioethics research committee became responsible for the evaluation of each of the local committees.

In addition, the founding of bioethics research committees in Panama in the public health installations was dependent upon the necessity of sponsored clinical research, but the administration of each institution has recognized the importance of these committees and has respected the autonomy of their decisions. However, the committees continue to be funded by the fees paid by the sponsors of proposed clinical research trials. There are no bioethics research committees in the private health sector, and for the National Committee, the evaluation of research protocols in the private sector depends on their sponsor and investigators.

The institutional bioethics committees (BC) exist only in the public hospitals in Panama. Actually, they are recognized in the classical model as the Hospital del Niño (HDN), or in a mixed one (BC and CBI) in the National Institute of Oncology (ION), and the National Institute of Mental Health (INSAM). They are consultative organizations, and their principal objectives are to protect the human rights of patients and to secure the protection of bioethical principles in the doctor–patient relationship (Martinez, 2005). Their functions are:

- To educate the members of the committees, the institution, and the public about bioethics. Each committee is responsible for developing this topic at their institutions through the regular offering of conferences and seminars, and, in addition, committee representatives should participate in public discussions about particular bioethical issues.
- To provide a recommendation for any case of ethical dilemma at the request of physicians, nurses, the patient, and his family. The inclusion of the family in the decision is a particularity of Latin America because of the poor development of adapted local structures (Luna and Salles 1996, p. 14). In a similar way and when necessary, representatives of the different indigenous groups have been invited. The ethical dilemmas depend on the specialty of the hospital:

    a. The institutional bioethics committee of the ION is working with the commission of palliative care, and the national recognition of the commission is more important than that of the bioethics committee.
    b. In the HDN, the institutional bioethics committee discusses pediatric topics. It also works with the commission of palliative care.
    c. In the INSAM, the institutional bioethics committee has to examine the ambulatory management of psychiatric patients and the administration of specific treatments.

- The establishment of guidelines for making recommendations pertaining to common bioethical issues and to institutional code of ethics.

Beginning in 2004, all public and private hospitals must present patients with a consent form for hospitalization and procedures. The consent forms are modeled after those used in American hospitals and for each surgical procedure there is a specialized form. At the Hospital del Niño, the committee published posters about Law 68 on Patient's Rights in all services opened to the public (2004); the consent form for hospitalization and procedures and the form for refusing treatment are the result of 2 years of discussion between the committee, physicians, nurses, directors, and representatives of the families of the patients (2005). In addition, students and visitors of the hospital are bound by confidentiality regarding the personal information of patients (2005). In September 2006, the Institutional Bioethics Committee of the Hospital del Niño presented the Regulation of the Functions of the Committee to the administration of the hospital, which were approved and published in the Official Gazette in June 2007.

The participation of the members of the bioethics committees (institutional or research) is honorific, and they have the authority to assist with bioethics courses. In all of the institutions, the members of the bioethics research committees (CBI) are given time to attend meetings and a budget for their establishment. These benefits do not apply to the members of the individual institutional committees (CBH).

The bioethics committees have members from a number of different disciplines and attempt to maintain some diversity of gender and age. In their establishment, the members of the national committee were nominated by the Minister of Health (2003) and the members of the local committees by the director of the institution. Research experience was a criterion for the members of the CBI. The members of the CBH of the Hospital del Niño were selected on the basis of their experience in Human Rights, and those of the National Institute of Oncology on the basis of their medical ethics. Over the years, new members were approached by active members of the committees and were later approved by the committee after a revision of their standards. During the first year, new members must take a foundational course in bioethics or research ethics. They have to be tolerant, open to dialogue and compromise, and they must not have any administrative or ethical warnings. The addition of a community member and a lawyer to the committee is the most difficult. The National Bioethics Research Committee included a lawyer and a university representative as members from the community. The bioethics committees of the Social Security Cash Desk of the public hospital of the Ministry of Health accepted representatives of the volunteer organization working with patients as members of the community; some included a lawyer (ION, INSAM, and Chiriqui). Since 2005, the Bioethics Research Committee of the Hospital del Niño has included a representative from the Department for the Protection of Children of the Ministry of Social Development; the first was a lawyer and in 2007 a psychologist. Until 2007, the member of the community on the Institutional Bioethics Committee of the Hospital del Niño worked for the volunteer association of the institution, and all other attempts to attract members of the community were unproductive. In 2007 the committee included a representative from the Children's Department of the People's Defender Bureau. This committee, in contrast with the committees of the ION and the INSAM, has had no permanent representative from the Catholic Church, considering the diversity of religions in Panama, and instead invites a representative from the patient's chosen church during a consultation; it also invites an external lawyer for regular consultations.

Interviews with some of the members of institutional bioethics committees have shown that the different models of moral justification defined by Beauchamp and Childress (see Beauchamp and Childress 2001, p. 39, pp. 337–413) are simultaneously employed among the different committees and even among different members of one committee in particular. Depending upon the individual's moral position, experience, and practice one may employ:

- The deductive model from a preexisting theory influenced by a deontological code and normative moral principles. This model is used by the religious fundamentalists for the discussion of problems within clinical ethics and, in particular, issues of the sexual and reproductive health of women.
- The model of induction which proceeds by analogy and makes a decision based on a specific problem. This pragmatic model responds to Anglo-Saxon utilitarianism, and is more adapted to the "transit culture" around the Panama Canal (Laurenza 1999); because it corresponds to the medical methodology for diagnosis, it is used by some committees. Luna considers that "its linear character evidences simplifications and concrete judgments and rules are derived from more general principles" (1996). Discussions under this model have resulted in approaching topics such as genetic enhancements and organ transplants with careful attention paid to the concepts of caution and responsibility.
- The model of coherence is an integrative model based on John Rawls' "reflective equilibrium" and "theory of coherence." It is necessary to practice "balanced or weighted judgments" of moral principles, which offer the least amount of bias possible (Casado 2005). The Institutional Bioethics Committee of the Hospital del Niño considers the Declaration on Human Rights and the Convention of the Rights of the Child to employ this model.

15.4 Bioethics in the Private Sector

In 2003, the National Medical Association (actually the College of Medicine of Panama) published its Moral Code, which dictates the rules for all physicians in the country (Picard Ami et al. 2003). The code emphasized in particular:

- Beneficence, no malevolence, respect for autonomy and patient confidentiality
- Respect for physicians in the health services
- Solidarity between physicians

In 2005, the creation of a hospital modeled after Johns Hopkins Hospital needed accreditation from this hospital. The creation of a bioethics committee is among the requirements for accreditation. As of 2007, the hospital had yet to form a bioethics committee, but if it does, it could have a domino effect on other private hospitals.

Dr. Picard Ami, with the aid of the Ministry of Health, created the National Association of Bioethics Studies in 2000. In 2003, this association won an award in Panama and Dr. Sousa Lennox became the president of the Third Congress of the Latin-American and Caribbean Federation of Bioethics Institutions (FELAIBE in Spanish, 2001) in 2003.

After the Third Congress of FELAIBE, the Association was divided into two different groups: the National Association of Panamanian Bioethics (ANBIOPA) with Dr. Sousa Lennox, and the Association of Bioethics in Panama *(ABIOPAN)* with Dr. Picard Ami. Dr. Sousa Lennox has remained president of FELAIBE since the Fifth Congress of FELAIBE in Panama in 2006. In this congress, ABIOPAN reinitiated its contacts with FELAIBE, and in 2007 Dr. Picard Ami formally participated in the Congress of FELAIBE in Argentina.

In 2005, ANBIOPA presented a project for the organization of the national bioethics committee to the Ministry of Health (Diaz, 2005). The members of the committee were the same as described for the CONABIO in 1999, but its role replicated that of the National Committee of Bioethical Research in Health. Thus, it created a heavy financial burden on the Ministry of Health. The Ministry asked for another proposal by ABIOPAN, and this association used the model of the French National Committee on Ethics with a broad representation from the government, the academy, religious representatives, and organized civil society, directly nominated by the President of Panama (ABIOPA, 2005). However, both projects were shelved by the Ministry and to date Panama has no national committee.

In October 2005, the Pediatric Panamanian Society (SPP) published its recommendations based on revisions in the literature and a discussion held by a group of pediatricians (Mizrachi et al. 2005).

15.5 Education in Bioethics

15.5.1 The Ministry of Health

In 1998, the Minister of Health accepted the proposition of PAHO to send Doctor Picard Ami (specialist in psychiatry, Chief of the Cathedra of Deontology and History of Medicine of the University of Panama) to a bioethics course in Havana, Cuba (1998).

In June 2004, Dr. Roberto Manzini, consultant of the Bioethics Unit of PAHO/WHO, (Drane 2004) and local professors organized a course entitled "Orientation for the Teaching of Bioethics." Nearly 30 academics and members of bioethics committees participated in the course, reviewing the curriculum for undergraduates and the options for graduate studies (Bioética Informa 2004).

15.5.2 The University of Panama

Since its establishment, the Faculty of Medicine of the University of Panama has included *Morality and Medical Ethics* in its medical career program, with 32 hours divided between two semesters. Its content, however, had no relation to anthropology, sociology, or philosophy. After his trip to Cuba, Dr. Picard Ami introduced new bioethical issues of the practice of medicine and new professors. In 2006, Dr. Picard Ami retired from the university and Dr. Claude Vergès took over his chair. She completely changed the curriculum, dividing it into two parts: one semester about deontology and the history of medicine, and the other semester about bioethics. The first semester was divided into three components:

- Analyzing the similarities and differences of the values employed in medical practice, research, and health politics
- Acknowledging the important events in the history of medicine
- Becoming familiar with moral and the ethical code of Panama

The second semester is dedicated to the study of bioethics: its history and fundamental theories, clinical relationships, bioethical dilemmas in medicine, research ethics, and ecology and health (www.telmeds.org).

In 2001, Dr. Picard Ami established the Center of Bioethics Studies in the Faculty of Medicine of the Panama University, with the authorization of the faculty. Dr. Claude Vergès, Dr. Raquel de Mock, and Dr. Jacinta de Almario were included on the staff of the center; other university professors and scientists also joined for specific collaborations.

In November 2005, the center offered the first Diploma of Bioethics, composed of 140 hours (two academic credits). The diploma was solicitated by the Ministry of Health and the topics included basic bioethics and research ethics for the members of the bioethics committees of the three academic hospitals in Panama. Eighteen persons participated in the program and 17 received their diploma. During this year, the center participated in conferences about bioethics committees in public hospitals under the supervision of Dr. Picard Ami.

In April 2006, the Social Security Administration required that the members of its bioethics committees receive a Diploma of Bioethics from the Faculty of Medicine; Dr. Vergès was designated to establish the curriculum and to supervise the students. Nineteen persons participated and received the diploma.

Following these courses, the participants developed research projects in a number of areas such as sexual and reproductive education for teenagers, palliative services, pain treatment in the emergency room, and the organization of bioethics committees in the Social Security services.

The training program for Emergency Medical Technicians included a course in bioethics in 2006, but it was later removed in 2007.

Dr. Picard Ami has been invited to speak at national and international conferences of psychiatry and bioethics (El Salvador, Argentina, Chile, Mexico, Spain, 2007–2009). Dr. Vergès has participated in two conferences of the International Association of Bioethics (2004, 2006) and has been invited to speak about bioethics at both national and international conferences for medical students (2005), pharmacists (2006), and clinical laboratory technicians (2007).

15.5.3 The University of Santa Maria La Antigua

The Catholic university of Santa Maria La Antigua established a Masters of Family Ethics and created the Institute of Ethical Studies in 1995. This institute has established contacts with the Gorgas Institute of Health Studies for the purpose of encouraging education in research ethics. The university offers a postgraduate course with a specialty in Human Rights, and is including ethical values in the Master's and post-graduate courses on Public Policy for Families, Children and Adolescents. These ethical values reflect the mission of the university: "The promotion of an essential culture for the formation of individuals with a great scientific and humanistic knowledge, a testimony of faith, and a true practice of Christian values through which they promote the creation of a more fair and humane society" ([Online] available: www.usma.ac.pa).

15.5.4 Other Universities

Two private universities, which offer health careers training, have also introduced bioethics into their curriculum.

15.5.5 The Teaching Hospitals

The training of medical residents in the national teaching hospitals has long established a research requirement since the first years of the program (around

1965). Students are supervised by a research committee whose members are designated by the director of the institution and generally include the chiefs of clinical services or professors of the research specialty. The requirements of the project are essentially technical, based on research methodology, and do not include the subject's information and/or his decisions. Initially, the research projects were clinical and epidemiological, but on occasion pharmaceutical companies have funded research projects. In 2007, all the teaching hospitals incorporated a course in research methodology for their medical residents and the research project have to be approved by the Bioethics Committees of Investigation (Martínez 2005).

15.5.6 Bioethics Associations

The Bioethics Association of Panama (ABIOPAN) has organized a symposium every 4 months about different topics within bioethics such as "Gender, Urbanism, Medical Education, and Euthanasia." During the monthly meetings of the association, a member presents a theme for discussion or research. In 2007, ABIOPAN created a Web site to promote bioethics in Panama. (ABIOPAN. Bioethics Association of Panama. Available: http://www.abiopan.pa/index.html). Some of its members are also members of the media and cover bioethical issues.

The National Association of Panamanian Bioethics (ANBIOPA) worked with the Nursing Faculty of the Panama University to organize weekly meetings and a 2-week course in bioethics taught by professors of the Complutense University of Madrid in 2006.

In 2005, a group of Catholic doctors founded an association to discuss topics in bio- and medical ethics and to organize opposition to issues such as sexual and reproductive health education for young people, contraception and abortion, stem cell research, and euthanasia as an alternative to palliative care. The association organizes meetings with obstetricians and specialists who are involved with these issues.

Glaxo-Wellcome and Pfizer, motivated by the clinical research they have been funding in Panama since 1985, have organized courses on good clinical practice for researchers and members of bioethics committees.

15.6 The Laws of Bioethics and Relative Themes

The laws, Ministerial Resolutions, and Decrees presented here are from 1995 to 2007 and pertain to the development of bioethics and patient rights (www.asamblea.gob.pa). They have been organized into four governmental periods. It is important

Year	Laws, resolutions, and decree	Publication	Observations
1995	The Deputy Assembly adopted Law 52 which "Regulates the achievement, preservation, storage, transportation, destiny and final disposal of organs or anatomic compounds and the procedures for transplantation in human beings" presented by the Ministry of Health (December 12, 1995)	Official Gazette Nº 22,929 (December 13)	The law is detailed and reflects the recommendations of WHO on this issue
1998	Resolution Number 0573 "Which created the Bioethics Committees in every public hospital under the administration of the Ministry of Health" (October 21, 1998)	Official Gazette Nº 23,663 (October 30)	Bioethics committees must function in both health systems of public health
1999	Ministerial Resolution on Bioethics Number 00496 (January 19, 1999): creation of the National Bioethics Commission (CONABIO) dependent on the Minister of Health	Not published in the Official Gazette	The CONABIO has never worked
	Law 40 "Special interpretations of penal responsibility for adolescents" (August, 26)	Official Gazette Nº 23,874 (August 28)	The rules for adolescents are less rigid
2000	The Deputy Assembly adopted Law 3 "Generalities on Sexually Transmitted Infections, HIV and AIDS" (January 5)	Official Gazette Nº 23,964 (January 7)	The law provides free treatment for pregnant women, children, and adults; the epidemiological report is obligatory
	The Deputy Assembly adopted Law 17 "Which approves the Convention on the minimal age of admission to work" (Convention 138 adopted on October 26, 1999) (June 15)	Official Gazette Nº 24,077 (June 19)	Not directly bound to bioethics; it has an impact on children's health
2001	The Deputy Assembly adopted *Law 17* "About the facultative Protocol of the Convention for the Elimination of all Forms of Discrimination against Women" (March 26)	Official Gazette Nº 24,272 (March 30)	The law emphasizes gender equity in all sectors of society
	The Ministry of Agriculture and Development published the Executive Decree Nº 137 (May 29, 2001) with the signature of the President, "Which created the National Commission on Biosecurity and Bioethics"	Official Gazette Nº 24,317 (June 6)	The Commission on Biosecurity is working independently
	The Deputy Assembly adopted Law 38 "About domestic violence and damages to children and adolescents" (July 10)	Official Gazette Nº 24,350 (July 23)	The law reforms the previous law (1995) and aggregates sexual violence under the Penal Code

2002	The Deputy Assembly adopted Law 29 "Which guarantees health and education of pregnant adolescents" (June 13)	Official Gazette Nº 24,575 (June 17)	The law allows pregnant adolescents confidentiality in health services and their inclusion in official schools
2003	The Deputy Assembly adopted Law 39 "Which modifies and completes the Family Code" (April 30)	Official Gazette Nº 24,794 (June 5)	Men have to pass an AND-test if they deny their paternity
	The Deputy Assembly adopted Law 68 "Which regulates the Rights and the Obligations of the Patients in the matter of Information and Free Informed Decision" (November 11)	Official Gazette Nº 24,935 (November 25)	Based on the Spanish Law on Patient Rights, it recognizes the right to refuse treatment and prohibits euthanasia
	The Ministry of Health published Resolution 390 "Operational Bioethics Guidelines for Research" (November 6)	Official Gazette Nº 24,938 (November 28)	Detailed guidelines based on the recommendations of the ICWHO
	The Deputy Assembly adopted Law 78, "Which organizes the Commemorative Gorgas Institute of Health Studies" and created the National Committee on Bioethics Research in this institution (December 17)	Official Gazette Nº 24,952 (December 19)	The institute is dedicated to research on health, and the national committee depends on the director
2004	The Ministry of Health adopted Executive Decree Nº 428 "Which orders the gratuity of health services and assistance for pregnancy, in all health services of the Ministry of Health" (December, 15)	Official Gazette Nº 25,199 (December 20)	Created to challenge poverty and to improve control of pregnancy; it has had minimal impact
	The Ministry of Health created the Department of Ethics and Security for Health Attention which depends on the Direction of Vigilance and Regulation in Health	Not published	The department was responsible for: bioethics, biosecurity and quality of services; it is dedicated to the last point
2005	The Ministry of Health adopted Executive Decree Nº 546 "Which orders the gratuity of attention for children under 5 years in all the services of the Ministry of Health" (November 21)	Official Gazette Nº 25,432 (November 24)	Created to challenge poverty and to reach the goals of the Millennium

(continued)

Year	Laws, resolutions, and decree	Publication	Observations
2007	The Deputy Assembly adopted Law 4 "Which creates the national program of neonatal screening and dictates other dispositions" proposed by the Ministry of Health (January 8)	Official Gazette Nº 25,708 (January 11)	The law establishes the provision of screening for six congenital diseases
	The Patronage of the Hospital del Niño adopted Resolution Nº 563 "Which approves the Regulation of the Bioethics Committee of the Hospital del Niño and the entire text of the Regulation" (March 28)	Official Gazette Nº 25,828 (July 5)	This resolution recognizes the functions of the bioethics committee in the Hospital
	The Patronage of the Hospital del Niño adopted Resolution Nº: "Which approves the Regulation of the Bioethics Research Committee on Health of the Hospital del Niño and the entire text of the Regulations"	Official Gazette Nº 25,791 (May 15)	This resolution recognizes the role of the bioethics research committee in the hospital
	The Deputy Assembly adopted Law 14 "Which approves the Penal Code" (May 18)	Official Gazette Nº 25,796 (May 22)	The new Penal Code increases the severity of charges for physicians and nurses participating in abortion
	The Deputy Assembly adopted Law 25 "Which approves the Convention on the Rights of Disabled Persons and the Facultative Protocol about the Rights of Disabled Persons, adopted in New York by the General Assembly of the United Nations" (July 10)	Official Gazette Nº 25,832 (July 11)	The law defines the societal obligations for the inclusion of disabled persons
	The Deputy Assembly adopted Law 26 "Which proclaims the Month of Sacred Writings and establishes the Day of their celebration" (July 10)	Official Gazette Nº 25,832 (July 11)	The law abrogates the separation of church and state

to observe that if the law, resolution, or decree was not published in the Official Gazette, it has no legal force.

15.7 Conclusion

With a history of nine years of promotion, achievements, and errors, Panamanian bioethics has produced a number of benefits and faced a number of setbacks.

The greatest benefit has been the recognition of the influence of bioethics on the quality of health services and the response to patient needs. The problems created by technological advances and the persistent issues of disease and poverty require the attention and recommendations of bioethicists and human rights advocates. The purview of bioethics has expanded in connection with ecological themes of concern to society. Panamanians have also begun to participate in Latin-American and international debates and conferences.

However, traditional political, religious, and associative interests obstruct democratic dialogue on bioethical issues (Drane, 2004). Particularly, religious fundamentalists are trying to dominate the bioethical debates and to fight against health rights pertinent to these debates.

Historically, the attraction of Panamanians to bioethical issues has been of considerable value to its development. The recognition of existing local institutional bioethics committees and bioethics research committees encourages the establishment of new ones. The cultural characteristics of the Panamanians, their search for modernity, their capacity to be open to changes, their acceptance of cultural diversity and their preference for dialogue and negotiation provide fertile grounds for bioethical debates and the formation of new bioethical practices.

References

ABIOPAN (2005) Propuesta de Comisión Nacional Consultora en Bioética. Panamá, September, copia en Archivos de ABIOPAN

Álvarez DJ, Lolas F, Outomuro D (2006) Historia de la ética en investigación con seres humanos. In: Lolas F, Quezada A. Rodríguez E (eds) Investigación en salud. Dimensión Ética. CIEB, Universidad de Chile, Chile, pp 39–46

Beauchamp TL, Childress JF (2001) Principles of biomedical ethics, 5th edn. Oxford University Press, New York

Bioética Informa (2004) Taller para Docentes en Panamá. Unidad Regional de Bioética. [Online] Available: www.paho.org/Spanish/BIO/boletin34.pdf. Accessed on 22 June 2006

Casado M (2005) La adquisición de un sistema propio de principios morales. Bases éticas para la bioética, bioética y derecho, Universidad de Barcelona. [Online] Available: www.bioeticayderecho.ub.es. Accessed on 27 Feb 2009

CEALP Centro Internacional de Investigaciones para el Desarrollo (1993) [Online] Available: http://www.idrc.ca/es/ev-1-201-1-DO_TOPIC.html

Drane J (2004) PAHO y bioética. Una relación accidental o un compromiso profundo? In: Lolas Stepke F (ed) Diálogo y cooperación en salud. Diez años de bioética en la OPS. Serie publicaciones, Unidad de bioética, IKM OPS/OMS, pp 15–22

Gabe M (1995) Pueblos Indigenas, Nustra Vision del Desarrollo. Ed. Icaria, Esp. ISBN 84–7426248-8, p 51–57

Laurenza RJ (1999) Panamá: República niña con retos adultos. El alma histórica del panameño, cited in Wynter Melo, C.O. (2004), Tablero N° 67, Jan.–Apr., pp 60–63

Lolas Stepke F (2006) Bioethics at the Pan American Health Organization. Origins, Development, and Challenges. Acta Bioética 12.1:113–119

Luna F, Salles A (1996) Develando la bioética. Sus diferentes problemas y el papel de la filosofía. Perspectivas Bioéticas en las Américas 1.1:10–22

FELAIBE (2001) Estatutos de la Federación Latinoamericana y del Caribe de Instituciones de Bioética, Caracas, 8 de febrero

Martínez MJ (2005) La relación médico-paciente. La bioética en las relaciones sanitarias Master en Bioética y derecho, Universidad de Barcelona. [Online] Available: www.bioeticayderecho.ub.es consultado 22-02-2009

Mizrachi A, Casal L, Ruiz F, de López CV, Villafañe G (2005) Manual de ética. Sociedad Panameña de Pediatría, Panamá

Picard Ami L, de Almario J, Macharaviaga L (2003) Código de ética. Asociación Médica Nacional, Panamá

Tealdi JC, Mainetti JA (1990) Los Comités Hospitalarios de Ética. Bioética: Temas y Perspectivas. Publicación Científica, 527, OPS, 54–61[2] Regulation of the Latin-American and Caribbean Federation of Bioethics Institutions, FELAIBE, Caracas, February 8, 2001

Chapter 16
The History and Development of Bioethics in Paraguay[1]

Marta Ascurra

16.1 Introduction

Bioethics first appeared in Paraguay during the late 1980s and the early 1990s within the context of medicine and research at the universities. Initially, Van Rensselaer Potter's principles were the main focus of study without much consideration for the cultural values of Paraguay or Latin America. Its growth has been slow but continuous, with the formation of hospital bioethics committees, training groups, annual courses, and the establishment of the National Commission for the Development of Bioethics in 2004. From the beginning, the pioneering groups and individuals in bioethics have all been related in some way to the field of medicine, because this is where their common concerns have been derived. Among these prominent figures were Dr. Julia Rivarola, pediatrics; Dr. Eduardo Aquino, specializing in hospital management; Dr. Rosalino Pinto, gynecologist; Dr. Enrique de Mestral, geriatrist; nurses Olga Lopez de Benítez, Julia Carmen Morel de Festner, and Deolinda Maciel; Father Alberto Leon, and Dr. Marta Ascurra, among others.

Before presenting an account of the development of Paraguayan bioethics and its many accomplishments, the relevant geographic and demographic information, as well as other indicators related to bioethics and human rights in the country, will be provided. This background information is necessary for one to get an accurate picture of a country where bioethical problems are due to a lack of access to health care, conditions of poverty, the destruction of the environment, and the lack of a sewage system and potable water – in summary, the lack of human rights. The subjects that

M. Ascurra (✉)
Biochemist specialized in Genetics, Researcher and professor of the Institute of Research in Health Sciences of Asunción (Paraguay). Advisor Member of the National Commission for the Development of Bioethics – Paraguay. Consultant of the Latin-American and Caribbean Bioethics Network – UNESCO
e-mail: mascurra@sce.cnc.una.py

[1] I would like to acknowledge Dr. Julia Rivarola, Dr. María Eugenia Montiel, Dr. Rosalino Pinto, Dr. Enrique de Mestral, Fr. Alberto Leon, and Guillermo Duarte, law expert, for their contributions to and corrections of this material.

L. Pessini et al. (eds.), *Ibero-American Bioethics: History and Perspectives*, Philosophy and Medicine 106, DOI 10.1007/978-1-4020-9350-0_16,

demand attention have been addressed from the beginning by Paraguayan bioethicists; however, the topics that receive the most attention are those incumbent on developed countries, not those peculiar to the developing ones.

16.2 Geographic Situation, Health, Demographics and Other Indicators

Paraguay is located in the central part of South America and is contiguous with Brazil in the northeast, Argentina in the south and Bolivia in the northwest. The total population, according to the 2002 Census, is 5,163,198 inhabitants, 89,169 of whom belong to indigenous communities. These communities, totaling 492, are found in remote and difficult-to-reach places and can be grouped into five linguistic families and 17 ethnic groups.

Paraguay is a country where geography itself demonstrates inequities. In the national territory, which includes 406,752 km^2 divided by the Paraguay River, there are two defined areas: the Chaco or Western Region, with 246,925 km^2, inhabited by 2.5% of the population, and the Eastern Region, with 159,827 km^2 and 97.5% of the population (58.5% live in the major urban area). The population forms a pyramid, the apex of which includes those individuals aged more than 60 years (7%), and the base of which includes the adolescent population (those less than 15 years old – 37%). The adolescent population is the most vulnerable, because they are most affected by problems like poverty, undernourishment, anemia, and a lack of access to health care and potable water. The child mortality rate is 19.7 for every 1,000 babies born alive to the general population and 93.9 for every 1,000 babies born to the indigenous population. About 4,000 children die every year before reaching the age of 5 years. Five percent (35,000) of the children under the age of five suffer from undernourishment and 20% (141,000) are on the cusp (DGEEC 2002). The maternal mortality rate, at present, is as high as 110.9 maternal deaths for each 100,000 newborns and 420.5 maternal deaths for every 100,000 newborns in rural areas. Only 60% of childbirths occur at health institutions. Thirty percent (45,000) of pregnant women suffer from undernourishment, 45% of the population (2,577,000 people) do not have access to potable water, about 75% of the population do not have access to a sewage system, and 27% of the population (1,527,000 people) do not have medical insurance, causing a reliance on traditional medicine for initial treatments, especially in rural areas (Paraguay 2003).

Paraguay is unique in having two official languages: the predominant language of Spanish in addition to its native language of Guarani. Spanish is the predominant language in rural areas and is spoken by 82.7% of the settlers, whereas in urban areas it is spoken by only 54.7%. While Guarani has been preserved as a national language, inhabitants of the country are far from proud of its use. Its study is considered to be a waste of time by most and therefore causes illiteracy, unemployment, larger families, and many forms of exclusion for the Guarani-speaking population (Paraguay 2003).

The demographics of religion include the Roman Catholics comprising 90% of the population, Christian churches accounting for 6%, and the other 4% is distributed among other religions and non-believers.

The economy of Paraguay relies primarily on agriculture and forest development for its stability; however, these practices cause many problems for the country. Even though there are express protection laws, many of their practices are carried out carelessly, leading to the increased contamination of waters as well as an increased prevalence of malformations at birth, attributable to the use of some herbicides.

16.3 Laws and Acts of the Executive Ministerial Resolutions

At the current time, there are no national laws explicitly addressing the realization of bioethical principles in the medical context; however, the constitution does provide the necessary resources to be able to create such legislation without constitutional reform. For example, Article 4 establishes the general protection of human life from the point of conception, as well as advocating for the protection of one's physical and psychic integrity by the State, including a mandate that there must be a law which regulates "... the freedom of the people regarding their own body within the scope of scientific or medical aims."

In addition, Chapter VI of the constitution proposes programmatic rules to protect the health rights granted in the constitution. Other programmatic norms relevant to bioethics can be found in the constitution, which addresses related issues such as freedom, equality among all citizens of the Republic, and the rights of all to a healthy atmosphere (Paraguay 1992).

In considering positive law, one must also mention those international treaties concerning issues of bioethics to which Paraguay is a party. For example, the Convention on the Rights of Children was signed by Paraguay in October 1989.

In this way, norms exist that directly realize those put forth in the constitution. Included among them are:

(a) Sanitary Code, established in 1980; and Decree 1635/99 that regulates Art. 175 of the Sanitary Code
(b) Act 369/72, creating the National Service of Environmental Defense (SENASA)
(c) Act 1340/88, which modifies and updates Act 357/72, preventing the illicit traffic of narcotics and other dangerous drugs in addition to other related crimes. It also establishes measures for the prevention of drug addiction and the recovery of addicts
(d) Law 70/91 creates the national organ bank
(e) Law 102/91 establishes rules for controlling AIDS dissemination
(f) Law 106/92 regulates organ extraction and transplantation
(g) Law 1,032/96 creates the National System of Health
(h) Law 1,119/97 regulates health products and others

The Penal Code has also established provisions against the frontal attack of those legal rights whose protection has been guaranteed by the constitution, the punishment of which would lead to fines and up to 25 years in prison. Some of the rules included in the Penal Code pertain to:

(a) Attacks on human life (Art. 105, 106, 107, 108, and 109).
(b) The prohibition of attacks on one's health or physical integrity (Art. 110, 111, 112, and 113), with only a few special permissions granted to physicians, for example, submitting a patient for surgery (Art. 114).
(c) Medical treatment without valid consent is subject to penal sanction (Art.123).
(d) Attacks on the natural bases of human life (Art. 197, 198, 199, 200, 201, and 202).
(e) Violations of medical privacy are also referred to in the Penal Code.

Several other groups of laws exist that are relevant to health, but do not explicitly address it. These laws include the Childhood and Adolescence Code, the Labor Code, and others. At this time, the Constitution does not provide for the regulation of scientific or technological research pertaining to health. The lack of such legislation allows researchers to solicit participation in research projects without any guidelines to prevent the exploitation of vulnerable groups, which is of special concern in biomedical research.

In the following sections, the development of bioethical activities at the national level will be considered. An attempt will be made to distinguish the different types of activities and organizations, but the fact remains that many of the contributions to bioethics in Paraguay have resulted from the combined efforts of many different institutions.

16.4 Civil Associations

The first civil institution was Pro-Bioética, a non-profit organization created in June 1995 (Pro-Bioética 1995). It was conceived as a permanent institution of study, analysis, and training that sought to establish norms for the behavior of health care workers, other professionals, and the population at large regarding bioethical issues. Some of the issues it addressed included respect for life, the right to the protection of health, integrity, autonomy, and human dignity, as well as the preservation of ecosystems. Some of its functions include elaborating educational programs; creating exercises to practice and encourage the discussion of problematic cases in areas such as medicine, the protection of nature, environmental preservation, ecology and respect for human dignity; organizing and supporting educational events pertaining to bioethics (congresses, courses, workshPAHO, and seminars); promoting the development of bioethics in health institutions, ministries, and centers; and supporting the creation of bioethics committees in hospitals. It also sought participation in organizations at both the national and international levels who were involved in the development, formation, and qualification of bioethics. The institution's involvement in higher education has revolved around the promotion of bioethics at centers and schools throughout the country by establishing bioethics as a distinct discipline in both undergraduate and graduate classes. The development of relationships with both public and private organizations (ministries, institutions, commissions, unions, groups, etc.) in addition to voicing opinions on general and controversial subjects of bioethics (e.g., AIDS, drug addiction, family planning, reproductive risks, ethics of sexual education, just and fair health legislation, transplantation and donation of organs) can also be included among its important functions.

One of the first actions of *Pro Bioética* was to establish the Information Center and Data Bank in Bioethics. The foundational act was signed on June 20, 1995, by Fr. Alberto Leon, Dr. Carlos M. Ramirez Boettner, Dr. Ramon Corvalan, Dr. Maria Eugenia Montiel de Doldan, Dr. Marta Ascurra de Duarte, Dr. Carlos Adolph Riart, Dr. Eduardo Aquino of the Port, Dr. Zenón González Romero, Dr. Miguel Sanchez González, Dr. Julio Montt Momberg, Dr. Fresh Manuel, Dr. Narcissus González Romero, Dr. Jose V. Altamirano, and Dr. Carlos Mersan Canale. The act was developed and endorsed during a bioethics conference at which Dr. Miguel Sanchez González was the keynote speaker. For more than four years, members remained dedicated to the study of bioethical subjects at monthly reading meetings. During the course of these meetings, two well-attended conferences were also organized. Unfortunately, after some time, members of the group who belonged to other organizations began failing to show up to the meetings and the group eventually disbanded.

In 2004, Our Lady of the Assumption Catholic University (Universidad Católica Nuestra Señora de la Asunción), on the initiative of Dr. Rosalino Pinto, Professor of Personal Ethics, established the Center for Bioethical Studies (Centro de Estudios Bioéticos), which institutionally depends on the Department of Theology and Pastoral Action of the university. The Center had among its main activities the promotion and study of bioethics with a personal approach. The members of the Center include professors from different disciplines at the Catholic University and people with experience in the field of bioethics, including priests Alberto Leon and Silvio Suárez; Dr. Miguel Fresco, psychologist; Dr. Antonia Benítez Rivas, pediatric physician and Professor of the Pedagogical Unit of Villarrica; Professor Ilde Silvero, journalist and Dean of the Philosophy and Human Sciences School at the Catholic University; Attorney Carolina Rodriguez; and Magdalena Genest, nurse and Director of the Nursing Graduate School (Escuela de Postgrado de Enfermería) of the Catholic University. The center was responsible for the publication of *Bioética* (Bioethics), which attracted submissions from national and international authors (Universidad Católica Nuestra Señora de la Asunción, Centro de Estudios Bioéticos 2005). The Center has also planned conferences specifically in the area of macro-bioethics.

In addition to those institutions mentioned, other groups and civil associations whose aims were not necessarily related to the health sector, but addressed topics of bioethics, were established, indicating the importance of the discipline within Paraguay.

16.5 Bioethics and Ethics Committees

Even though the creation of bioethics and ethics committees has not been stimulated or recognized by the government, there are three different types of committees in Paraguay which have been established primarily by health professionals who are self-taught bioethicists. The hospital committees of bioethics were created for the analysis of patient dilemmas in the clinical setting as well as the establishment of protocols to address issues of frequent conflict occurring in increasing numbers in public and private health organizations. There are also research ethics committees that evaluate research protocols and a National Commission for the Development of Bioethics in Paraguay (Comisión Nacional para el Desarrollo de la Bioética en el Paraguay). All of these committees are also responsible for the teaching and diffusion of bioethics, inside and outside of their institutions, for which seminars, symposia, and other bioethics events are organized, both with national and foreign speakers. In some cases, they also coordinate activities related to professional ethics.

The first hospital ethics committee to be established was that of the Mother-Infant Hospital "Reina Sofía" of the Paraguayan Red Cross created on August 2, 1993. Its primary responsibilities were the consideration of ethics cases that arose at the hospital, in addition to developing yearly discussions and courses for their health professionals.

On March 8, 1994, the Chair and Service of Pediatric Medicine at the Hospital of Clinics at the Medical Sciences School (UNA) created a bioethics committee. The founder was Jose Luis Delgadillo, Ph.D., and his committee was dedicated to the analysis of ethical dilemmas in the area of pediatric medicine, requiring the participation of members in discussions related to clinical cases. In 1998, with the arrival of Dr. Elena Lugo and many meetings on self-education, the Bioethics Committee of the Hospital of Clinics was officially founded and directed by Enrique de Mestral, Ph.D.

In October 1999, the Committee of Ethics of the Paraguayan Circle of Doctors was created. Among its founders were Fr. Alberto Leon, Dr. Julia Rivarola, Dr. Maria Eugenia Montiel de Doldan, and Dr. Ignacio Iramaín Ch. The main functions of the committee were the discussion of specific ethical situations at the request of Welfare Services and the analysis of laws and regulations related to the subject. The committee met regularly and recently sponsored two courses in bioethics: an analysis of welfare services and a study of proposals relating to the national law on the ablation and transplantation of organs, as well as the rules regarding the criteria for the admission of patients (both children and adults) to intensive care units.

The Cancer Institute, after attending a bioethics course sponsored by members of the Bioethics Committee of the Hospital of Clinics, officially founded its own bioethics committee on June 23, 2003, although it was not recognized by the authorities of the institution. Dr. Elena Osnaghi, biochemist; Dr. Riechert Robert, expert in palliative medicine; Deolinda Benitez de Maciel, nurse; Dr. Walter Cáceres, physician; Laudelina Borja, nurse; Dr. Gustavo Gugiari, oncologist; Raquel Molinas, psychologist; were the initial members of the committee. Included in its normal functions was advocating for the right to a dignified death that was free of pain and therefore also supporting the use of medications, such as morphine, in the process.

In 2004, the Bioethics Committee of the Hospital Barrio Obrero was established. Dr. Ricardo Riveros, surgeon, became the committee's director and its members included Dr. Jerónimo Baudo, pediatrics; Dr. Miguel Rolón Angel, pediatrics; Paulina Culzoni, nurse; and Maria Santander, psychologist. This hospital was located near one of the main poverty belts in the country and therefore serviced the least advantaged members of society who had limited access to resources.

The Social Welfare Institute (Instituto de Previsión Social) is the primary organization responsible for the social security of private organization workers in Paraguay. After several meetings and years of work, the Institute developed a bioethics group that gained recognition in May 2006. In this group, the names of Dr. Sara Florentín, Dr. Carmen Frutos de Almada, Dr. Carlos Ortiz, Dr. Estela Elías, Olga Benítez, Dr. Imelda Martinez de Núñez, Dr. Francisco Perrota, and Dr. Vicencia Tejera stand out. One of its recent projects has been the humanization of its services.

The National Hospital of Itaugua is a highly complex hospital, dependent on the Ministry of Health. Dr. Magdalena Tatter, who received a Master's in Bioethics from the PAHO in Santiago, Chile, advocated for the institutional acceptance of a bioethics committee. The population served by the hospital is culturally diverse and consists primarily of those existing in situations of poverty, making imperative the hospital's participation in the prevention and resolution of social conflicts that may affect the rights of patients.

In March 1993, the first research ethics committee was established by the Institute of Research in Health Sciences (Instituto de Investigaciones en Ciencias de la Salud-IICS/UNA), an organization linked to the National University of Asunción, by a resolution of the Director of UNA, at the time Dr. Martín Chiola. The committee became known as the "Bioethics Committee" and among their functions were the analyses and approval of research protocols, the revision of articles for presentation at congresses or submission for publication, as well as the coordination of seminars and courses with guest speakers on topics of bioethics (one of the invited lecturers was Fr. Leo Pessini) for professionals at the institute. Members of the committee also served as faculty for the graduate course on the methodology of research at the institution.

A second research ethics committee, constituted by Dr. Esteban Ferro, Dr. Antonio Cubillas, and Dr. Agueda Hair in 1998, as part of the Medical Sciences School (Facultad de Ciencias Medicas) of UNA, was restructured by a resolution of the school's Honorable Board of Directors in 2006: Dr. Imelda Núñez, Dr. Fátima Ayala, Dr. Enrique de Mestral and Dr. Cristina Jiménez.

The National Institute of Health, part of the Ministry of Public Health, is dedicated to the education of professionals and relies on its bioethics committee for the evaluation of research protocols in addition to many other functions. The committee is composed of Dr. Jose Marín Massolo, surgeon; Gustavo Cristaldo, Luis Simancas, and Luis Pavetti, all sociologists; and, lastly, a professor at the Catholic University's Chair of Ethics for the Evaluation of Research.

It is worth remembering that from the creation of the Regional Program of Bioethics of the Pan-American Health Organization in 1995, Dr. Julio Montt Momberg, the first director of this program, was able to stimulate a remarkable number of bioethics activities. He was followed by Dr. Hernán Malaga, a sanitarian, who, during his term as representative of PAHO-OMS in Paraguay, together with the National Institute of Asunción, an agency of the Ministry of Public Health and Social Welfare (Ministerio de Salud Publica y Bienestar Social – MSPyBS), organized a workshop on "The Analysis of the Situation and Elaboration of a Project for the National Development of Bioethics." The event was held in June 2001 and involved different Paraguayan institutions. Later, representatives of the attending institutions decided to continue meeting for the next three years, until being recognized (considering the relevance of the subject as a fundamental aim in developing bioethics in Paraguay) as members of the National Commission for the Development of Bioethics, by the Resolution of MSPyBS Nº 1.140 in October 2004 after a request from Dr. Malaga to the then Minister of Health Dr. Julio Cesar Velasquez. The commission's members include Dr. Marta Ascurra, Secretary of the Commission, representative of the Institute of Research in Health Sciences, Committee of Ethics in Research (IICS); Dr. Estela Elías, pediatrics, of the Bioethics Committee of the Instituto de Previsión Social; Olga de Lopez, nurse, of the Bioethics Committee of the Instituto de Previsión Social; Fr. Edgar Bobadilla, Master in Bioethics and theologian; Dr. Maria Magdalena Tatter, pediatrics, Master in Bioethics, National Hospital of Itaugua; Ascención Deolinda Benítez de Maciel, nurse and obstetrician, of the Bioethics Committee of the National Cancer Institute; Dr. Elena Osnaghi Doria, biochemist, of the Bioethics Committee of the National Cancer Institute; Dr. Julia Maria del Pillar Rivarola, pediatrics, of the Bioethics Committee of the Hospital of Clinics and the Bioethics Committee of Paraguayan Circle of Doctors; Julia Carmen Morel de Festner, nurse and obstetrician, of the Nursing School of the Institute "Dr Andrés Barber," a member of the Scientific Society of Students of Medicine, the National University and a representative of the Ministry of Public Health and Social Welfare. The commission's primary task is the elaboration of national guidelines pertaining to research, which are currently being constructed. This task is essential, considering the increasing number of people who work in research and the volume of research projects soliciting human subjects and, in many cases, securing the participation of vulnerable groups.

16.6 Specialists in Bioethics

To date, the country relies on the Regional Program of Bioethics for Latin America and the Caribbean for the presence of a Master's program in bioethics. The program is directed by Dr. Magdalena Tatter and Fr. Edgar Bobadilla who holds a Master's in theology with an emphasis in bioethics, as well as Dr. Julia Rivarola, who studied bioethics at the University of Rome, Dr. Enrique de Mestral, who studied bioethics at the Pontifical Catholic University of Chile, and Dr. Imelda de Núñez, who studied bioethics at the Free University of the Americas (Universidad Libre de las Américas). The members of the different bioethics committees can also be considered, in their majority, to be self-educated persons in bioethics who formed their education through different graduate courses, national and international workshPAHO, and conferences and seminars which they attend.

16.7 Education

Currently, in undergraduate education, the presence of bioethics is sporadic, and the loss of values constitutes a serious problem for this population. At the graduate level, some courses touch on bioethics, especially those related to the health sciences. As members of the academic world, individuals have an ethical responsibility to develop the education of various professionals, and of the general public, in such a way that it will help assure and promote respect for human rights. In 1989, at the National University, medical ethics became a part of the medical curriculum and was considered one of the subjects within the chairs of Legal Medicine and Medical Deontology. In the same year, at the nursing school of the Catholic University, the chairs of Professional Ethics, General Ethics, Medical Ethics and Bioethics, were created in graduate courses. In 1992 the Chair of Bioethics as curricular subject matter was included in the nursing and obstetrics school of the "Instituto Andrés Barbero," an organization linked to the National University.

In 1996, graduate courses in bioethics were developed for the resident physicians of the chair of Pediatric Medicine at the School of Medical Sciences of UNA, as well as for the residents in Pediatric Medicine at the Instituto de Previsión Social, coming from the Catholic University of Villarrica, Department of the Guaira. Courses at the private universities of Paraguay have also flourished. Although it is difficult to determine the precise level of education in bioethics in Paraguay, it is known that at the curricular level, the subject of bioethics is developed as a discipline in one of the semesters. This information was deduced from the author's discussions with individuals in charge of the national universities. With the curricular reform of 2005 in the School of Medical Sciences of the National University of Asunción, and impelled by the Bioethics Committee of the Hospital of Clinics, the disciplines of medical ethics and bioethics were introduced into the curriculum of the second course with 40 hours of study.

16.8 Literature

In this section, details of some of the national publications on Bioethics will be given. Most of the publications are from the second half of 1995 and are selections from edited volumes on health. To begin, it should be mentioned that Fr. Montero Tirado has been publishing articles relevant to values in the written press, in anecdotal form, for several years. It is also worth noting that in the previous 2 years, journals and books were established that were solely dedicated to bioethics.

Dr. Gilda de Fatima Burgstaller de Justiniano published in 1995 a book titled *The Legal Responsibility of Doctors: Legislation, Doctrine and Jurisprudence* (*Responsabilidad penal de los médicos. Legislación, doctrina y jurisprudencia*), in which several chapters discussed bioethical subjects such as abortion, euthanasia, eugenics, assisted suicide, and consent. While many of these subjects are not currently encoded in Paraguayan law, Dr. Burgstaller considered them not only from a legal standpoint, but also from a bioethical standpoint (Burgstaller 1995).

In June 2005, the Center of Bioethical Studies at Our Lady of the Assumption Catholic University established the first specialized publication, titled *Bioethics*, which was distributed biannually and included submissions from both national and international authors. At the Sixth Brazilian Congress of Bioethics, the First Congress of the MERCOSUR, and the Forum of the Bioethics Network (RedBioética) of UNESCO, the first scientific publication was launched: *The Epistemologic Statute of Bioethics*, edited by Volnei Garrafa from Brazil, Miguel Kottow from Chile and Alya Saada, responsible for the Program of Bioethics of the Office of UNESCO in Mexico. In this publication, Marta Ascurra wrote the commentary for León Olivé's contribution (Ascurra 2005).

In July 2005, from the Ministry of Public Health and Social Welfare, a book titled *Public Health: A Bioethical Approach* (*Salud pública. Enfoque bioético*) by Dr. Hernán Malaga and his collaborators was published. This book was heavily based on the contributions of Dr. Juan Carlos Zanotti, a Paraguayan industrial chemist. Chapters written by Marta Ascurra and Dr. Carlos Rosales, the Argentinean consultant of PAHO in Paraguay, include: Chapter 15, "Personal and Communitarian Bioethics"; Chapter 16, "Analysis and the Bioethical Profile of Research in Public Health"; and Chapter 17, "Formation and Qualification of Human Resources in Public Health" (Ascurra and Rosales 2005a, b). In 2006, a third volume from the Bioethics Network for Latin America and the Caribbean, UNESCO, titled *An Overview of the Legislation Pertaining to the Human Genome in Latin America and the Caribbean* (*Panorama sobre la legislación en materia de genoma humano en América Latina y el Caribe*), under the coordination of Alya Saada and Diego Valadés, was published. This volume contained the contribution: "An Overview of the Legislation Pertaining to the Human Genome in Paraguay" by Jorge Seall-Sasiain, a Paraguayan university professor of national and comparative constitutional rights at the law schools of the National University of Asunción and the Catholic University of Asunción (Seall-Sasiain 2006).

Later, in March 2006, a *Manual of Bioethics* was published, written by Enrique de Mestral, based on the undergraduate program of bioethics (de Mestral 2006). Chapters in the book addressed various issues related to the beginning and end of life, family planning, palliative care, the human genome, ecology, and research ethics.

16.9 Courses, Symposia, and Congresses

The first bioethics gathering occurred in Paraguay in 1990; since then, similar events have occurred with increasing consistency. Most of the activities are organized by ethics and bioethics committees throughout the country and are meant to fulfill the common goal of the continuous advancement of bioethics education. Initially, these functions were designed specifically for health professionals, but over the last few years they have been more and more inclusive of the general public. A participant of these events over the years, whether as an attendee or an organizer, would have noticed a steady increase in the number of participants, as well as the growing interest of both professionals and citizens.

In June 1990, the Department of the Guaira at the Medical School of Villarrica offered the first course on bioethics in Paraguay. The class was taught by Dr. Julia Rivarola, Dr. Daniel Domini, and Fr. Alberto Bertaccini and was designed for the education of medical students, obstetricians, and nurses. The first bioethics conference, intended to draw the attendance of many health professionals, was held on November 21–25, 1994, and was organized by the Research Ethics Committee of the Institute of Research in Health Sciences – U.N.A.

The Medical Academy, an organization recognized for its dedication to the dissemination of knowledge to practicing doctors, strongly endorsed bioethics during the years between 1998 and 2000 through the development of conferences focused on bioethics.

In 1998, the Association of Professors of the Medical Sciences School invited Dr. María Elena Lugo to be the keynote speaker at their annual bioethics event. In the following years, she participated annually in the seminars and symposia organized by the Bioethics Committee of the Hospital of Clinics pertaining to the formation of bioethics committees, controversial issues in bioethics (clinically related or not), and those events designed to assist in one's self-education in bioethics. Other invited speakers included Profs. Carlos Diaz and Jose Domínguez from Spain, who participated in the August 5–6, 2004, seminars including those titled "Bioethics and the Value of Human Life," "Human Genetic Manipulation and Research on Human Beings," "Cemetery of Consciences," and "Professional Ethics." The event was organized by the Emmanuel Mounier Institute of the Catholic University of Asunción, the Bioethics Committee of the Hospital of Clinics, and the National Commission for the Development of Bioethics.

On July 22–23, 2002, an 8 hours bioethics course was held for the purpose of strengthening and developing the methods of the research ethics committee of the Baptist Hospital of the city of Asunción. During the course, the University of New Mexico and the Office of Human Research Protection provided information about the standards and methods necessary for an institutional review board.

The National Commission for the Development of Bioethics in Paraguay organized the first and second National Symposia of Bioethics, on November 5, 2004, and October 23, 2005, respectively. Both events drew the attendance of more than 300 participants, which included health professionals, college students, and the general public. The first symposium included the following lectures: "Euthanasia: Knowledge, Attitudes and Practices," "Palliative Care: Bioethics for Terminal Patients," "The Ethics of Geriatrics," "Nursing Ethics," and "Unwanted Pregnancies and the Objection of Conscience." The theme of the second symposium, "Humanism in Health Care," was developed within the following lectures: "Humanism and Treatment: Patient Rights," "Technology and Humanization," "Divine Providence: A Humanized Medical Experience," "Bioethics and the Environment," and "Bioethical Reflections on Equality." When bioethics first became a topic of discussion at conferences and symposia is unclear, although it was several years ago when the word "bioethics" began to be incorporated into discussions at conferences of pediatric medicine, gynecology, oncology, and nursing.

Paraguay was one of the organizers for the Sixth Brazilian Congress of Bioethics and the MERCOSUR Congress. In addition, Paraguay also contributed to the organization of the forum of the Bioethics Network for Latin America and the Caribbean–UNESCO on the topic of "Bioethics, Environment and Human Life," held in Foz de Iguaçú, Brazil on August 30–September 3, 2005. Many Paraguayans participated in the events pertaining to both the central theme and other subjects, in addition to Dr. Marta Ascurra's acceptance as an advisory member of the network.

The First International Congress of Bioethics held in Paraguay was titled "Personal Bioethics in a Globalized World" and was organized by the Partnership of Catholic Doctors and the Pontifical Academy for Life. The congress was held on July 5–7, 2006, and included over 500 participants, many from religious or educational institutions, in addition to health professionals of all specialties. The keynote speakers for this event were Dom Elio Sgreccia, Ph.D., President of the Vatican's Pontifical Academy for Life (PAV – Pontifícia Academia para a Vida); Dom Mauricio Calipari, Ph.D., study official of PAV; Dom Fernando Chomali, representative of the Center of Bioethics of the Catholic University of Chile; and Rubén Revello, Ph.D. from Argentina.

16.10 The Universal Declaration on Bioethics and Human Rights

On November 6, 2004, the regional seminar, "Bioethics: An International Challenge. Towards a Universal Declaration," was convened by the Ministry of Justice and Human Rights of Argentina. During this event, the "Letter of Buenos Aires on Bioethics and Human Rights" was elaborated. The letter was a statement on fundamental bioethical issues within the context of Latin American and the Caribbean, approached from political, socioeconomic, and cultural perspectives. It was sent to the Secretary of the International Bioethics Committee of UNESCO on the grounds of establishing that any universal bioethical instrument that failed to secure a right to health, access to potable water, or to appropriately address the issue of poverty would legitimize the practices of inequality and exclusion, two major problems for Latin American countries. The Letter of Buenos Aires was accompanied by others sent by the chancelleries of other countries within the region to the UNESCO headquarters. The Universal Declaration on Bioethics and Human Rights was approved unanimously by the 191 member countries of the organization on October 19, 2005, during the General Conference of UNESCO in Paris, France (UNESCO 2006). The declaration included 28 articles, some of which address the modifications asked for in the Letter of Buenos Aires, making apparent a commitment to vulnerable populations and human rights.

16.11 Conclusion and Challenges

In recording the development of Paraguayan bioethics, the main facts and actors have been mentioned, although there is much more that could be said. To conclude, after almost 15 years of development, Paraguayan bioethics still requires more significant diffusion in rural areas, the elaboration of additional educational resources, more hospital bioethics committees, governmental recognition, the development of a national system for the evaluation of research, and so forth. It has, however, begun to confront important issues such as undernourishment, poverty, the destruction of the environment, and high infant and maternal mortality rates, as well as responding to those challenges that require the preservation of human rights.

References

Ascurra MA (2005) Comentarios a la ponencia de León Olivé. In: Garrafa V, Kottow M, Saada A (eds) Estatuto epistemológico de la bioética. UNESCO, Mexico City, pp 161–163

Ascurra MA, Rosales C (2005a) Análisis y perfil bioético de la investigación en salud publica. In: Málaga H (ed) Salud pública. Enfoque bioético. Disinlimed C.A., Caracas, Venezuela, pp 207–219

Ascurra MA, Rosales C (2005b) Formación y capacitación de recursos humanos de la bioética en salud publica. In: Málaga H (ed) Salud pública. Enfoque bioético. Disinlimed C.A., Caracas, Venezuela, pp 223–239

Burgstaller de Justiniano G. de F (1995) Responsabilidad penal de los médicos. Legislación, doctrina y jurisprudencia. Graphis, Asunción

De Mestral E (2006) Manual de bioética. Edição do Autor, Asunción

Paraguay (1992) Constitución Nacional del Paraguay, June

Paraguay (2003) Exclusión Social en Salud, October

Pro-Bioética (1995) Acta de Fundación de Pro-Bioética, June

Seall-Sasiain J (2006) Panorama sobre la legislación en materia de genoma humano en Paraguay. In: Saada A, Valadés G (eds) Panorama sobre la legislación en materia de genoma humano en América Latina y el Caribe. Publicación Científica N° 3, Red Latinoamericana y del Caribe Bioética, UNESCO, pp 343–376

UNESCO (2006) Declaración Universal sobre Bioética y Derechos Humanos

Universidad Católica Nuestra Señora de la Asunción (Centro de Estudios Bioéticos) (2005) Bioética, 1, Junio

Bibliography

PAHO (Área de Análisis de Salud y Sistemas de Información Sanitaria) (2005) Iniciativa regional de datos básicos en salud. Sistemas de Informaciones Técnicas en Salud, Washington, DC

Dirección General de Estadísticas, Encuestas y Censos (DGEEC) (2002) Principales Resultados. Encuesta Integrada de Hogares, Fernando de la Mora

Paraguay (2004) Resolución del Ministerio de Salud Pública y Bienestar Social, October 5

Chapter 17
Bioethics in Peru

Roberto Llanos Zuloaga

17.1 Introduction

The advent of bioethics as a discipline concerned with the systematic study of human behavior in the health and life sciences, and grounded by a set of moral principles, initially began as a simpler medical ethics. Bioethics in Peru has not yet developed its own Peruvian identity, but its content has developed far beyond the traditional issues of medical ethics. Although it has not been established as an autonomous discipline, it has found its place within the educational offerings of medicine, psychology, philosophy, and theology. The increasing salience of bioethics education has allowed it to develop a certain character related to its concern with the important subject matters of philosophy of medicine, medical anthropology, and medical epistemology. With the initial foundations of bioethics in place, now is the appropriate time to begin encouraging its dissemination. The first book in bioethics was written in 1996 by Montori Tudela from the Cayetano Heredia Peruvian University and dealt specifically with the topic of euthanasia.

One of the main objectives of bioethics in Peru thus far has been to establish hospital ethics committees (Comitê de Ética Hospitalar - CEH) within all major health organizations. Nevertheless, the majority still expects that the medical school's ethics committee will solve all problems that arise, and that the National Commission to Combat AIDS will solve all problems related to this pandemic. However, there has been a push by the media for the population to abandon prejudices about organ donation and to focus on its ability to save lives. For organ donation to be successful, its related practices must be regulated, and, therefore, the development of bioethics committees is required. These factors, in addition to many others, demonstrate the realization of the preliminary stage of recognizing bioethics as a discipline.

R.L. Zuloaga
Psychiatry, Psychotherapist. Specialized in clinical psychiatry. Founder and current president of the Peruvian Association of Bioethics. Professor and coordinator of doctorate programme in psychology at the University of the Sacred Heart
e-mail: rollanos@rcp.net.pe

L. Pessini et al. (eds.), *Ibero-American Bioethics: History and Perspectives*, Philosophy and Medicine 106, DOI 10.1007/978-1-4020-9350-0_17,

The development of modern medical technologies has become a topic of significant debate in countries throughout the world due to its extreme cost and the uncertainty of its effectiveness and potential for social aid. The intensity of the disagreement on these issues has generated a modern bioethics, which demands a conscience in its development and emphasizes the need for its regulation. Peru has adopted this approach and has recognized the urgency of establishing regulations (Llanos 1990).

However, there are many issues waiting to be addressed by bioethics, including organ transplantation laws, informed consent, quality of life, and the promotion and creation of institutional and research ethics committees. Of serious concern for preventative ethics are those problems inherent to a country with an increasing population and decreasing economic resources. Efforts are being made to encourage responsible paternity and family planning, although the results are not yet optimal. The number of pregnant adolescents remains around 15%, and, often times, by the time they have reached adulthood, girls have had three children and a couple of abortions. Contraceptives and the morning-after pill continue to be controversial, and a women's right to choose is not yet preponderant. Illegal abortions continue to be practiced, carrying the serious risks of infection or death for young women. Additionally, academic and social circles continue to keep silent on the possibilities of vasectomy and fallopian tube ligation or sectioning. Unfortunately, women do not speak about these issues.

In relation to another major topic, euthanasia, various issues are being discussed. Questions are being raised about whether a compassionate killing causes more problems than those it seeks to solve, and the complexities and complications of advance-directives are being discussed. These conversations are sporadically organized and often take place within the context of a roundtable or scientific forum.

Other issues of bioethical concern include the education of special-needs children, whose integration into common schools has been difficult, due to a lack of acceptance and social aid, and the assistance and treatment of individuals with AIDS, who still suffer from social discrimination motivated by fear and ignorance.

17.2 Honorio Delgado: A Precursor

Honorio Delgado, a Peruvian professor of psychiatry, the first President of the Cayetano Heredia Peruvian University, former President of the Greater National University of San Marcos, and former Minister of Education in Peru, represented medicine's humanistic vision and European ideas of health during the period 1930–1960. He frequently paraphrased the work of Friedrich Schiller and ultimately applied Schiller's moral analysis to the study of the psychiatric patient.

Delgado deeply identified with German culture and psychiatry, which is reflected in his essay, "Around the Core of Other People" (En torno al alma ajena) in which, quoting Schiller, he states: "If you want to understand yourself, watch how others behave" (Delgado 1992, p. 11). He also believed that medicine comprised three dimensions – scientific, professional, and supportive – which he always explained in his classes, books, and personal communications as playing a decisive role in the technological and axiological development of one's culture.

These principles espoused by Delgado were coherent with the humanistic perspective of his time, which provided the basis for the controversial development of bioethics. As such, bioethics has become the area of scientific knowledge that studies the technological transformations of medicine and provides rational answers to the moral, political, and social questions that arise when considering the benefit and impact of biomedical interventions on human health.

In Delgado's courses and books, he provided the information necessary for one to identify what are now the three levels of bioethics, namely:

1. Macrobioethics: environmental, ecological, and planetary ethics
2. Mesobioethics: the ethics of biotechnical interventions affecting human life, including issues of birth, human development, abortion, and euthanasia, among others
3. Microbioethics: medical ethics proper, including issues related to the doctor–patient relationship and medical care

In his lessons, Delgado illuminated the interconnections between philosophy, medicine, epistemology, and medical anthropology. The establishment of these interrelations enters the territory of bioethics, chiefly at the meso- and micro-levels, because some of his primary lessons focused on the connections between medicine and philosophy.

When philosophy enters medicine, it passes through the domains of ontology, nosology, and ethics as they are related to clinical and therapeutic pathology. Delgado promoted education in the philosophy of medicine and charged Peruvian universities with its continuation.

Delgado's understanding of medicine promoted an approach involving meditation and treatment. A life of medicine without meditation was not a life, according to Delgado. Medical life must be metaphysical, logical, and moral, that is, it must be medical philosophy in action. As technology advances, the more important critical thought and meditation will be. The less one engages in critical thought, the more dangerous and expensive medicine will become.

17.3 The Beginnings of the Peruvian Bioethics Movement

The beginning of Peru's bioethics movement occurred in 1988, when the Medical School's Board of Directors began calling to roundtable discussions some 20 doctors with professional backgrounds in ethics, bioethics, and deontology. This led to the founding of a commission whose membership included Guillermo Contreras and Salomón Zavala, among others.

In June 1988, the Latin American Confederation of Bioethics Institutions (Federación Latinoamericana de Instituciones de Bioética – FELAIBE) was established in Caracas by Dr. Pablo Pulido, a Venezuelan physician and Executive Director of the Pan-American Confederation of Medical Schools and Colleges; Dr. José Alberto Mainetti, an Argentine humanist and Director of the Oncology Excellence Center (COE); and Dr. Alfonso Llano Escobar, S.J., Director of the National Bioethics Center (CENALBE) in Colombia. Until 1988, Peru was not represented at this level. In that year, at the Chilean Congress of Psychiatry, Dr. Mainetti, with the recommendation of Fernando Lolas Stepke and other Chilean specialists, invited me to attend the next meeting of FELAIBE.

In December 1988, I attended the first meeting of FELAIBE, which was sponsored by the COE in Argentina and marked its official establishment, because the necessary statutes had been approved and registered, thus acquiring legal status. At this meeting, PAHO (Pan-American Health Organization) asked me to write an article on bioethics in Peru to be published in the Bulletin of PAHO (1990) in both English and Spanish. I was also later asked to promote bioethical conversations in Peru and to organize a bioethics group.

In 1992, the second meeting of FELAIBE occurred in Villa de Leyva, Colombia, where a triennial agenda was written. At this meeting I was asked to coordinate the next meeting and, as a result, I established the Peruvian Association of Bioethics (ASPEBIO), an organization that came to serve as Peru's official representative for FELAIBE.

In 1993, the third meeting took place at the University of the Sacred Heart (Universidad del Sagrado Corazón) in Lima and was a pleasant affair with a high degree of scientific expertise.

In 1994, Dr. Gabriel Cortés Gallo organized the fourth meeting, and in 1995 Dr. Alfonso Renato Meira coordinated the fifth meeting where the First Congress of Latin American and Caribbean Bioethics took place, meetings of which were to occur at least biannually.

17.4 The Peruvian Association of Bioethics (ASPEBIO)

The Peruvian Association of Bioethics (ASPEBIO - Associação Peruana de Bioética) promotes the interdisciplinary study of ethical problems created by the development of modern technology and their solutions. ASPEBIO promotes, supports, and propagates bioethics education in medical schools and institutions of health. From 1998 forward, it has encouraged the creation of institutes and centers of bioethics, in addition to the furtherance of bioethical research.

17.4.1 The History of ASPEBIO

In March 1993, the first preparatory meeting of the Peruvian Association of Bioethics (ASPEBIO) took place, and of the 70 professionals invited, 35 were in attendance. After several additional meetings, on May 2, 1993, it was decided that ASPERBIO would be affiliated with FELAIBE and the International Bioethics Association.

Beginning in March of 1993, an uninterrupted series of monthly scientific conferences was sponsored. These conferences were initially held at the auditorium of

Santa Isabel Clinic (Clínica Santa Isabel) and in 1994 at the Ricardo Palma Clinic (Clínica Ricardo Palma) and the Laboratories Glaxo, Tecnofarma, and Farmindustria. The keynote speakers at the international conferences included Dr. Joaquin Clotet (Brazil), Ruth Macklin, Ph.D. (USA), Mahal Dacosta (Chile), Fernando Lolas Stepke (Chile), Roberto Manzini (Chile), Dafna Feinholz (México), and Eduardo Souza Lennox (Panama).

The subjects addressed include: "Reproductive Techniques in Genetic Engineering"; "Patient Rights"; "Bioethics and End-of-Life Issues"; "Organ Transplants"; "Bioethics and Disability"; "Bioethics in the 21st century"; "Contraception"; "Drug Addiction and Recreational Drugs"; "The Foundations of Bioethics"; "Bioethics, Violence, Psychosis and Mental Health"; "Ecology, Philosophy and Bioethics"; "Human Life and Bioethics"; "Psychotherapy"; "Autonomy, Informed Consent, and Bioethics"; "Abortion"; "Psychiatric Diagnosis"; "Dante's *The Divine Comedy*"; "Bioethics in the Institutionalized Psychiatric Patient"; "Medical AutPAHOy"; "Third Age"; "Research Involving Human Beings"; "AIDS"; "Medical Ethics and Thanatos"; "Dialogues of the Body and Bioethics"; "Honorio Delgado and the History of Bioethics"; "Assisted Reproduction"; "Deplorable Humanism, Subversion and Development"; "Violation and Bioethics"; "Amazonian Peoples"; "Professional Secrecy"; "Dignified Birth"; "The Human Genome Project"; and "Infant Mental Health."

In September 1993, the Third Latin American Bioethics Meeting took place in Lima and included the following subjects: "Medical Ethics and Psychology," "Abortion," "Cognitive Impairments," "Organ Transplants," "Euthanasia," "Genetic Engineering" and "Death with Dignity." The Peruvian Association of Bioethics relied on the support of the German-Peruvian Medical Association, the University of the Sacred Heart and the Medical College of Peru. Invited speakers were Reyna de Klotik, Celia Bordim, Marta Fracapani, Liliana Gianncarini, Juan Carlos Tealdi, and Alberto Bochatey from Argentina; Alfonso Renato Meyra, J. Francisconi, and Joaquin Clotet from Brazil; Alfonso Llano Escobar, César Sanchez, María Marchand, María Mercedes Hackespiegel, Ricardo Cely, and H. Seminario from Colombia; and Jorge Hernandez and Luis Diaz from Mexico.

17.4.2 ASPEBIO: Projections

The Peruvian Association of Bioethics has established relations with a diverse group of foreign organizations and receives important journals, such as *Medicine and Ethics* (*Medicina y Ética*), published by the University of Anahuac in partnership with the University of the Sacred Heart, Rome; *Bioética*, published by the University of Rio Grande do Sul, Brazil; and *Bioética*, published by the Federal Council of Medicine, Brasilia. The Bioethics Commission of the United States Senate also receives periodic information about ASPEBIO's activities.

17.5 Historical Events

17.5.1 International Bioethics Course: "Bioethics and Health" (1996)

In August 1996, the Episcopal Department of Pastoral Health (DEPAS) sponsored an international course on bioethics in Lima, Peru, entitled, "Bioethics and Health." The aims of the course were to study the different paradigms of bioethics that had emerged in Peru and Latin America, to analyze the bioethical issues related to the beginning, development, and end of human life from a Latin American perspective, and to reflect on what fundamental human values require for a basic program of health. In attendance and actively participating were 156 attendees, a number of whom were health professionals, including physicians, medical school directors, and pastoral health representatives. As a result of this event, the Episcopal Pastoral Commission of Peru published a book entitled, *Life Is Worth It: New Approaches to Bioethics* (*La vida vale: bioética: nuevos caminos*) (1996). This publication serves to record communications pertaining to three fundamental aspects of bioethics:

1. The general principles and foundations of bioethics in Latin America as discussed by specialists such as Leo Pessini (Brazil), Christian de Paul de Barchifontaine (Brazil), Robert Mancini (representing the Regional Bioethics Program of Latin America and the Caribbean of PAHO/OMS [Chile]), and Ludolfo Ojeda (Peru).
2. The socio-political and economic factors of the Peruvian reality, with a presentation by Christian de P. de Barchifontaine on health in Peru; an interview with Francisco Sanchez Moreno, Dean of the Medical School of Peru; and a presentation by Felipe MacGregor on ecological experiences and reflections on the relationship between life, health, and violence.
3. The significance of pastoral support in medicine, as presented by Maria van Der Linde (Peru).

17.5.2 Seminar and Workshop of PAHO/OMS (1999)

In June 1999, the PAHO/OMS sponsored a seminar and workshop in Lima, Peru, entitled, "Foundations for the Systematic Planning of Courses and Methodologies for the Study of Bioethical Questions." The seminar was led by Marlen Oliver Vásquez, Ed.D., adviser to PAHO/OMS, who presented the appropriate teaching methods for developing bioethical concepts and skills. The course was geared towards educating the faculty of the Greater National University of San Marcos (Universidad Nacional Mayor de San Marcos), where an undergraduate bioethics course had been created three years earlier.

17.5.3 *First Ethics and Medicine Day (2000)*

The Dos de Mayo National Hospital, the Medical School of Peru and the Teaching, Research and Qualification Unit jointly coordinated the First Ethics and Medicine Day on October 6, 2000. The agenda included: "Ethics and Medical Teaching," "Research Ethics," "Dilemmas in the Human Genome Project," "Euthanasia and Life Support," "The Humanization of Medicine," and "Medical Ethics, Medical Rights, Negligence, and Medical Responsibility."

17.5.4 *International Bioethics Course: Controversies and Challenges (2000)*

On September 28–30, 2000, the MSC Cristoforus Denyke Institute of Health (Instituto de Salud MSC Cristoforus Denyke – ISDEN) and the Stella Maris Clinic offered an international course in bioethics. Its aims included: the promotion of bioethical reflection and debate concerning current issues in medicine and human rights; the establishment of ethical guidelines for professional practice; the presentation of the concepts of bioethics, their origins, evolution, and perspective; the promotion of the value and dignity of life as the foundation of bioethics; the analysis of ethical questions generated by technological developments; and an exploration of the ethical issues and challenges of research involving human beings. Among others, Susana Vidal (Argentina), Marcio Fabri (Brazil), and Eduardo Souza (Panama) participated as guests.

17.5.5 *First International Bioethics Course (2003)*

The institutional research ethics committee of the María Auxiliadora General Hospital organized the First International Course of Bioethics 2003 on research ethics and ethics committees. The course took place March 14–16, 2003, and had invited guest lecturers Ruth Macklin (USA), Florence Luna (Argentina), Sigfrido Orchard (Mexico), Patricia Saidón (Argentina), Ignacio Maglio (Argentina), and Solitude Diaz (Chile) in attendance. The subjects addressed included: "The Transcultural Character of Bioethics and its Paradigms"; "Bioethics and the New Century"; "The Bioethical Implications of AIDS"; "Challenges for Research Ethics Committees"; "The Development of the Chilean Institute of Reproductive Medicine's (ICMER) Ethics Committee"; "Ethical Controversies in International Research"; "Responsibility of Researchers in Developing Countries"; "Frontiers of the Medical Act in the Chronic Patient"; "Principles of Research Ethics"; and "Contraception and Planning."

17.5.6 International Bioethics Week (2003)

The International Bioethics Week took place September 12–20, 2003, at the University of Lima, organized by the Archbishop of Lima and Pro Ecclesia Sancta in coordination with the Catholic University of Chile and the University of Lima, with the support of the Scientific University of the South (Universidad Científica del Sur), the Medical School of Peru, and the Lima Law School.

The Congress had a program of 35 presentations and four plenary sessions with the following themes: (1) the person; (2) the beginning of life; (3) the end of life; and (4) the doctor and the health professional. The aims of the Congress were to promote awareness of bioethical questions pertaining to the person and life and their solutions and to eliminate conceptual ambiguities by encouraging more precise language and communication.

17.5.7 Tenth Pastoral Day of Health (2004)

On July 16–17, 2004, the Tenth Pastoral Day of Health took place with the theme, "Suffering: A Mystery that Speaks." It presented four simultaneous sessions addressing the bioethical topics of family violence and HIV-AIDS. It closed with the declaration "In favor of life."

17.5.8 Ethical and Legal Aspects of the Medical Act

The Institute of Forensic Medicine and the Medical School of Peru organized a panel on May 19–20, 2005, to discuss a variety of professional themes. Among them were included: "Professional Ethics"; "Informed Consent"; "Forensic Sciences and Human Rights"; "Blood Transfusions"; "Error and Malpractice"; "Dignified Death"; "Euthanasia and Assisted Suicide"; "Organ Transplants"; "Ethics and Media Propaganda"; "Rights and Duties of the Doctor"; "Professional Responsibility: The Invasive Component of the Medical Act"; "Ethics and Forensic Sciences"; "Moral Conscience and Corruption"; and "Ethics and Administrative Disagreements."

17.5.9 International Symposium of Bioethicists

The "Carlos Vidal Lavseca" Faculty of Public Health and Administration of the Cayento Heredia Peruvian University organized the International Symposium of Bioethics with the support of the Ethics of Science and Technology Unit of

UNESCO and the Pan-American Health Organization (PAHO). It took place April 19–20, 2006, and was divided into the following three panels:

- The Status of Bioethics in Peru
- Specialized Education in Bioethics
- Bioethics Qualifications for Professionals and Researchers

Two workgroups were established:

1. The Condition of Bioethics in Peru: Research, Clinical Assistance and the Normative Framework
2. Necessities for the Development of the Field: Specialized Teaching, The Qualification of Professionals and Researchers, and Operating Mechanisms

The international guests in attendance included: Henk ten Have, Armanet Pillar, Gabriel D'Empaire, and Maria Dolores Vila-Coro.

17.6 Legal Aspects

In the last decade, a number of laws pertaining to bioethics have been approved in Peru. However, the Latin American Proposal for Indigenous Legislation for the Collective Consultation on Genetic Studies, which emphasizes the rights of indigenous peoples to the protection and enjoyment of their cultural heritage as it is guaranteed by the Universal Declaration of Human Rights, the International Covenant of Economic, Social and Cultural Rights, The International Covenant of Civil and Political Rights and the International Labor Organization Agreement 169, will be the only one mentioned here.

Act Nº 27811 of the proposal, created on July 24, 2002, establishes a protection system for the biological resources of indigenous people. The law defines informed consent as authorization granted by the representative organization of the indigenous people, understood as possessors of the collective knowledge, that must be solicited in accord with their recognized norms, and must be used for the accomplishment of a specific activity that requires access to their collective knowledge. Informed consent must be obtained by any individual wishing to secure access to the collective knowledge for the purpose of scientific, commercial, or industrial applications. The information provided will be limited to the biological resources to which the collective knowledge refers.

17.7 Research Ethics Committees in Peru

The National Research Ethics Commission of Peru was established in 1995 and has a diversified membership of 20 who are appointed for two-year terms. The Commission's purpose is to promote the establishment of research ethics committees and to register all institutional research ethics committees.

Additionally, there are 50 individuals who have committed themselves to the development of bioethics in Peru and have distributed themselves into five work-groups, each addressing different topics. They include:

1. Political Action: the Medical School of Peru
2. Professional Training (Academic): Dr. Alberto Perales
3. Health Services: Dr. César Molero, a Camillian priest
4. Research: Dr. César Molero and Dr. Roberto Llanos
5. Bioethics and Communication: Engineer Elsa Benavente

The institutions that have agreed to make a joint effort in research ethics include: the Universities of San Marcos (Engineering); Cayetano Heredia, Sagrado Corazón (Catholic); the Medical College of Peru; the Order of Saint Camillus; the Peruvian Association of Bioethics; Edgardo Rebagliati, Guillermo Almenara, Dos de Mayo, and Arzobispo Loayza Hospitals; the Peruvian Bioethics Center, the Merck, Sharp and Dohme Laboratories; and the NGOs PRISMA San Christophorus, and Ethics for Life.

The members of the Peruvian Research Ethics Group include: Dr. Roberto Llanos, Rafael Arce, Pedro Ruiz, Francisco Rivera, Berta Reyes, Carmen Bravo, Gustavo Araujo, Roberto Espinoza, Manuel Paz, and Alois Kennernecht.

Since the establishment of the National Bioethics Commission in 2001, Peru has seen the number of ethics committees grow from nine to 20 (in 2003) to the current 40. In the same way, in 2001, there were six research ethics committees, which, in 2003, when the Peruvian Chapter of the Latin American Forum of Research Ethics Committees (Foro Latinoamericano de Comités de Ética de Investigación en Salud – FLACEIS) was established, became 10. Consequently, there are now 23 research ethics committees in Peru. The history of some of them is recounted below.

17.7.1 Research Ethics Committee of the Edgardo Rebagliatti Martins Hospital

The Edgardo Rebagliatti Martins Hospital belongs to the Social Security Network of Hospitals (ESSALUD) and offers 38 medical services to those occupying their 1,300 beds. In 2003, the hospital conducted 59 research projects. The research ethics committee was established in August 1998 and is comprised of 11 members, five of which are physicians, two nurses, a lawyer, a priest, a social worker, and two community representatives. In addition, in 10% of its sessions, it has reviewed research protocols for other institutions.

17.7.2 National Institute of Health

Established in February 2000 and restructured in June 2002, the National Institute of Health has 13 members, has reviewed 39 research protocols, and has approved 24 of the proposals reviewed. The Institute is bound by the guidelines of the

International Registry and publishes the *Peruvian Journal of Experimental Medicine and Public Health* (*Revista Peruana de Medicina Experimental y Salud Pública*), which has been indexed in LILACS (Literatura Latino-americana e do Caribe de Informações em Ciências da Saúde) 2003 and MEDLINE 2004.

17.7.3 Peruvian Bioethics Center (CEPEBIO)

The CEPEBIO's ethics committee was founded on June 14, 2001, and is comprised of five members. It has participated in three of CEPEBIO's congresses (1999, 2001, and 2002) and has also participated in the Volunteer's Qualification Workshop attended by 27 laypersons and 14 priests. In addition, it has organized four research ethics courses (1999, 2000, 2001, and 2002) and a foundational course with 30 participants.

17.7.4 RENACE: General Office of Epidemiology (OGE)

The General Office of Epidemiology's (Oficina General de Epidemiología, OGE) committee has four members and, as of 2002, it had reviewed 1,495 financed research projects and has promoted 129 activities (8.6% of which were dedicated to research).

17.7.5 PRISMA (A Non-governmental Organization)

PRISMA was established in 1986, but it was not until 1994 that its research ethics committee was founded. Additionally, since 1999 it has undertaken a private study of research protocols, consulting, and monitoring.

17.8 The Journey of the Cristóforis Deneke Health Institute (ISDEN) Through the Pathways of Bioethics (1998–2006)

17.8.1 Antecedents

The ISDEN was established in 1998 and has been under the directorship of Sister Maria Van der Linde ever since. Her account of the beginnings of the ISDEN follows.

> In light of the sanitary reality of the country, restlessness for the humanization of health in ethics and bioethics was evident even after the establishment of ISDEN. At that time, we worked at the Pastoral of Health of the Peruvian Episcopal Conference, and in our position we realized the concern with patients of tuberculosis in the years 1992–1993. As a result,

> we sponsored eight formative and experiential workshPAHO in partnership with health professionals from the Tuberculosis Control Program in the Territorial Health Units of Comas and the Sergio E. Bernales Hospital, including about 50 institutions of health and five districts of Lima Northe and Canta of MINSA with the theme "The Study of the Values of Basic Assistance Regarding Tuberculosis."

In 1992, Dr. Paolo Mocarelli, an Italian bioethicist, was invited by the project "Education and Culture of Peace," developed by the Pontifical Catholic University of Peru, to deliver a lecture at a conference forum entitled "Ethics of Life," which had been organized in partnership with the Association of Catholic Doctors. Dr. Mocarelli made his presentation in the auditorium of the Municipality of Jesús Maria with 60 people in attendance. His presentation opened up a bioethical perspective for us, with which we were already very much in tune. He considered ethics not only in relation to technology and medical ethics, but also concerning important communitarian and social aspects. He provided a summary of his presentation, which we later used as a guide for different activities.

We also knew of Dr. Leo Pessini from Brazil who had worked on questions of bioethics from a Latin American perspective and considered public health and social questions mandatory topics for consideration. This encouraged us to coordinate an event for health professionals and others where they could reflect on these issues, because there was very little discussion or debate of these issues within the country at that time. As a result, in February 1995, we sponsored the First Forum on the Introductory Aspects of Bioethics, held in the auditorium of the Stella Maris Clinic. Dr. Leo Pessini (Brazil) and Fr. Ludolfo Ojeda (Peru) participated, in addition to many others.

Motivated by the sustained interest in bioethics activities since 1992, echoing the call of the First Forum on Bioethics, the First International Course: "Bioethics and Health" was organized in Lima in August 1996. During the same period (1992–1995), workshPAHO on "The Study of the Values of Health Professionals for Quality Assistance" were provided in several areas of Lima and other cities, through an agreement with the Peruvian Social Health Security Agency (today called ESSALUD), which extended the workshop to MINSA staff in those cities included in the agreement. With the production of more than 40 workshPAHO, we managed to engage over 2,000 people, including members of disciplinary groups, professionals, and technical and administrative personnel. All these individuals came to occupy the same reflective space. From the evaluations of the workshop, we were able to determine that the participants enjoyed the opportunity to reflect on their work from a humanist perspective.

17.8.2 Current Work

In 1998, in the already named MSC Cristóforis Deneke Health Institute (ISDEN), we established a special area dedicated to ethics and bioethics training called the "Humanization in Health Area."

17.8.3 Ethics Training in Undergraduate Nursing Courses

Following the suggestion of many government health professionals who had participated in our workshPAHO, we decided to work with health professionals in pre-service training and invited all of the professional schools and those programs for the health and social sciences professions from the different universities in Lima to attend a meeting. Not all responded to the invitation, although there were medical professionals, obstetricians, nurses, and social workers in attendance who engaged in a dialogue about the teaching of ethics in undergraduate courses. There were opinions, contributions, and concerns voiced by the participants, and in the end it was agreed to hold a second meeting. The group of nurses appeared to be most engaged, so we decided to work primarily with them at that time. The progression from that point forward can be summarized as follows:

1997: Prior to the formal establishment of ISDEN, we conducted a study of the status of "Humanist and Ethical Education in Undergraduate Nursing Courses," which served as the foundation for an intervention plan involving the participation of nurses throughout Lima and the country as a whole.

1999: "Nursing: An Ethical Formation of Life" was written and published under the auspices of PAHO, in which the human and ethical formation as a transversal axis was set out throughout one's nursing career.

2000 to the present: Work was continued with universities and nursing schools (FAENs); the establishment of about 30 professional nursing centers was meant to encourage, advise, and monitor the formation of undergraduate nursing courses.

With these aims, we engaged in:

1. Visits to FAENs: Providing workshPAHO for the qualification of teacher and consulting services for organizing local events.
2. Two Days of Annual Reflection: (One of the days was for first-year students and the other was for those in their last years and residents.) Students representative of 12–18 universities from around the country participated. The events were developed and prepared with the active participation of educational professionals from the FAENs in Lima.
3. Seminar/Workshop and Annual Meeting with the Deans and Directors of FAENs: These meetings also include the participation of educational coordinators in the areas of ethics and bioethics at the universities who are involved in the agreement with ISDEN.
4. Publication and Diffusion of Annual Bulletin: "Qualification in Bioethics."

17.8.4 Graduate Education in Bioethics

In partnership with the Cayetano Heredia University Nursing School, we developed an interdisciplinary graduate course in bioethics during the 2002–2003 academic year, which had participants from Lima and other provinces.

17.8.5 Publications of ISDEN

The nursing publications of ISDEN include: "Ethical Formation of Life" (Formación Ética para la Vida); *Fundamental Knowledge of Bioethics and Ethics* (*Nociones fundamentales de ética y bioética*). *Fundamental Knowledge of Bioethics and Ethics, Vol. I.* (*Nociones Fundamentales de Ética y Bioética* – a compilation); *Fundamental Knowledge of Bioethics and Ethics, Vol. II;. Fundamental Subjects of Bioethics and Ethics* (*Temas fundamentales de ética y bioética*); *Fundamental Knowledge of Bioethics and Ethics, Vol. III (Nociones fundamentales de ética y bioética*); *Questions of Social Ethics* (*Temas de ética social*, a compilation); *The Dwelling of Man* (*La Morada del hombre*), by Miguel Polo Santillán, co-published with The Greater National University of San Marcos (UNMSM).

17.8.6 National and International Bioethics and Ethics Events

2000: The International Bioethics Course took place over the course of three days and was worth one academic credit. Its theme was "Controversies and Challenges" and was organized by ISDEN and the Stella Maris Clinic. Participants included: Dr. Susana Vidal (Argentina), Dr. Marcio Fabri (Brazil), Dr. Eduardo Sousa Lennox (Panama), and Dr. Miriam Falla, Dr. Enrique Varci, Dr. Patrick Wagner, Dr. Demetrio Molero, Dr. Mario Ríos, Dr. Alfredo Benavides, Dr. Pilar Bandrés, Dr. Fierro, and Sonia Flores from Peru.

2002: An Ethical Reflection Meeting was held over the course of three days with "Diversity, Ethics and Religion" as its theme. The meeting was organized by the Institute of Ethics and Development at the Antonio Ruiz de Montoya, S.J., Undergraduate School (Instituto de Ética y Desarrollo – Escuela Superior Antonio Ruiz de Montoya, S.J.) and ISDEN. Dr. Adela Cortina (Spain), Dr. Fidel Tubino (Catholic University of Peru), and Dr. Paul Valadier (France) participated, in addition to the 230 people in attendance.

2002: A roundtable discussion was organized by students from seven nursing schools and coordinated by ISDEN. Its theme was "Ethics Cures" and over 600 young people attended from the different universities in Lima.

2002: A nine-month course entitled "Ethics and Community" was held for community leaders.

2003: A course running from May to October entitled "The Place of Bioethics in Healthcare" was organized by the Stella Maris Clinic and ISDEN. The lecturers were from the Master's program in bioethics developed by PAHO and included Dr. Diego Grácia and Dr. Azucena Crucero from Spain.

2002–2005: Seminars and workshPAHO organized by ISDEN in coordination with FAENs and local nursing schools were held in Lima, Chiclayo, Iquitos, Trujillo, Arequipa, Cuzco, Puno, and Cajamarca.

17.9 Conclusions

Bioethics in Peru has made significant advances. This is demonstrated by the establishment of several institutions that work intensively within the field, the existence of a group of more than 50 people that serve as the leadership of bioethics in Peru, and the fact that at least half of these individuals have taken it upon themselves to engage in independent study and to attend a Master's course in Peru, South America, or Europe. However, despite these advances, there are challenges still to be overcome.

- In the social sphere, one hopes that social groups will participate and advocate for discussions pertaining to issues such as organ donations for transplant, abortion, euthanasia, the environment, and assisted reproduction, among others.
- In the academic sphere, there is a need for greater academic responsibility and organization within educational institutions. At present, the University of San Marcos and the Pastoral of Health of the Brothers of Saint Camillus are the only institutions at this stage of organization; great things are expected of their future work.
- In the scientific sphere, there have been 23 research ethics committees established and the Peruvian Chapter of the Latin American Forum of Research Ethics Committees now has 15 members. This is foundational for achieving great future work, including what has already begun with the organization of seminars; the approval, teaching, and study of research protocols; and the provision of monitoring, counseling, and consulting services.
- The language of bioethics has become more readily used in the mass media as it gains recognition. Some newspapers, radio stations, and television channels have begun asking for interviews, commentaries, and articles presented in this language, which means it will be progressively diffused throughout the community.
- Regarding civil society participation, we are hoping that the work of the National Commission of Bioethics will engage institutions directly and indirectly concerned with life and demonstrate the importance of bioethics.
- At present, other than some self-help groups, the community has not been motivated and informed about bioethics. Much work remains to be done. However, with the increasing education of community leaders, the possibility of starting and sustaining communication and dialogue is assured.

Works Cited

Alcala-Zamora J et al (1994) Obtención del consentimiento informado (CI) en medicina intensiva. In: Anales del II Congreso Internacional de Bioética. Kirón, Buenos Aires, pp 4–5

Bunge M (1997) Medicina y filosofía. El Comercio [Lima], Sección Dominical (7 de Septiembre), 6

Cely G (1997) Bioética y universidad. Centro Ed Javeriano, Bogotá, pp 176–179

Clotet J (1994) Que tipo de consentimiento informado puede ser usado para las personas de los países en vías de desarrollo? In: Anales del II Congreso Internacional de Bioética. Kirón, Buenos Aires

Dias M (1999) Bioética, uma nova visão interdisciplinar. Jornal do CFM, Brasília

Fins J (1997) Experiencia norteamericana de la enseñanza de la Bioética. In: Cuadernos de Bioética. Programa Regional de Bioética para América Latina, OMS-PAHO, Santiago, pp 32–35

Gevers S (1994) Physician-assisted suicide: New developments in the Netherlands. In: Anales del II Congreso Internacional de Bioética. Kirón, Buenos Aires, p 15

Grácia D (1994) Principios de la bioética. In: Anales del II Congreso Mundial de Bioética. Kirón, Buenos Aires, pp 29–31

Gros H (2000) Report of the Legal Commission of the IBC. In: International Bioethics Committee of Unesco, vol 1. UNESCO, Paris, p 39

Leon Barua R (1998) Bases biológicas de la ética. *Diagnóstico*, 37.5 (September–October). Alafarpe, Lima, pp 311–116

Novoa F (1996) Consideraciones éticas en pacientes con daño cerebral. In: Extensiones. Ed. Interamericana, México

Perales A, Rivera F, Wu D (1997) Civilización y medicina. UNMSM, Lima, pp 77–81

Sartorius N (1998) The mental health programme of the World Health Organization. In: Anales de Salud Mental, vol 2. UNMSM, Lima

References

CEP (Centro de estudios y publicaciones) (1996) La vida vale. Bioética: nuevos caminos. Universidad del Pacífico, Lima

Clotet J (1994) Que tipo de consentimiento informado puede ser usado para las personas de los países en vías de desarrollo? In: Anales del II Congreso Internacional de Bioética. Kirón, Buenos Aires

Delgado H (1992) El médico, la medicina y el alma, 3rd edn. UPCH, Lima

Llano A (1990) El morir humano ha cambiado. Boletín de la Oficina Sanitaria Panamericana, 108.5–6 (May–June). PAHO, USA, pp 465–472

Llanos R (1990) Bioética en el Perú. Boletín de la Oficina Sanitaria Panamericana, 108.5–6 (May–June), pp 179–183

Miro Quesada O (1998) Bioética: momento de definiciones. El Comercio [Lima] (November 28), p 1

Chapter 18
Bioethics in Portugal

Jorge Biscaia and Walter Osswald

18.1 Introduction

During the early developmental stages of bioethics as a new area of science and ethics, its impact reached far beyond America, quickly pervading other countries. Portugal was an exception to the common occurrence of a fast and immediate incorporation of bioethics which many countries experienced. In fact, the first organized group devoted to the study of bioethics in Portugal was not formally established until 1988 when the Center of Bioethical Studies (Centro de Estudos de Bioética) in Coimbra, a non-profit, independent organization which had evolved from an informal discussion group, was founded. Since then, there has been a remarkable evolution and rapid expansion of bioethics in Portugal, with a relatively large number of students enrolling in graduate programs and Master's courses in bioethics. This has led to a significant number of individuals, coming from diverse backgrounds (doctors, nurses, philosophers, theologians, teachers, and so forth), to consider themselves bioethicists.

The aim of this essay is not to give a historical perspective or an exhaustive review of the development of bioethics in Portugal, but rather to address select topics that have been and remain prominent issues of bioethical debate – some of which have gained significant attention from the general population. To achieve this aim, consideration of the institutions where bioethics is discussed, taught, or researched is necessary. In addition, one will be able to see how these institutions and their activities have increased public awareness of the controversial topics in bioethics, allowing for the opinions of the citizenry to have an impact on political

J. Biscaia (✉)
MD, Director of Coimbra Center for Bioethics Studies (Centro de Estudos de Bioética de Coimbra), Portugal
e-mail: jorgebiscaia@netcabo.pt

W. Osswald
Former-director of the Institute of Bioethics, Portuguese Catholic University (Porto), Former-President of the World Association of Catholic Doctors
e-mail: ib@porto.ucp.pt

L. Pessini et al. (eds.), *Ibero-American Bioethics: History and Perspectives*, Philosophy and Medicine 106, DOI 10.1007/978-1-4020-9350-0_18,

and legal processes of paramount importance. The consideration of institutions of importance in this essay will focus primarily on the last decade, since information concerning earlier years has already been reviewed in previous articles (e.g., Nuñez and Abel 1992; Biscaia and Osswald 1995).

18.2 Institutions

The main forums of bioethical debate in Portugal are academic institutions and those independent societies with relevant interests. Curiously enough, the university at large was slow to recognize the need for bioethics to become a part of the internal structure of its institutions. The first and most prominent institution responsible for the acceptance and diffusion of bioethics in Portugal was the Center of Bioethical Studies (Centro de Estudos Bioéticos, CEB), which was the sequel to an informal think-tank in existence for two years prior (i.e., since 1986). The CEB is an independent, non-confessional, non-profit organization with a long roster of activities (see below) which, since its founding in 1988 in Coimbra, has made significant contributions to the positive acceptance and evolution of bioethics in Portugal.

The National Council for Ethics in Life Sciences (CNECV - Conselho Nacional de Ética para as Ciências da Vida) is the advisory board responsible for making recommendations to the Government, National Parliament (Assembléia da República), and the President on pertinent issues in bioethics. Founded in 1990, many of its members (including three chairpersons) were recruited from the CEB's membership. At present, the CNECV has produced 49 opinions on a variety of themes, ranging from medically assisted reproduction (MAR) or the use of embryos in scientific experiments to the obligatory testing of HIV-AIDS; from the management of genetic data to end-of-life issues; and from drug abuse policy to the criteria of death, among others. The advisory board is well esteemed and has demonstrated appreciable influence on the laws passed by Parliament. The chairperson of CNECV is nominated by the Prime Minister, while the other 20 members are nominated by 19 different entities, including Parliament, ministries, and the associations of physicians, lawyers, and biologists, as well as science academies and citizens' organizations.

The Center for Biomedical Law (Centro de Direito Biomédico, CDB), a research institute established by the law faculty of the University of Coimbra, has a significant history and, since 1988, has worked to aid in the resolution of those problems arising from conflict between the interests and codes of medical and pharmaceutical professionals and the strict legal rules governing the profession.

The medical schools of the University of Lisbon, the University of Coimbra, and the University of Porto have always taught some form of medical ethics, but it was not until 1996 that the University of Porto's medical school created a Service of Bioethics and Medical Ethics (Serviço de Bioética e Ética Médica, SBEM), marking the first time the word 'bioethics' appeared in the curriculum and structure of any Portuguese medical school. The University of Lisbon followed suit in 1998 by creating the Center of Bioethics (Centro de Bioética).

The only university department to address bioethics without conceptual or institutional links to the education of medical students is the Institute of Bioethics at the Portuguese Catholic University, which evolved in 2002 from a pre-existing bioethics research group (originally founded in 1995). This is not to exclude consideration of other university departments that have made significant contributions to the field of bioethics. For example, it should be mentioned that the philosophy departments of the University of the Azores in Ponta Delgada and the Portuguese Catholic University in Braga both include bioethics in their postgraduate curriculum, and their faculty members have published books on relevant topics. The department at the University of the Azores has also provided support for ethics committees and nursing organizations.

The Portuguese Association of Bioethics (Associação Portuguesa de Bioética) was established in 2003 at a relatively late stage of development, but maintains close personal and institutional links with the Service of Bioethics and Medical Ethics mentioned above.

In the following section, the development of significant activities that have contributed to the evolution of Portuguese bioethics by the aforementioned institutions will be discussed.

18.3 Main Activities

It is impossible to detail the numerous activities developed by the aforementioned institutions in the context of the short overview provided here. Instead, a brief examination of the most important initiatives will be provided.

The Center of Bioethical Studies (CEB) and the Institute of Bioethics both organize large meetings focused on issues of national concern with important implications for public policy. These meetings are paradigmatic of how bioethics has to be approached for the benefit of the general population. In addition, the CEB has organized the European Congress of Medical Ethics Centers (in 1997) and has held a number of smaller meetings to address specific questions in bioethics. The CEB has a seat in Coimbra and delegations in Lisbon, Porto, Azores, Évora, Madeira, and Braga.

Additionally, the *National Congress of Bioethics* is now in its seventh year with the last four meetings having been organized by the Portuguese Association of Bioethics. The National Council on Ethics for the Life Sciences also organizes annual seminars that are important and well-attended events. Various smaller meetings and workshops that deal with specialized issues in bioethics commonly attract the attendance and delivery of lectures by select scholars (e.g., vulnerability at the beginning and end of life, the teaching of bioethics in secondary schools, problems in the care of premature babies, terminal patients and palliative care, conservation of water resources, etc.). Other meetings and congresses of scientific societies, lawyers associations, and lay or confessional organizations often address bioethical questions that are of special interest to their members. To assist in the discussion of these issues as well as to deliver presentations, such organizations invite bioethicists to participate in their meetings. As is clear, there are numerous occasions for individuals to advance their knowledge of bioethics or to familiarize themselves and perhaps take an interest in the pertinent questions.

18.4 Publications

Given the substantial number of activities and events sponsored by the relevant organizations, it comes as no surprise that these activities have led to a growing number of publications in the area of bioethics.

Cadernos de Bioética (Revista Portuguesa de Bioética), edited by the CEB, is the only journal dedicated to bioethics published in Portugal and has produced an impressive array of articles in its 41 volumes. While the journal remains the only major Portuguese publication, a number of articles addressing issues of bioethics are published regularly in medical journals, the publications of physicians and lawyers associations, confessional journals, and cultural magazines. Newspapers and television shows cover (sometimes sensationally) cases considered to be exemplars of certain bioethical issues – for example, the Terri Schiavo case or the alleged cloning of human beings. Even though bioethicists are often interviewed about these cases, the majority of this type of coverage is of poor quality.

Over the last decade, almost 70 books have been published directly addressing issues of bioethics. These works range from textbooks to more specialized books and deal with various themes like nursing ethics or institutional review boards (the existence of which is obligatory in every Portuguese hospital). Some of the themes that have been addressed include the ethics of genetics, cloning, the common good and individual interest, clinical trials, eco-ethics, and assisted reproduction.

Two volumes were the result of workshops organized by the Institute of Bioethics and provided commentary on the European Convention on Human Rights and Biomedicine, which discussed the legal documents and their implications for medical care and cures (the conventions were adopted by Portugal). Lastly, collections of monographs, either presented at congresses or representing the work of a sole author, conclude the list of these publications. In this style, the National Council of Ethics for the Life Sciences has launched an impressive series of eight books (in addition to another nine books recording the opinions of this body) which are each a compilation of the lectures given at a seminar organized by the CNECV.

18.5 Teaching Bioethics

As previously mentioned, the universities have been rather slow in recognizing their responsibility to teach and disseminate the knowledge of bioethics. In fact, it was not until the academic year of 1986–1987 that the first postgraduate course in bioethics (dealing with the theme of MAR) was offered by the philosophy department of the Portuguese Catholic University in Braga. Since then, postgraduate and Master's courses of much larger scope, addressing the whole gamut of bioethical issues, have been organized by the above-mentioned universities where bioethics has become an important part of the academic fabric. This includes the direction of seven Master's courses by both the Institute of Bioethics of the Portuguese Catholic University and the Service of Bioethics and Medical Ethics of the Medical School of Porto University. In addition, the philosophy faculty of the Portuguese Catholic University and the Center of Ethics at the University of Lisbon's medical school each direct five courses. As a result, a number of students (an estimated 70) have successfully defended a Master's thesis and have earned a Master's degree.

At the postgraduate level, medical schools and a majority of law schools and nursing schools have included bioethics in their curriculum. Surprisingly, biology faculties and other related sciences only include bioethics in some of their courses and their respective curricula.

A number of studies have addressed the need to teach introductory bioethics in some capacity at the level of secondary school education. As a result, concrete proposals to this effect have been made to the Ministry of Education, although no advancements have been made. The hope is that the government will recognize the benefit of providing students with initial contact with bioethics' main questions in an interdisciplinary manner that would allow for their contemporaneous consideration within the contexts of biology, philosophy, and religion. However, this innovative pedagogical approach is far from being actualized.

18.6 Biomedical Research

Research projects at the national and international level have and are being conducted by the Institute of Bioethics (Portuguese Catholic University) and the Service of Bioethics and Medical Ethics (Porto University School of Medicine). Some issues being addressed by these research projects include: the death of premature babies, burnout syndrome in palliative and intensive care departments, stem cell research, teaching bioethics at the high school level, nature and ethics, deaf–mute recuperation and its ethical problems, xenotransplantation, and resource allocation.

In addition, the determination of an appropriate topic for a Master's thesis requires a certain degree of research, which deepens once a proposal has been approved. The standard of research quality is high for those schools offering a doctoral program in bioethics and can be considered contributions to biomedical research. Currently, the Institute of Bioethics at the Portuguese Catholic University is the only Ph.D.-granting institution in Portugal.

Taking into consideration the progressive involvement of Portuguese bioethicists in different research projects at different levels, especially for the younger generation, it appears that an optimistic view of the development of bioethics is justified.

18.7 Laws of Biomedical Relevance

While one can argue for the relevance of all laws directly or indirectly affecting health or the environment to bioethics, the focus of this section is only on those laws that appear to be of primary importance to the field and/or have been submitted to the CNECV for consideration (in the current legal framework, any legal project that pertains to the life sciences has to be submitted to the CNECV for review). Since the CNECV is only an advisory council, its opinions and recommendations do not determine the law, but its significant influence has been witnessed in the past. Some examples of such laws follow.

Abortion has been determined to be a crime punishable by imprisonment (from two to eight years) except under certain excusing conditions (the risk of physical or mental harm to the pregnant woman; the presence of a severe and incurable disease of the fetus; or a pregnancy resulting from the act of rape).

Organ transplantation is allowable when donors are either deceased (brain death has been determined) or are close living relatives. In addition, there is a registry of non-donors which allows individuals to declare their desire not to have their organs harvested postmortem for the purpose of transplantation. If one is not on the non-donor registry, then it is presumed that one does not object to the donation of one's organs.

Clinical trials are strictly regulated and the European Directive has recently been adopted by Portugal (Act 46/2004 is a transcription of the European Directive 2001/90/CE).

The use of human cadavers in medical education or research projects is allowable in limited contexts and requires the consent of the individual *ante mortem*.

MAR has been regulated after being practiced for many decades without any legal restrictions. Current law restricts MAR to heterosexual couples (married or not) but allows, in exceptional cases, heterologous fecundation and surrogate motherhood. Surplus embryos may be used for research if parental authorization is secured and only after the embryo has been in a frozen state for a few years.

The adoption of the European Convention of Human Rights and Biomedicine into Portuguese law is an important milestone in Portuguese bioethics. The convention emphasizes the importance of informed consent, human dignity, autonomy, and the prohibition of the production of human embryos for the sole purpose of research, while also conveying a number of important bioethical notions that will strongly influence future legislation.

18.8 International Links

The nature of bioethics and its concern with distinctively human issues allows for its treatment at the international level. The goal of achieving a universal bioethics to guide the appropriate actions and attitudes of individuals in the spheres of life science and, more specifically, in preserving the biosphere is considered to be a utopian ideal by some. What is true is that without the international exchange of ideas, requiring the discussion and realization of differing cultural backgrounds, no common ground will be established and the goal of a universal bioethics will be unattainable. Given this context, it is not surprising that, since the beginning of the "bioethical era" (which in Portugal really took place in the mid-1980s), Portuguese scholars have tried to establish and maintain relationships with colleagues and institutions in other countries. Due to cultural and linguistic similarities, regular contacts were established with Brazil and other Latin countries such as Spain and Italy. Portuguese and Brazilian scholars have attended and delivered lectures at conferences and courses in each other's countries and, as a result of this cooperation, a conference (Encontro Luso-Brasileiro de Bioética) has been established whose fourth session recently (September 2006) took place in São Paulo (previously held in Lisbon, Brasília, and Ponta Delgada). The conference fosters important exchanges of different viewpoints and the discussion of varying approaches, with the added benefit of a common cultural and linguistic background. In addition, international connections are made by the travel of postgraduate students, although in small numbers, to other cities such as São Paulo (and in Europe: Barcelona, Rome, Padua, Paris).

Links to the United States, the United Kingdom, and other European countries also exist and are maintained by those individuals who have received their degrees in these countries or through collaboration with foreign scientists on research projects funded by the European Union. As previously stated, the CEB has been a member of the board of the European Association of Medical Ethics Centers, and Portuguese bioethicists have been regularly appointed to the specialized groups of the European Council, the European Union, and UNESCO which focus specifically on bioethics (respectively: Comité Directeur pour la Bioéthique; European Group on Ethics of Science and New Technologies; International Committee on Bioethics).

In addition, a significant number of bioethicists from other countries have been invited to attend and present at conferences and seminars in Portugal and have also contributed to the education of postgraduate students preparing their theses. Furthermore, Portuguese scientists are board members of international societies and associations of bioethics, and one scientist has even secured membership to the prestigious Pontifical Academy for Life.

An important factor for the international recognition of Portuguese bioethics is the level of publication of Portuguese scholars in international journals. Publication at this level is occurring on a modest scale but needs to be increased; therefore, additional publications should be encouraged and fostered.

18.9 Contacts

For additional information about the institutions and/or their activities mentioned above please contact:

Centro de Bioética – Faculdade de Medicina da Universidade de Lisboa (Director: Prof. Doutor A. Barbosa) Av. Professor Egas Moniz, 1649-028 Lisboa. Telefone: (+351) 217 985 100. Fax: (+351) 217 985 110. E-mail: fml@fm.ul.pt

CDB – Faculdade de Direito da Universidade de Coimbra (Director: Prof. Doutor G. de Oliveira) Pátio da Universidade, 3004-545 Coimbra, Portugal. Telefone: (+351) 239 859 801/02. Fax: (+351) 239 823 353. E-mail: fduc@fd.uc.pt

Centro de Estudos de Bioética (Director: Dr. Jorge Biscaia) Rua General Humberto Delgado, 444, 7ºD, 3030-327 Coimbra. Telefone: (+351) 239 712 806. E-mail: jorgebiscaia@netcabo.pt.

Conselho Nacional de Ética para as Ciências da Vida (CNECV – Presidente: Dra. Paula Martinho da Silva), Prof. Gomes Teixeira, Edifº PCM, 4º, 1350-265 Lisboa. Telefone: (+351) 213 927 978. Fax: (+351) 213 927 629. E-mail: pres.cnecv@sg.pcm.gov.pt

Instituto de Bioética da Universidade Católica Portuguesa (Director: Prof. Doutora Ana Sofia Carvalho) Rua de Diogo Botelho 1327, 4169-005 Porto, Portugal. Telefone: (+351) 226 196 216. Fax: (+351) 226 196 291. E-mail. ib@porto.ucp.pt.

Faculdade de Filosofia da Universidade Católica Portuguesa, Bioética Geral (Director: Prof. Doutor J.H. Silveira de Brito), Praça da Faculdade 1, 4710-297 Braga. Telefone: (+351) 253 201 200. Fax: (+351) 253 201 210. E-mail: secretaria.facfil@braga.ucp.pt

SBEM da Faculdade de Medicina da Universidade do Porto (Director: Prof. Doutor Rui Nunes) Alameda Prof. Hernâni Monteiro, 4200-319 Porto, Portugal. Telefone: (+351) 225 513 625. Fax: (+351) 225 513 697. E-mail: ruinunes@med.up.pt

Universidade dos Açores, Departamento de Filosofia (Director: Prof. Doutora Maria do Céu Patrão Neves) Campus de Ponta Delgada, Apartado 1422, 9501-801 Ponta Delgada, S. Miguel, Açores, Portugal. Telefone: (+351) 296 650 000. Fax: (+351) 296 650 005. E-mail: patrao@notes.uac.pt

References

Biscaia J, Osswald W (1995) Bioethics in Portugal: 1991–1993. In: Lustig BA (ed) Bioethics year book, vol 4. Kluwer, Dordrecht, pp 285–289

Nuñez MP, Abel F (1992) Bioethics in Portugal: 1989–1991. In: Lustig BA (ed) Bioethics year book, vol 2. Kluwer, Dordrecht, pp 265–271

Bibliography[1]

Almeida F (2004) Ética em Pediatria: uma nova dinâmica num relacionamento vital?. Edição do Autor, Porto

Antunes JL (2005) Sobre a mão e outros ensaios. Gradiva, Lisboa

Archer L (2006) Da genética à biótica. Gráfica de Coimbra, Coimbra

[1] A short list of books that might be useful for scholars and bioethicists; this list does not aim to be comprehensive or complete.

Archer L, Biscaia J, Osswald W (eds) (1996) Bioética. Editorial Verbo, Lisboa
Archer L, Biscaia J, Osswald W, Renaud M (eds) (2001) Novos desafios à bioética. Porto Editora, Porto
Biscaia J (ed) (1998) Bem da pessoa, bem comum. Gráfica de Coimbra, Coimbra
Biscaia J (2004) Perder para encontrar. Gráfica de Coimbra, Coimbra
Biscaia J (2005) Ao encontro da ternura. Gráfica de Coimbra, Coimbra
Brito JHS (ed) (2001) Bioética: questões em debate. Faculdade de Filosofia da Universidade Católica Portuguesa, Braga
Cabral R (2000) Temas de Ética. Universidade Católica Portuguesa, Braga
Carvalho AS (ed) (2000) Clonagem: o risco e o desafio. Gabinete de Investigação de Bioética da Universidade Católica Portuguesa, Porto
Coutinho V (2005) Bioética e Teologia: Que paradigma de interacção?. Gráfica de Coimbra, Coimbra
Cunha JT (2002) Bioética breve. Paulus Editora, Apelação (Portugal)
Leone S, Privitera S, Cunha JT (2001) Dicionário de bioética. Editorial Perpétuo Socorro, Vila Nova Gaia
Neves MCP (ed) (2002) Comissões de Ética: das bases teóricas à actividade quotidiana. Gráfica de Coimbra, Coimbra
Neves MC Patrão, Pacheco S (eds) (2004) Para um ética da enfermagem. Desafios. Gráfica de Coimbra, Coimbra
Neves MC Patrão (ed) (2005) Bioética ou bioéticas. Gráfica de Coimbra, Coimbra
Nunes, R. (1995). Questões éticas do diagnóstico pré-natal da doença genética. Editora do Autor, Porto
Nunes R, Melo H, Nunes C (eds) (2002) Genoma e dignidade humana. Gráfica de Coimbra, Coimbra
Nunes R, Melo H, Nunes C (eds) (2000) Genoma e reprodução humana. Gráfica de Coimbra, Coimbra
Nunes R, Melo H, Nunes C (eds) (2001) A ética e o direito no início da vida humana. Gráfica de Coimbra, Coimbra
Nunes R, Rego G (eds) (2002) Prioridades na saúde. McGraw Hill, Lisbon
Oliveira G (1999) Temas de Direito da Medicina. Coimbra Editora, Coimbra
Osswald W (ed) (2003) Direitos do homem e biomedicina. Universidade Católica Editora, Porto
Osswald W (2004) Um fio de Ética. Gráfica de Coimbra, Coimbra
Pinto JR Costa (2004) Questões actuais da ética médica, 4th edn. Editorial A.O., Braga
Serrão D, Nunes R (eds) (1999) Ética em cuidados de saúde. Porto Editora, Porto
Silva JR, Barbosa A, Vale F (eds) (2002) Contributos para a bioética em Portugal. Cosmos, Lisbon

Chapter 19
Historical Development of Bioethics in Puerto Rico

Leonides Santos y Vargas

19.1 Introduction: The Present

On September 5, 2006, the Governor of the Commonwealth of Puerto Rico, the Honorable Aníbal Acevedo Vilá, issued an executive order by which he authorized the establishment of the Bioethics Advisory Board of Puerto Rico (BAB). The nine members of the BAB were meant to advise the Office of the Governor in areas having to do with the bioethical implications of legislation and government policies in matters of health, science, and environment. The BAB began meeting officially in May 2007.

The BAB of Puerto Rico is comprised of four physicians, a gerontologist, a lawyer, a professor of pharmacy, a philosopher, and a theologian-bioethicist. The board appointed a Coordinator of Research and Projects (a philosopher-bioethicist) to coordinate the activities that will carry out the mission of the BAB, the members of which will be in charge of promoting and organizing the research and public outreach activities sponsored by the board.

The decision to establish the BAB was the result of several recommendations that were included in the final report of a commission in charge of evaluating the health system of Puerto Rico. That commission was created by the governor of Puerto Rico in 2005, and was commissioned to evaluate the Puerto Rican health system in terms of its financial resources, administrative structures, effects on the education of health professionals, and the ethical dimensions and implications of the health reforms that were implemented beginning in 1993.

Evaluating the health system was a result of the public uproar that caused the privatization of the prior public health system in 1993, which had been in place since the beginning of the 20th century. The reform was allegedly geared towards the health needs of the medically indigent population of Puerto Rico. Since 1993, the governmental budget for health care has been distributed among competing

L. Santos y Vargas
Physician Director of the Institute of Bioethics Medical Sciences,
Universidad de Puerto Rico, San Juan, PR
e-mail: leosanvar@yahoo.com

L. Pessini et al. (eds.), *Ibero-American Bioethics: History and Perspectives*,
Philosophy and Medicine 106, DOI 10.1007/978-1-4020-9350-0_19,

private health maintenance organizations and private health insurance corporations, which intervene in the recruitment of individual providers and group providers for health care services. One reason the former system required reform was its need to contain the spiraling tendency of the public health system's expenditures due, allegedly, to the inefficiency of the state health agencies.

Cost containment was one of the basic justifications for the adoption of the new privatized system. Another of the reform's salient features was the adoption of the managed care approach in 1993, as a better way to distribute and control scarce public resources and as a strategy to implement cost containment measures. The managed care approach assigned primary physicians the role of gatekeepers in accessing the new system. As gatekeepers, they would bear the responsibility of channeling the care needs of the medically indigent population. It was believed that this control would ensure a better utilization of the resources appropriated by the state. No patient under this model can directly access services from a medical specialist, pharmacy, or laboratory, nor can one be hospitalized without prior authorization and referral by the primary physician assigned to the patient.

The ethics committee of the evaluation commission decided to evaluate the system from the perspective of the four principles typically associated with clinical bioethics: autonomy, beneficence, non-maleficence, and distributive justice, in addition to other considerations, such as the impact of the new model on the virtues and professionalism of caregivers, especially physicians. The use of bioethics as a needed frame of reference from which to evaluate a public health system is, undoubtedly, the highest recognition that this discipline has achieved a socially relevant position in our milieu.

The generalized acceptance of bioethics in Puerto Rico has been further evidenced by the fact that since February 23, 2007, the Medical Sciences Campus of the University of Puerto Rico (UPR) (under the leadership of the Hostos Institute for Bioethics) has been training a group of 22 professors in the field of bioethics. The institutional goal of the training is to prepare a critical mass of university professors who, after intensive study, will be capable of conducting bioethical research, teaching bioethics, and participating in hospital ethics committees, as well as in the many universities' institutional review boards (IRBs). After the completion of the training session (12 months), the participants will receive a Professional Certificate in Bioethics. For this year-long training session, several courses were designed, including: Foundations of Bioethics, Clinical Bioethics, Social Bioethics, Bioethics and Research, Special Topics in Bioethics, and a Seminar in Research Bioethics.

Besides the participation of qualified Puerto Rican bioethicists and philosophy professors (like Drs. Jorge Ferrer, Sandra Fábregas, Héctor Huyke, Rafael Ruiz Quijano, and Leonides Santos y Vargas), the teaching activities have been enriched by the presentations of guest lecturers from Spain, Argentina, México, Venezuela, Brazil, and Chile. Professors Juan Carlos Alvarez (Spain), Delia Outomuro and José A. Mainetti (Argentina), Volnei Garrafa (Brazil), Gilberto Cely Galindo (Colombia), and Fernando Lolas Stepke (Chile) have all contributed valuable international and diverse perspectives.

The faculty development initiative has been possible because of a grant from the Pan-American Health Organization (PAHO)'s office in Puerto Rico and appropriations from the institutional budget assigned to the Hostos Institute for Bioethics of the Medical Sciences Campus at the UPR. Both the Office of the Chancellor and the Dean of Academic Affairs at this campus have been very supportive of this initiative.

The official recognition of bioethics as an intellectual and practical assessment of social policies in Puerto Rico and its growing acceptance as part of the university mission are due to the patient, rigorous, and anonymous work of a small group of individual academics, private professionals, and university departments that have been promoting a bioethics culture through public conferences, congresses, public lectures, newspaper interviews and publications, and radio and television appearances.

19.2 The Pioneering Phase: The UPR, Mayagüez Campus

In 1979, the UPR, at Mayagüez (a large city at the Western extreme of Puerto Rico), received a grant from the Fundación Puertorriqueña de las Humanidades (the Puerto Rican branch of the USA National Endowment for the Humanities, NEH), to sponsor a series of symposia on medical ethics. The project was designed and organized by Elena Lugo, Ph.D., a member of the philosophy department at the Mayagüez campus. These symposia were initially intended to serve the needs of undergraduate pre-medical students, but the organizer and participants felt that something else was also needed for the students enrolled in the newly established industrial microbiology program. As a result, a bioethics course was developed with a focus on research ethics, university–industry relations, and the relation of the life sciences to social issues.

Later, the UPR-Mayagüez campus established the Center of Philosophy in its Interdisciplinary Function (CEPHIF). The director of the center was Dr. Elena Lugo. CEPHIF endeavored to achieve its purpose by sponsoring regular academic courses, short courses, workshops, discussion sessions, colloquia, and international congresses and conferences. Since its creation, it has sponsored two inter-American congresses, in which participants from 24 nations have come together to discuss the relationship between technology and theoretical and practical knowledge, as well as the complex interplay between technology, politics, economics, and social institutions in North, Central, and South America from a philosophical perspective.

After various years of successful initiatives, CEPHIF evolved and is now known as the Center for Ethics in the Professions. As such, this center has promoted the establishment of trans-curricular courses for the various faculties from different professional programs offered at the UPR-Mayagüez campus. For example, it offers courses on engineering ethics (for engineering students) and clinical bioethics (for pre-medical students). Surrounding hospitals in the city of Mayagüez have also benefited from the consultation services offered by, above all, Dr. Elena Lugo.

Professor Lugo has significantly contributed to the bioethics literature and its cognates in Puerto Rico. As evidence of her intellectual work, a bibliography of her works is provided at the end of this essay. In addition to her pioneering efforts in the promotion of bioethics, Dr. Elena Lugo was also one of the founding members of the Puerto Rican Federation of Bioethics (PRFB) and one of its past presidents.

19.3 The Medical Sciences Campus of the UPR

The earliest encounter with bioethics at the Medical Sciences Campus (MSC) of the UPR was when Edmund D. Pellegrino, M.D., and David Thomasma, Ph.D., two prominent bioethicists, were invited to deliver public lectures at the beginning of the 1980s. Several efforts to promote the study of the medical humanities and bioethics were made during the 1980s and early 1990s, including the establishment of an ethics committee at the university hospital; the appointment of a medical humanities committee by the Academic Dean; and the establishment of the journal, *Health and Culture* (*Salud y Cultura*), at the College of Health Related Professions (one of the academic entities affiliated with MSC).

An important step was taken in 1993 with the unofficial establishment of the Hostos Bioethics Center (Centro Hostosiano de Bioética), under the leadership of Dr. Leonides Santos y Vargas, a philosopher who had been connected with the MSC for several years as Dean of the College of Health Related Professions (1986–1993). In 1995, due to the vision of Dr. Jorge Sánchez, then Chancellor of the MSC, the "Eugenio María de Hostos" Institute for Humanistic Studies and Bioethics (Instituto de Estudios Humanísticos y Bioética "Eugenio María de Hostos") was established as a way to officially endorse the idea behind the former Hostos Bioethics Center. Since 1995, the Institute has developed into a more visible and accepted institutional establishment. The name of Eugenio María de Hostos had been associated with the Institute in homage to the famous nineteenth century Puerto Rican philosopher who wrote extensively about ethics and law, emphasizing the role of ethics in the professions. In March 2006, the Institute was renamed the Hostos Bioethics Institute (Instituto Hostosiano de Bioética-IHB).

Functioning under the Dean of Academic Affairs, the IHB is provisionally located at the MSC main library. The mission of the Institute includes the teaching and research of bioethics in its humanistic origins (history, philosophy, history of medicine, and critical thinking), as well as in relation to the education of scientists and medical practitioners. Throughout its history, the IHB has promoted bioethical discussions throughout the wider community and has organized activities to facilitate a dialogue between literary and scientific humanism for liberally educated persons who seek to do more than master a particular domain of specialized knowledge.

One of the achievements of the IHB was its receipt of a $187,000 grant from the National Endowment for the Humanities in Washington for 1998–2000. This grant was utilized to make possible the training of 32 university professors (from mainland America and Puerto Rico) in the contents and method of bioethics. International scholars participated in the teaching process during the months of June and July at the 1998, 1999, and 2000 summer sessions. Among those prominent scholars were

Edmund Pellegrino, Diego Gracia Guillén, Javier Gafo, Baruch Brody, and Joseph Fins – all of whom spent a week sharing their knowledge and experience with participants. The proceedings of those summer training sessions were published in a book titled *Humanities and the Health Sciences*.

Another great achievement of the IHB was the successful organization of the Fourth Congress of FELAIBE (Federación Latinomericana y del Caribe de Instituciones de Bioética), which took place at the Wyndham Conquistador Hotel in Fajardo, Puerto Rico, on September 24–27, 2003. This congress is still remembered as one of the best academic events because of its intellectual quality and institutional impact on the university's acceptance of bioethics.

During the time Dr. Santos y Vargas was in charge of the IHB, he authored several publications. A list of these is given at the end of this essay.

19.4 Initiatives Outside of Academia: The Bioethics Seminar

In 1993, the Bioethics Seminar (Círculo de Bioética) convened, following the initiative of a group of friends interested in bioethics. The idea originated with Dr. Jorge Ferrer, a Jesuit priest and moral theologian interested in bioethical issues. Dr. Ferrer shared his idea with two physician friends: Rafael Ruiz-Quijano, a urologist and member of the Council for Ethico-Judicial Affairs (CEJA) of the Puerto Rican Medical Association (PRMA), and Ernesto Frontera, a psychiatrist. Both physicians were in private practice. The basic idea was to convene a small interdisciplinary group interested in holding a monthly seminar. The Bioethics Seminar has held numerous meetings since 1993 and has been a truly interdisciplinary group by including physicians, philosophers, nurses, a microbiologist, a pharmacist, and other health professionals. The seminar was a stimulating forum and a training opportunity for professionals interested in bioethics. Many members of the seminar have played key roles in the initiatives of the PRMA and in the founding of the PRFB and, subsequently, in the creation of the Hostos Institute for Bioethics.

19.5 Initiatives Taken by the Puerto Rico Medical Association

On November 13, 1993, Dr. Jorge Lastra, one of the founding members of the Bioethics Seminar, was inaugurated as President of the PRMA. A main platform of his presidential program was the promotion of bioethics through the PRMA. Dr. Lastra appointed a sub-committee for education in bioethics that was to work under the CEJA. Dr. Ruiz-Quijano, another founding member of the seminar, was appointed as chair of the sub-committee. This sub-committee was asked to develop a program for the continuing education of medical professionals, as well as supporting the development of curricula for medical schools and premedical programs in

Puerto Rico. On August 28, 1994, an entire day was devoted to the study of bioethics, the "Day of Bioethics" ("Jornada de Bioética"). The program took place at the San Juan Hotel in Isla Verde and was followed by a series of weekly lectures held at the Association's headquarters.

More important than these public activities was the coming together, for the first time, of several people interested in bioethics. The sub-committee had also invited people who were interested in the field but were not yet working together. Among the members of the subcommittee were Dr. Elena Lugo, Dr. Eduardo Santiago Delpín, Dr. Rafael Burgos Calderón, Dr. Ramón Isales, Dr. Jorge Ferrer, and many others.

It is worth mentioning that since the 1990s, Dr. Rafael Burgos Calderón (a nephrologist) has been the president of the ethics committee at the UPR University Hospital, and for several years was Puerto Rico's representative at the PAHO. In addition, he was an advisor to the Department of Health. Due to his leadership, since 1995, the ethics committee of the University Hospital has organized many training activities on bioethics for more than 500 professionals, including: nurses, residents in training, medical faculty and hospital administrators. The director of the Hostos Institute for Bioethics (who, for more than 10 years, has been a member of University Hospital's ethics committee) has frequently been in charge of the educational and case analysis activities that the hospital ethics committee has organized.

Dr. Santiago Delpín, Professor of Surgery at UPR and a leading transplant surgeon, has also been interested in bioethics for a number of years and had been working to establish a bioethics curriculum at UPR School of Medicine. Aside from being a world renowned transplant surgeon, he is also a recognized poet and has published several collections of his poems.

19.6 Additional Efforts

As a continued and combined effort, initiated by CEJA (of PRMA) with other members of the PRFB, the week of February 26 through March 5, 1995, was officially declared "The First Week of Bioethics in Puerto Rico" by the Secretary of Health, Dr. Carmen Feliciano-Melecio.

Several agencies from the public and private sectors joined in this effort, namely, the Puerto Rico Department of Health, the PAHO, and all three local accredited medical schools in addition to the recently created PRFB. Prominent international figures in bioethics participated during the week's educational activities. Dr. Diego Gracia (a leading Spanish bioethicist and professor at the Universidad Complutense in Madrid) visited under the sponsorship of PAHO. In addition, three prominent U.S. educators in bioethics (Nancy M.P. King, J.D.; James J. McCartney, Ph.D.; and Stuart F. Spicker, Ph.D.) conducted a five-day touring workshop on Educating Healthcare Ethics Committees (EHEC), supported in part by the Fund for the Improvement of Postsecondary Education (FIPSE) of the U.S. Department of Education. Their participation was also sponsored by CEJA of PRMA through an educational grant provided by Rhone-Poulenc Rorer Caribbean, Inc. The workshop began with a one-day plenary conference devoted to discussions of the philosophical, legal, and religious aspects of HECs in American health institutions. The plenary session was held at the PRMA's Past Presidents Auditorium. Physicians, lawyers, health care professionals, academicians, and philosophers, as well as the general public, from all over the island, participated in the first session. During the remainder of the tour, the three EHEC faculty members met with health care ethics committees from different private and public hospitals on the island. The local arrangements committee was formed by Professor E. Lugo, Ph.D., Dr. J. Ferrer, and Dr. R. Ruiz-Quijano, President of PRMA's CEJA. It was a very productive week, which served to motivate all of the island's medical schools to formally include topics from the medical humanities and bioethics in their curriculum.

During the August 1995 PRMA Board of Directors meeting, a motion presented by Dr. Rafael Ruiz-Quijano, seeking to formally include at least one topic in bioethics in all of their continued scientific medical education programs, was unanimously approved. A similar resolution was also approved at the assembly of PRMA's House of Delegates, held in October of the same year.

Recognizing the limitations of a voluntary association in dealing with the different influences affecting the medical profession, as well as the patient's best interests over the past 20 years, PRMA began lobbying with the island's government to create a College of Physicians. In August 1994, Law 77, creating the Puerto Rican College of Physicians (PRCP), was passed, requiring mandatory membership for all physicians. On September 10, 1995, the first Board of Directors of the PRCP was elected and its general by-laws were approved. The elected President of the college asked the PRFB to assist in the formulation of its Code of Ethics.

19.7 The Puerto Rican Federation of Bioethics

The final effort to establish the Federation of Bioethics came from within the Bioethics Seminar, due to the fact that Dr. Ernesto Frontera took the initiative to call a meeting of interested persons. A good deal of enthusiasm was generated by the coming together of people working in the field. In January 1995, the Federation's core group attended its first meeting. Dr. Frontera was elected coordinator and a series of meetings was held to develop a document that would reflect the federation's basic philosophy. Since its creation, it has been an autonomous, non-profit organization committed to the promotion of ethical and humanistic values in biomedicine, health, and the environment. Its intentions are to promote the open discussion of ideas in the field of bioethics, understood as an interdisciplinary enterprise, in addition to promoting research and scholarship in the field. In this spirit, its founding members have participated in public debates whenever appropriate.

Among its activities, the federation began to offer consultation services for the development of a bioethics program at the Ponce School of Medicine, located in Southern Puerto Rico. Several members of the core group also worked as consultants to the School of Medicine in Bayamón (a private institution) in order to develop a program in the medical humanities. Dr. Ernesto Frontera, the federation's coordinator at the time, was a faculty member, as well as President of the Medical Humanities Committee at that institution.

Since the creation of the PRFB, the founding members of the Federation (Ernesto Frontera, Elena Lugo, José M. García-Castro, Leonides Santos y Vargas, the late José R. Echevarría, R. Ruiz-Quijano, and Jorge Ferrer) have been actively involved in multiple professional and academic activities geared toward the promotion of a bioethical culture in Puerto Rico.

Dr. Jorge Ferrer, for example, has not only been a scholar in the field of Puerto Rican bioethics but has also been an inspiring force, due to his personal traits and undisputed intellectual brightness. Everyone who now holds a leadership role promoting a culture of bioethics within the Puerto Rican community and institutions has had Dr. Ferrer as a reference model. His devotion to bioethics as an academic discipline and as a social movement can be attested to by his intellectual production and publications, some of which are required reading in Puerto Rico. Some of his many publications are listed at the end of this essay.

There is still another initiative that deserves mention. The Inter-American UPR (IUPR), the largest private university in Puerto Rico (founded in 1912), for several years has served as a forum for the promotion of bioethics, especially at its San German campus. Unfailingly, every October since 1987, it has sponsored a public lecture dedicated to topics relevant to bioethics. This activity is held in memory of Dr. Boyd D. Palmer (a late biology researcher and professor at IUPR). The first lecture was offered in 1987 by the late David Thomasma under the title "Bioethics in the Modern World." Since then, other lecturers have followed, some of whom can be mentioned as evidence of the high intellectual quality of this activity: Richard Zaner, Edmund Pellegrino, Javier Gafo, Thomas D. Murray, Robert Veatch, Warren Reich, and many others.

19.8 The Future

In spite of the growing institutional acceptance of bioethics at the universities, as evidenced above, there is still a pressing need to establish departments and chairs in bioethics and the medical humanities at every institution where health professionals and scientists are trained. This process of institutionalization is necessary not only to guarantee the full liberal education of future health professionals and scientists, but also to facilitate the production of creative scholarship in the field.

In summary, we can reasonably affirm that the early 1990s witnessed the birth of the bioethics movement in Puerto Rico. Since that time, a number of initiatives and activities have been organized: public congresses (with international representation), public conferences, and interviews on television and radio. In addition, the publication of articles and opinions in newspapers, and new books and articles in professional journals of diverse academic rigor have contributed to the public acceptance of bioethical discourse as a credible approach to understanding and analyzing many of the innovations in biomedical technology and public policy.

The bioethical movement in Puerto Rico has developed a momentum that is difficult to stop. What began with the initial steps of the establishment of the PRFBs, the Institute of Medical Humanities, the establishment of the Hostos Institute for Bioethics at the Medical Sciences Campus, and the creation of the Advisory Board on Bioethics by the Governor of Puerto Rico, is now proof that bioethics will be a decisive force in suggesting enlightened public policies to direct the developments in health services, scientific research, and environmental concerns.

Over the short term, the bioethics agenda of Puerto Rico will have to address the following topics: the reevaluation of the ethical foundations of the health care system (within the public and private sector), the bioethical implications of Puerto Rico's conversion to a Mecca of biotechnology (the "Bio Island," as our governor has labeled this policy), the crisis of professionalism, and the demise of the natural environment due to uncontrolled urban and corporate developments.

Based upon the developments achieved, bioethics in Puerto Rico should be taken to the public sphere. That is, bioethics should not be interpreted as a new academic paradigm solely relevant to university professionals. We must work to translate bioethics into a popular language that the people can utilize to make sense of the challenges posed by science, health reforms, and our relationship to the environment. Bioethicists should strive to empower civic society, because after all is said and done, it is the people who will either enjoy or regret the results of those challenges.

Publications by Elena Lugo[1]

Lugo E (2006) Bioética personalista según la visión orgánica del Padre Jose Kentenich. Editorial Patris, Cordoba, Argentina

Lugo E (2003) Filosofía de la medicina. Revista de Cardiologia, Buenos Aires

Lugo E (2002) Relación médico-paciente: ética y espiritualidad. Agoras, Bogota

Lugo E (2001) Error y certeza en el juicio clínico: implicaciones éticas de los errores en medicina. QUIRON 32(2/3):78–89

Lugo E (2000) Naturaleza y funciones de los Comités Institucionales: experiencias en USA. Publicación de la Academia Nacional de Medicina, Buenos Aires, Argentina

Lugo E (1999a) Empatía e intersubjetividad: modelo fenomenológico de la relación médico-paciente. Revista de Médicos Católicos, Buenos Aires

Lugo E (1999b) Edith Stein y su concepto de Dios. Revista de Psicoterapia Simbólica, Buenos Aires

Lugo E (1998a) Anthology of Conferences: Filosofía de la Medicina, Espiritualidad y ética clínica. Universidad Tecnológica del Cibao, Dominican Republic, Relación de intersubjetividad entre médico y paciente

Lugo E (1998b) Temas de bioética. Editorial Schoenstatt, Buenos Aires

[1] Drs. Elena Lugo and Jorge Ferrer Negrón submitted much of the information that has been included in this article. Some of the historical details reviewed here were published in *HEC Forum*, 1996.

Lugo E (1998c) Filosofía de la medicina y otros temas. Universidad Técnica del Cibao, Dominican Republic
Lugo E (1995) Reflexiones sobre el Proyecto del Genoma Humano. Temas de Enfermería Actualizados, Buenos Aires
Lugo E (1995) Proyecto del Genoma Humano. Antiguas y nuevas responsabilidades éticas, Atenea, Mayagüez, Puerto Rico
Lugo E (1995) The being of personhood in Mary and her role before the 'Technological Man.' In: RP and JE Francis (eds) Christian humanism. Peter Lang, New York
Lugo E (1995) Joseph Kentenich: Social, moral integration of the person. In: RP and JE Francis (eds) Christian humanism. Peter Lang, New York
Lugo E (1994) Reflections on philosophy, spirituality and mariology. In: Astell A (ed) Divine presentations. Paulist Press, New York
Lugo E (1992a) Woman and violence. Proceedings from the 2nd World Congress on violence and human coexistence. Montreal, Canada
Lugo E (1992b) "New dimensions for action", new worlds, new technologies, new issues. Lehigh University Press, PA, Research in Technology Issues
Lugo E (1990a) Concepto de la enfermedad y de la enfermedad mental. Universidad de Costa Rica, Revista de la Filosofía
Lugo E (1990b) Ethics in academic research. Sigma, Mayagüez, Puerto Rico
Lugo E (1989) Manual de ética fundamental. Editorial de la Universidad de Puerto Rico en Mayagüez, Puerto Rico
Lugo E (1985a) Ética profesional de la ingeniería. Editorial Riqueñas, Mayagüez, Puerto Rico
Lugo E (1985b) Philosophy of technology. Atenea, Mayagüez, Puerto Rico
Lugo E (1987) Psiquiatría y ética. Editorial de la Universidad de Puerto Rico en Mayagüez, Puerto Rico
Lugo E (1984) Ética médica. Editorial Riqueñas, Mayagüez, Puerto Rico

Publications by Jorge José Ferrer

Álvarez JC, Ferrer JJ (2005) Bioética. In: Tamayo JJ (ed) Nuevo diccionario de teología. Trotta, Madrid
Álvarez JC, Ferrer JJ (2003) Para fundamentar la bioética: teorías y paradigmas teóricos en la bioética contemporánea. Editorial Desclée de Brouwer, Bilabo
Ferrer JJ (2007) Deber y deliberacion: una invitacion a la bioetica. CEPA-UPR, Mayagüez
Ferrer JJ, Santory AO (2004) Hacia una bioética global. In: Alarcos FJ (ed) La moral cristiana como propuesta. San Pablo, Madrid
Ferrer JJ (2004) Genética y bioética. Milenio 7:64–81
Ferrer JJ (2003) Historia y fundamentos de los comités de bioética. In: Martínez JL (ed) Comités de bioética (Dilemas éticos de la medicina actual). Universidad Pontificia Comillas, Madrid, pp 17–42
Ferrer JJ (2002a) Medicina y espiritualidad: redescubriendo una antigua alianza. In: Ferrer JJ, Martínez JL (eds) Bioética: un diálogo plural. Universidad Pontificia Comillas, Madrid, pp 891–917
Ferrer JJ (2002b) El debate etico sobre la clonación humana. Razón y Fe 245:523–539
Ferrer JJ (2002c) La clonación de seres humanos: ciencia y conciencia. Sal Terrae 90(7):587–603
Ferrer JJ (2001a) El porqué y el qué de los Comités de Etica en Santos. In: Ferrer JJ, Damiani B (eds) Humanities and the health sciences. Scripta Humanistica, Potomac, MD, pp 117–132
Ferrer JJ (2001b) Ecoética. In: Santos L, Ferrer J, Damiani BM (eds) Humanities and the health sciences. Scripta Humanistica, Potomac, MD, pp 156–166
Ferrer JJ (2001c) Agenda bioética para Puerto Rico: un diálogo abierto. In: Santos L, Ferrer J, Damiani Bruno (eds) Humanities and the health sciences. Scripta Humanistica, Potomac, MD, pp 167–178

Ferrer JJ (2001d) Treinta años de bioética en el centenario de 'Razón y Fe'. Razón y Fe 243:591–596
Ferrer JJ (2001e) Javier Gafo: Bioeticista y teólogo. Revista Latinoamericana de Bioética 1:68–87
Ferrer JJ (2000a) Identidad profesional y compromiso ético en los tiempos del "managed care. Puerto Rico Health Sci J 19(1):83–86
Ferrer JJ (2000b) Needle exchange in San Juan, Puerto Rico: A traditional roman catholic casuistic approach. In: Keenan JF, Fuller JD, Cahill LS, Kelly K (eds) Catholic ethicists on HIV/AIDS prevention. Continuum Publishing Group, New York, pp 177–191
Ferrer JJ (2000c) Quod Omnes Tangit ab Omnibus Tractari Debet: una 'questio disputata' de epistemología moral en la teología católica. In: Gafo J (ed) Bioética y religiones. Universidad Pontificia Comillas, Madrid, pp 127–152
Ferrer JJ (2000d) El SIDA y los pobres del mundo. Jurisprudencia Argentina 6218:24–30
Ferrer JJ (1999a) Los trasplantes de órganos en la teología moral católica. In: Santiago Delpín E, Ruiz-Spearle JO (eds) Trasplante de órganos, 2nd edn. JGH Editores, México, pp 172–180
Ferrer JJ (1999b) Identidad profesional y compromiso ético: binomio irrenunciable. Hola M.T., 15.3, 18–19
Ferrer JJ (1998a) Reflexiones éticas a propósito de la clonación. Gregorianum 79:129–148
Ferrer JJ (1998b) Los principios de la bioética. Cuadernos del Programa Regional de Bioética 7:37–62
Ferrer JJ (1997a) Teorías éticas y principios bioéticos. Puerto Rico Health Sci J 16(1):81–86
Ferrer JJ (1997b) La reforma del sistema de prestación de los servicios de salud: consideraciones éticas. El Galeno, Puerto Rico
Ferrer JJ (1995) Los trasplantes de órganos ante la ética cristian. Boletín AMPR 87:94–97

Publications by Leonidas Santos y Vargas

Santos y Vargas L (2004) Hacia una bioética hostosiana. Exégesis (Revista de la UPR en Humacao) 17:48–50
Santos y Vargas L (2003) Valuación bioética del Proyecto Genoma Humano. Acta Bioética (Programa Regional de Bioética, OPS, Chile) 8 (1) (also published in *Ethos Gubernamental,* 1, 1, julio-diciembre)
Santos y Vargas L (ed) (2001a) Humanities and the health sciences. Scripta Humanistica, MD
Santos y Vargas L (2001b) Meditación sobre el genoma humano. Puerto Rico Health Sci J 20(1):63–7
Santos y Vargas L (2001c) Aproximación casuístico-inductiva a la bioética. Puerto Rico Health Sci J 20(3):
Santos y Vargas L (1999) Necesidad de la enseñanza de la bioética como una disciplina crítica. Puerto Rico Health Sci J 18(1):
Santos y Vargas L (1998) Bioética y sociedad. Puerto Rico Health Sci J 17(2):
Santos y Vargas L (1997a) Implicaciones éticas de las nuevas tecnologías reproductivas. Puerto Rico Health Sci J 16(3):
Santos y Vargas L (1997b) La justicia sanitaria como prioridad para América Latina. Puerto Rico Health Sci J 16(14):
Santos y Vargas L (1996a) Reflexión bioética en torno a pacientes renales. Salud Renal, Revista del Consejo Renal de PR 8
Santos y Vargas L (1996b) Implicaciones éticas del modelo de cuidado dirigido. Puerto Rico Health Sci J 15(2):
Santos y Vargas L (1994) Bases filosóficas de la bioética. Prensa Médica, Asociación Médica de PR, San Juan

Santos y Vargas L (1992b) Formación ética en la universidad. University of Puerto Rico, San Juan, Diálogo

Santos y Vargas L (1991) Integración social, salud y educación. In Educación y marginación urbana y modernización. Universidad Pedagógica Nacional, México, pp 683–701

Chapter 20
The Dynamics of the Bioethical Dialogue in Spain

Francesc Abel and Núria Terribas

20.1 Introduction

In this essay, the birth and development of bioethics in Spain are presented by distinguishing three historical periods. The first period extends from 1976 to 1984. In those years, the Borja Institute of Bioethics (Instituto Borja de Bioética), the first institute of its kind in Europe, was founded in Sant Cugat del Vallès (Barcelona). In 1984, the third meeting of the International Study Group on Bioethics of the International Federation of Catholic Universities (FIUC/IFCU) was held, also organized in Sant Cugat and with extensive repercussions for different Spanish universities. The second period spans from 1985 to 2000. These were years of expansion, development, and consolidation in Spanish bioethics, when significant legislation pertaining to medical–biological advances and their use was generated. During this time, jurists and philosophers also became acquainted with and interested in bioethical debates. Starting in 1990, diverse approaches and schools of bioethics began to define themselves: the emergence of apparent differences in attitudes and approaches to ethics and legislation could be seen, in addition to the growing division between the approaches of lay and faith-based ethics. The third period extends from 2001 to the present. This period can be considered one of review, projection, and integration, with different propositions being generated from those with polarized political views and strongly determined by techno-scientific, economic, and ethical–religious factors. This period also denotes a situation of greater complexity than in previous periods, due to the unlimited possibilities for scientific and technological advances.

F. Abel (✉)
Jesuit. Ph.D, Medicine (USA). President of the first European Institute of Bioethics, Instituto Borja de Bioética (Borja Institute of Bioethics) Barcelona, Spain
e-mail: fabel@ibb.hsjdbcn.org

N. Terribas
Jurist. Professor of the Borja Institute of Bioethics (IBB)
and Coordinator of IBB's MA in Bioethics
e-mail: fabel@ibb.hsjdbcn.org

L. Pessini et al. (eds.), *Ibero-American Bioethics: History and Perspectives*,
Philosophy and Medicine 106, DOI 10.1007/978-1-4020-9350-0_20,

20.2 The Birth of the Borja Institute of Bioethics

The Borja Institute of Bioethics (Instituto Borja de Bioética – IBB) was founded in 1976 on the initiative of its founding president, Dr. Francesc Abel, after his return from a 5-year stay in the United States. The Institute's development drew heavily on Dr. Abel's experiences and the knowledge he acquired while working under the direction of Dr. André Hellegers to complete his dissertation on fetus-placental physiology (a process that lasted more than 3 years) at Georgetown University. Dr. Abel witnessed the creation and growth of the first and most important two bioethics centers in the world: The Kennedy Institute (KI) and The Hastings Center. He returned to Spain determined to establish a bioethics institute modeled as closely as possible to the ones he had known in the United States, allowing for suitable adaptations and guided by three operative objectives: (1) to create a specialized library in bioethics; (2) to establish forums for bioethical dialogue in hospital settings by creating bioethics committees; (3) to maintain institutional independence from ecclesiastic and civil institutions. All of these objectives were gradually achieved. In 2000, the IBB was incorporated into the Universidad Ramon Llull (Barcelona).

Although the beginnings were difficult due to lack of resources, the founding members of the Institute maintained a strong conviction that the recognition of the fruitfulness and necessity of bioethical dialogue between health sciences and ethics was urgent. Above all, this required the introduction of the term "bioethics" into society in addition to conveying the concept and requirements of bioethical dialogue.

In Spain, the term "bioethics" came into use in 1976 and was easily accepted for a number of reasons, e.g.: (1) it distanced itself from a perception of ethics as religious, negative, authoritarian, and dogmatic, shaped by the hierarchy of the Catholic Church and the State; (2) the socio-political climate in Spain, from the death of Francisco Franco in 1975 and the approval of the 1978 Constitution by Parliament, was one of transition, as democracy and its teachings were introduced; (3) the prevailing intellectual climate of Spain's universities, and in particular the Society of Jesus (Compañía de Jesús), was one that easily accommodated interdisciplinary dialogue, because a large number of Jesuit professors were educated at universities in England, France, Belgium, Germany, Italy, and America, giving them diverse backgrounds on which to draw. In fact, IBB was created almost simultaneously with two other institutions, both of which were also founded by Jesuits and a group of university professors: Christianity and Justice (Cristianismo y Justicia – C&J)[1] and the Interdisciplinary Association of José Acosta (Asociación Interdisciplinar José de Acosta – ASINJA).[2]

---

[1] Founded and recognized simultaneously with the IBB. P. Ignacio Salvat, mediated in the approval of both statutes. C&J published a monthly issue on current controversial topics. Up to date, 141 titles have been published. The last five refer to: 141. Teresa Forcades i Vila. *Los crímenes de las grandes compañías farmacéuticas* (The crimes of Big-Pharma); 140. Lluís Magriñà. *Refugiados en el siglo XXI* (*Refugees in the XXI Century*); 139. Alfredo Marhuenda Fluixá. *¡Coge la lupa!* (*Use the magnifier!*); 138. José Ignacio González Faus. *Símbolos de fraternidad* (*Symbols of brotherhood*); 137. Óscar Mateos. *África el continente maltratado* (*Africa, the abused continent*).

[2] The Interdisciplinary Association José de Acosta was founded in 1984 and has been directed by Professor Albert Dou. Up to date, 32 volumes have been edited by various authors who specialize

The first definition of "bioethics" was adopted from the *Encyclopedia of Bioethics*: the systematic study of human conduct in life sciences and health care, insofar as this conduct is examined in the light of moral values and principles (Reich 1995). Nevertheless, the Institute enriched this definition by emphasizing the necessity of dialogue between the sciences and the humanities:

> Bioethics is the interdisciplinary (transdisciplinary) study of ethical decision-making for the solution of problems arising in different ethical systems due to medical and biological advances occurring in the microsocial and macrosocial, and micro- and macroeconomic environment and their impact in society and its value system, both in the present and in the future (Abel 2001, pp. 5–6).

This definition has the advantage of linking the ideas of the first bioethics institutes with the issues addressed by bioethics which, on the initiative of Dr. Van Rensselaer Potter (1911–2001) in 1985, can be classified as *clinical bioethics* and *global bioethics* (see, e.g., Potter 1970, 1971). During 1985, Potter had become annoyed with the clinical direction of bioethics at the KI and as a result coined the term "global bioethics" to emphasize his interest in ecological or environmental bioethics.

In 1976, Dr. Abel began to collaborate in the formation of the Clinical Ethics Committee (Comité de Ética Asistencial – CEA) of Sant Joan de Déu Hospital in Esplugues (Barcelona), continuing the work of a previous committee (1974). The CEA was the first ethics committee to be established and, despite its anonymity, was the only CEA in Spain for several years; it was also a forum for bioethical dialogue in a clinical setting, as had been envisioned by Dr. Hellegers.

The IBB began to establish an international presence in 1976 by participating in a debate on "Biology and Ethics" at the invitation of the organizers: "Fondation Internationale Humanum" of Lugano (Switzerland) and the "Fondation Prospective" of Brussels. The debate took place on September 2–4 among a restricted group of 40 scientists, moralists, and representatives from the hierarchy of the Catholic Church. Dr. Hellegers was among the guests, along with his followers and good friends from the KI. The debate unveiled the challenge of reconciling the different positions generated by bioethical issues, such as: hormonal contraception, assisted procreation (two years before Lesley Brown was born, thanks to in vitro fertilization and embryonic transference), the status of the human embryo, and other fundamental moral issues. The dialogue became highly controversial when representatives of the American bishops, to the surprise of European scientists and moralists, rejected European concepts of a secularized society and general ethics, interpreting the Europeans as supporting the laicization of society and the denial of God.

Pedro Arrupe (1907–1991), Superior General of the Society of Jesus, recognized from the very beginning the importance of bioethical dialogue at the international level. He also encouraged the creation of the International Group for the Study of Bioethics (GIEB/IEGB), by an independent statute, inside the International Federation

---

in different topics. The last volumes include: 28, *El pensamiento alternativo. Nueva visión sobre el hombre y la naturaleza* (Alternative thought. A new vision of mankind and nature) 2002; 29, *Nuevas tecnologías y futuro del hombre,* (New technologies and the future of mankind) 2003; 30, *Bioética: la cuestión de la dignidad,* (Bioethics: the issue of dignity) 2004; 31, *Investigación, desarrollo e innovación: cuestiones éticas* (Research, development and innovation: ethical issues) 2005; 32, *Ideologías: conflictos y tensiones* (Ideology: conflicts and tensions), 2006.

of Catholic Universities. The group was established in 1980 with Dr. Abel, president of the "Steering Committee," and P. Edouard Boné S. J. and Dr. John C. Harvey playing a crucial role in the coordination of 20 international meetings (Abel 2001, pp. 108–114). Sant Cugat was the site of the first three meetings that took place between 1982 and 1984. The discussions revolved around the following themes:

1. The expectations of genetic engineering and its risks for man and the environment
2. Policies to guide and monitor research
3. The beginning of human life and its manipulation
4. The concept of nature and the epistemological revolution

The need for profound interdisciplinary dialogue was recognized for the purpose of discussing the meaning of concepts that, when used by scientists, philosophers, or theologians, have different connotations and occasionally produce opposite meanings. More specifically, the importance of scientific or philosophical backgrounds in shaping the perceptions and significance of fundamental words such as "life," "dignity," and "person" was acknowledged.

A large group of Jesuit scientists with degrees in the humanities (philosophy, theology, anthropology) held professorships at public and private universities and experienced the possibilities of bioethical dialogue when their positions were challenged by the positions of other Jesuits, professors of philosophy or theology, or secular scientists. The international dimension of cooperation between the Church and the world, and the narrow collaboration between Jesuits and laypeople, did not need to be emphasized because such was clear.

Some of the participants of the first two IEGB meetings creatively promoted the dynamics experienced in bioethical dialogue. These participants included Spanish theologians, scientists, and philosophers. Among the Spanish theologians were Manuel Cuyás, Javier Gafo, and Juan Masiá (who created the Sophia University, Tokyo), and Eduardo López Azpitarte; among the scientists were Carlos Alonso Bedate, Manuel García Doncel, Ramón Mª Nogués, Juan Ramón Lacadena, Ignacio Núñez de Castro, Julián Rubio Cardiel, Jacobo Cárdenas, and Josep Egozcue; and among the philosophers were Arturo Juncosa, Augusto Hortal, and Eusebio Colomer. Moreover, among the foreign participants in the initial IEGB meetings, the theologian Klaus Demmer should be highlighted along with the scientists Edouard Boné, Luis Archer, Thomas J. King, and Angelo Serra. The physicians deserving special mention include Dr. John C. Harvey, Víctor Conill, Jordi Font, Josep Mª Dexeus, Xavier Iglesias, Antonio Tejedo, Luís Campos, Joaquín Plaza, Pere N. Barri, and Josep M. Carrera. Also actively present at these meetings was the Hno. Gabino Gorostieta, of the Hospital Order of St. John of God (Orden Hospitalaria de San Juan de Dios), who made contributions from the perspective of nursing and pastoral medical assistance, and who was an advocate for the creation of the health care ethics committee in Barcelona.[3]

[3] The creation of ethics committees for medical care has always received the firm support of the Order and especially the current support of Hno. General Pascual Piles. In Barcelona, the collaboration of Brothers Jose Luis Redrado and Miguel Martín, among others, has also been added.

During this initial period, these meetings had an extensive international impact but did not resonate as much within the Spanish community.

The IBB was a charter member of the European Association of Centers of Medical Ethics (EACME/AECEM), whose foundations were conceived between 1984 and 1986. The creation of EACME was due to the initiative of Dr. Maurice de Wachter, who had been working from 1978 until 1984 at the Center for Bioethics at the Clinical Research Institute of Montreal. This center was created at the same time as the IBB by Dr. David Roy and became a reference center for ethical consultations to the 26 research laboratories in Montreal (Abel 2001, p. 40). In 1984, Dr. de Wachter was nominated as the Director of the Maastricht Institute for Bioethics. These bioethics centers began to exchange opinions about how to promote the development of bioethics in Europe. Other centers that might have been interested in the exchange were also invited to participate at various meetings and, today, the association is comprised of more than 70 centers. The constituent Assembly of the Association was held September 26, 1986 (De Wachter 2006).

It is very clear that the reflections that occurred during 1960–1977 had as a frame of reference the ethical responses to different scientific discoveries and innovative technologies of undoubted social importance, including intensive care units (1960); hormonal contraception (1960); renal (1960) and cardiac transplants (1967); prenatal-karyotype diagnosis (1969); and ultrasound scans (1975). But, the most profound change in medicine consisted of recognizing the rights of patients as autonomous moral agents which guided the transition from a paternalistic to a contractual approach to medicine.

20.3 The Second Period

Many significant events occurred during what has been defined as the second period of bioethics. For example, the discovery of restriction enzymes in the 1970s enabled the controlled recombination of DNA particles (genetic engineering), and Professor J. R. Lacadena wrote an interesting essay about the Nobel Prizes in genetics, "Historia Nobelada de la Genética: Concepto y método" (Lacadena 1995). Also during this time, the diagnosis of fetal malformations was perfected; advancements in immunology and surgical skills facilitated improvements in organ and tissue transplants; and agreements were reached about the definition of brain death and the description of persistent vegetative states. In 1978, the first successful in vitro fertilization and embryo transference (IVF-ET) was achieved. In the same year, the Belmont Report was published, identifying three basic bioethical principles that influenced the Western world: respect for persons, beneficence, and justice.

In this period (1) bioethical dialogue spread and became more complex; (2) Spanish bioethicists from diverse backgrounds such as philosophy, law, economics, and politics were brought together and conducted themselves in a brave and responsible manner; (3) in the search for human progress, the differences among the three primary rationalities (techno-scientific, legal–political, and faith-based ethics) were stressed.

This allowed one to distinguish three practical–theoretical approaches (Barreau 1989, pp. 194–216) to bioethical discourse, depending on their foundation: (1) ethics, (2) theology, or (3) law. Furthermore, this period was characterized by a search for the most appropriate and essential applications of new knowledge and biomedical technologies for humans, which was more precisely expressed in the concept of "quality of life" as a basis for all medical research and bioethical discussion.

This period closed with the signature of The European Convention on Biomedicine and Human Rights in Oviedo (Spain). It was ratified by Parliament on October 19, 1999, and became law on January 1, 2000,[4] bringing an end to a period of evolution, for better or worse, in which bioethics tended towards the development of bioethical law.

The different trends in bioethics will be explained from the perspectives of (1) the ethical foundation of bioethics; (2) the theological foundation of bioethics; (3) the legal foundation of bioethics; and (4) testimony and narrative in bioethics.

20.3.1 The Ethical Foundation of Bioethics

A. University Ramón Llull (Barcelona) and Borja Institute of Bioethics

The initiative and personal effort of Dr. Francesc Abel, S. J., led to the founding of the IBB in 1976. Serving as director until 1999, Dr. Abel's contact with the Institute contributed to the continuity and development of his work, particularly in four fields:

1. Teaching and training in bioethics.[5]
2. Research in bioethics: The IBB participated in different research projects, at the European, international, and Spanish levels. The IBB participated in projects financed by the European Union, including: (1) The Biomed II Project on "Human Embryonic and Fetal Tissue Transplantation," coordinated by professors Guido de Wert and Ron Berghmans (de Wert et al. 2002); (2) a joint publication (IBB and the Centre for Ethics and Law) of two volumes on "Basic Ethical Principles in European Bioethics and Biolaw," coordinated by Dr. Peter Kemp, director of the Center for Ethics and Law (Copenhagen) (Rendtorff and Kemp 2000). The IBB was also developing its own research projects on different issues related to bioethics. Some of the projects resulted in publications and there are now more than 30 related titles. In addition, since 1995, the IBB has begun producing a quarterly journal, *Bioethics & Debate* (*Bioética & Debat*), which addresses current bioethical topics using clear and didactic language.
3. Advising: The IBB contributes to and staffs health care ethics committees – many of which were started by the IBB – as well as the research ethics committees for different centers and public health institutions, promoting the use of bioethical

---

[4] BOE 1999, num. 251, Wednesday, October 20.

[5] Cf. www.ibbioetica.org; www.campus.ibbioetica.org; www.biotica-debat.org.

dialogue in clinical cases. The IBB participates in the Bioethical Committee of the Autonomous Government of Catalonia (in Spain) and its different commissions and workgroups to advise the government on bioethical questions that will subsequently be discussed by the legislature.

4. Documentation Center and Library.[6]

Clearly, the development of all of these activities requires a full-time commitment and in 1999, when Dr. Abel left his position as the executive director of the IBB, Mrs. Núria Terribas took his position. Currently, Dr. Abel is president of the Institute in addition to being an outstanding research and teaching member.

Núria Terribas, a practicing attorney with excellent legal training, became interested in bioethics in 1992 when she first contacted the IBB. Currently, Núria Terribas provides legal representation for the Institute in those cases involving sensitive bioethical issues with the potential of legal repercussions, such as the preparation of the euthanasia document by the IBB (Abel et al. 2005) or the preparation of a similar document by the Catalonia government (Armengol et al. 2006).

Inside the IBB council, special reference should be made to Dr. Juan Viñas, a surgeon responsible for introducing medical schools to bioethics conferences (Jornadas de Bioética). As Dean of the medical school at the University of Lerida, he has worked in collaboration with the IBB over the last 20 years to introduce bioethics into the curriculum. At present, he is the president of this university and a full academic member of the Royal Academy of Medicine of Catalonia (see Viñas 2004).

B. Complutense University (Madrid)

Diego Gracia is the Chair of the History and Medicine Department at Complutense University. The inclusion of bioethics at this university is undoubtedly due to his presence. A productive and creative physician and philosopher, he entered the field of bioethics in 1986 while visiting various American universities in an attempt to find the foundations and methodology of ethical decision-making in the clinical setting. His experiences generated some foundational works: *Foundations of Bioethics* (*Fundamentos de la bioética*) and *Decision-Making Procedures in Clinical Ethics* (*Procedimientos de decisión en ética clínica*) (Gracia 1989, 1991). In addition to his masterful classes, Diego Gracia has extraordinary skills in synthesizing information, as demonstrated in his most recent articles, e.g., "From Clinical Bioethics to Global Bioethics: Thirty Years of Evolution" ("De la Bioética clínica a la Bioética Global: Treinta años de Evolución") and "The Contribution of the Medical Humanities to the Formation of the Doctor" ("Contribución de las Humanidades Médicas a la formación del médico") (Gracia 2004, 2006).

Many physicians and philosophers have become specialists under the chairmanship of Diego Gracia. Amongst the first group can be mentioned Dr. Pilar Núñez Cubero, who collaborated with the IBB for 11 years; Dr. Abizanda, Dr. José Sarabia; Dr. Isolina

---

[6] Cf. http://www.udd.cl/prontus_udd/site/edic/base/port/biblioteca.html.

Riaño; Dr. Azucena Cruceiro; Dr. Manuel de los Reyes; Dr. Juan Carlos Alvarez, and Dr. Pablo Hernando; and to single out some of the philosophers: Dr. Lidia Feito; José Ramon Amor Pan; José García Férez; and Dr. Fabio Alberto Garzón.

Dr. Juan Ramon Lacadena, Chair of Biology at Complutense University (Madrid), also deserves special mention: as a biologist, he was already a teacher of bioethics and a point of reference for all the Spanish schools of bioethics, but he chose to formalize his knowledge of bioethics with a Master's Degree from the Complutense University.

C. University of Valencia

Adela Cortina is Chair of the Ethics Department at the University of Valencia. Her book, *Minimum Ethics: Introduction to Practical Philosophy* (*Ética Mínima: Introducción a la filosofía práctica*) (1986), awakened a new perspective that was intuitively present but had not yet been sufficiently articulated; to be able to overcome the impact of natural law on philosophical thought. Her theory requires one to practice ethics and to participate in dialogue as an attempt to do justice to autonomous beings by opening man up to dialogue. Necessarily, this demands a moral minimum: the only norms considered just are those which are desired by the affected, and these can only be determined after a dialogue has taken place in an atmosphere of equality. Therefore, a universal and deontological ethic is adopted which protects the solidarity of the autonomy of man and serves as a strong foundation for just rights, legitimate politics, and a religion that in its content submits to the criticism of reason.

D. Autonomous University of Barcelona

Victoria Camps is the acting Chair of the Ethics Department at the Autonomous University of Barcelona and President of the Bioethical Advisory Committee at the Autonomous Government of Catalonia. As a well-established philosophy professor, her most recent book, *The Will to Live* (*La Voluntad de Vivir)* (Camps 2005), is an exemplar of her superior communication skills and teaching experience. Her book is a mandatory reading for individuals interested in penetrating the essence of bioethical questions. In this work, Camps firmly establishes for bioethics the requirements of being interdisciplinary and secular. With H. Tristram Engelhardt, Jr., she admits that one cannot discover a secular canonical morality gifted with content, which forces one to fine-tune one's decision procedure so that the most appropriate decision can be reached. She suggests a process consisting of dialogue, discussion, and deliberation with the avoidance of positions that cannot be accepted by all. Finally, bioethics aspires to adopt a "minimal morality" whose nuclear value is the dignity of persons, expressed in the basic values of modernity: freedom, equality, and brotherhood, which are also the basic principles of human rights.

E. Bioethics as a Promoter of International, Political, Social, and Cultural Dialogue

Marcelo Palacios is a physician, politician, and promoter of global bioethics. He is the founder of the Society of International Bioethics, President of its Scientific Committee, Director of the magazine SIBI, and one of the elaborators of the

European Agreement on Human Rights and Biomedicine. As evidenced by his accomplishments, he is one of the most significant figures of bioethics in Spain.

F. Bioethics and Primary Attention to Health

At this point it is necessary to render due homage to those physicians – many of them affiliated with *SEMFIC* (Spanish Society of Family and Community Medicine) – and the health teams who dedicate their work and effort to primary health care, with special reference to all those working in assisted-living programs and palliative care (PADES). These health care professionals are the future of bioethics, as they are capable of supporting the best spirit of the Hippocratic tradition, necessary bioethical knowledge, and closeness to patients and citizens. In a very concrete way, these characteristics have been observed in the following physicians: Martín Zurro, Rogelio Altisent, and Xavier Busquet, who are those the author has known and with whom he has collaborated.

20.3.2 The Theological Foundation of Bioethics

A. Universidad Pontificia de Comillas (UPC) – Madrid

The Chair of Bioethics at UPC was created by Javier Gafo (1936–2001), priest of the Society of Jesus, biologist, and theologian. In his lifetime, he did not see the publication of *Theological Bioethics* (*Bioética Teológica*) (Gafo 2003), which grouped the scientific and theological knowledge that he had prepared, condensed, updated, and developed in his classes, books, and articles, all of which are testimony to his extraordinary abilities.

In 1987, as the Chair of Bioethics, Javier Gafo institutionalized yearly seminars to discuss questions of bioethics. Thanks to his followers, these seminars have survived him and with good reason can be considered the foundations of Catholic bioethical dialogue. The collection he inaugurated, *Current Dilemmas in Today's Medicine* (*Dilemas Éticos de la Medicina Actual*), published by UPC in 1991, continues to be a reference for all the topics covered in the book. Assisted reproductive technologies and genetic biotechnology were some of his favorite subjects, as is evidenced by the related topic of his doctoral dissertation: abortion and the beginning of human life ("El aborto y el comienzo de la vida humana") (Gafo, 1979), which he defended in 1976 at The Pontifical Gregorian University in Rome.

The schools of fundamental theology and morality of Granada followed the same path and direction as Javier Gafo. These schools have collaborated with the Hospital Order of St. John of God and the school of the Redentoristas of Madrid through the Master's program and other courses. They have as main representatives Marciano Vidal and Javier Elizari, who also collaborated with the Universidad Pontificia de Comillas and with the Complutense University of Madrid. With different overtones, the four authors adopt an ethical system focused on the value of autonomy within the context of the Christian faith.

B. Hospital Order of St. John of God

This Order has always made a strong effort to educate their health care professionals working in the hospitals in bioethics. This interest was decidedly promoted by the General, Brother Pascual Piles, who was instrumental in publishing in 2000 the document Identity Card of the Hospital Order of St. John of God (Carta de Identidad de la Orden Hospitalaria), in which the author had the privilege of collaborating. It is worth mentioning that in Spain there are many who have followed such initiatives: physicians, nurses, and public health professionals; and in all the health care centers of the Order there are brothers and public health professionals with a Master's degree in bioethics. Since 2001, the Betic province of the Hospital Order of St. John of God has organized a Master's program in bioethics under the title, "Bioethics and the Humanization of Health Care" (Bioética y Humanización de la Asistencia). Its Director, Dr. José Mª Galán, and Dr. José Mª Rubio, professor of the School of Medicine of Seville, have maintained high standards in designing the program and have also collaborated with and drawn on the resources of other ethics institutes, such as the IBB, Complutense University, and the UPC. In 2000, Dr. Bosco Cordeiro organized a national conference in Pamplona on palliative care, and in 2003 Dr. Francisco Javier Obis organized a similar conference in Zaragoza, both of which were attended by the IBB.

C. Private University of Navarra

At the University of Navarra, the teaching of bioethics is linked to the institution "Opus Dei" and depends deeply on an individual affectionately bound to a normative dimension of ethics: Dr. Gonzalo Herranz, Professor of Histology and Pathology since 1970 and Dean of the School of Medicine (1974–1978). He has also worked hard and well for the Spanish Medical Association (Organización Médica Colegial de España) from 1984 to 1995. He is a member of the International Bioethics Committee of UNESCO and the Pontifical Academy for Life.

20.3.3 The Legal Foundation of Bioethics

A common characteristic of all of the foundations of bioethics is the importance they grant to law without disregarding basic ethical principles. One must be careful to distinguish the school of Professor Maria Casado, which teaches that law shapes bioethics; that of Professor Antonio Beristain, S. J., which specializes in criminal law, criminology, and victimology; and that of Professor Romeo Casabona, which specializes in legal questions regarding the human genome.

It is important to note the excellent contributions to bioethics and biolaw by Dr. María Casado, Director of the Observatory in Bioethics and Law (Observatori de Bioètica i Dret), Director of the Master's program of Bioethics and Law at the University of Barcelona, and Professor of Philosophy of Law, Morality, and Politics. The observatory was created with the aim of becoming a participant in dialogues at the university and within society for the purpose of making its voice heard to public, administrative, and political organizations involved in the regulation and control of research activities and new technologies. Dr. Casado has published with other specialists, in both Spanish and English, the detailed and well-written "Opinion Documents" ("Documentos de opinión"), which have been widely distributed in university circles.

The work of Dr. Carlos Mª Romeo Casabona, Professor of Criminal Law at the University of the Basque Country and the Director of the Interuniversity Chair in Law and Human Genome, can be considered a model. His services are often required by international organizations such as WHO and UNESCO and he has trained first-rate jurists who now constitute a second generation of professors in biolaw (Aitziber Emaldi; Pilar Nicolás; Sergio Romeo). Javier Sánchez Caro, Director of the Unit of Bioethics and Health-Care Orientation of the Autonomous Community of Madrid (Unidad de Bioética y Orientación Sanitaria de la Comunidad de Madrid) must also be recognized for his excellent research and teachings.

In the dialogue between law and bioethics, professors of criminal law have also had a prominent role: Antonio Beristain, from the Basque Institute of Criminology; José Luís Diez Ripollés, from the University of Málaga; Esther Giménez-Salinas, President of the University Ramon Llull, and Dr. Encarna Roca, Professor of Civil Rights in Barcelona and Supreme Court Judge.

Finally, Dr. Francisco Javier Blázquez Ruiz, Professor of Philosophy and Law at the Public University of Navarra, should be mentioned for his exploration of bioethical problems by approaching them from the unique perspective of supporting the relevant legal components via ethics, as well as from the complementary perspective of trying to justify the relevant ethical principles within a legal framework.

Recognizing that everyone mentioned has written and continues to write important documents in the field of health care law, the author would also like to mention the jurists with whom special ties of friendship and collaboration exist: The Emeritus Supreme Court Judge José Manuel Martínez-Pereda, whose direction and performance in the Bioethics Commission of SEGO (Sociedad Española e Ginecología y Obstetricia) has been and continues to be crucial; Manuel Amarilla Gundín, President of the European Pharmaceutical Group Law; Ricardo de Lorenzo, President of the Spanish Healthcare Law; and the Judge Xavier Abel Lluch, Professor of the Law School.

20.3.4 Testimony and Narrative in Bioethics

There are many physicians whose lives are exemplary and serve as models in the practice of medicine, based on clear ethical criteria, for the generations that follow them. Among them should be recognized Dr. Jordi Sans, Dr. Jordi Gol, Dr. Antonio Tejedo, Dr. Moisés Broggi, Dr. Francesc Vilardell, Dr. Ciril Rozman, Dr. Marius Foz, Dr. Estanislao Boren, Dr. Francesc Ma. Doménech, Dr. Jordi Setoain, Dr. Domingo

Ruano, Dr. Josep Ma. Laïlla, Dr. Sagrario Mateu, Dr. Lydia Buisan, and Dr. Carmen Cuadrado. In the opinion of the author, without prejudice to so many other names that cannot all be mentioned here, they indisputably remain models.[7]

20.4 A Period of Review, Projection, and Integration

The analysis of this period can be considered a necessary review of Spanish bioethics. The period requires that one accept a universal minimum ethics, while attempting to integrate an ethics of maximums, aimed at those who require more due to personal, family, or group obligations. The primary objective is the selection of values at a social level that will allow the construction of a better and healthier world, which tries to overcome the embarrassing differences between rich and poor or powerful and excluded. This section will summarize the development of these issues up through the current time from the perspective of the three rationalities previously mentioned.

A. Techno-Scientific Rationality

The last two decades of the twentieth century witnessed the enthusiasm of scientific discovery, which was duly magnified by the media, and related particularly to the sequencing of the human genome and the possibility of regenerating damaged or degenerated human tissues from "stem-cell" research. The possibility of one day preventing or even curing degenerative diseases of the central nervous system not only generates enthusiasm, but also engenders hope as people begin to believe that "if we want it, we will achieve it." More than ever, the danger of subordinating human dignity to the attainment of scientific achievements is present. The obligation of thinking seriously about the type of society one would want to have when making ethical and legal decisions is now of critical importance. The ethical approach that has been agreed upon by those who trust the axiological neutrality of science and those who embrace social responsibility as the correct ethical principle of professional conduct is the principle of precaution, which requires weighing the consequences of a hasty application of new biogenetic technologies. This attitude, whether attributable to either conviction or to a fear of new discoveries being employed for military aims, is hopeful. In addition to this principle, all levels of society should receive appropriate and sufficient information in an attempt to make them aware of what is at stake when researching or developing new technology. This includes providing the advantages, disadvantages, and possible risks; furthermore, it is necessary to specify who will benefit from the new discoveries.

[7] The author admires the second generation of physicians, who strive to cope with the unpleasantness of daily problems, who struggle to act in the best possible manner in almost insurmountable conditions. They are a multitude and that is why the author was only able to recall those who became acquainted with bioethics at the very beginning and who promoted the art of bioethical dialogue: Marius Morlans; Marc A. Broggi; Lidia Buisán. These individuals also encouraged the author to found the Catalonian Society of Bioethics.

B. Faith-Based Rationality

The biogenetic possibilities that technology can offer create restlessness. The further possibility of their scientific, social, ethical, and legal legitimization compounds this feeling further. However, engaging in bioethical dialogue requires openness to other perspectives and reviewing previous judgments as, due to the passing of time, conceptual changes or cultural evolutions can occur, rendering such judgments anachronistic. It is necessary to update periodically the relationship among scientific knowledge, ethics, and theology.

In all of the rationalities discussed, it is not unexpected that citizens are often polarized in their opinions, as was evidenced by the results of the election for the representatives of the Spanish Courts. What is surprising is that the strongest polarization is related to the resistance of some citizens to the separation of Church and State. A sector of the episcopate supports this resistance because they are nostalgic for national-Catholicism and fearful of technology and its potential abuse. Consequently, this is observable in discussions of legal projects and those projects that may impact human life or the family.

C. Legal–Political Rationality

In recent years, there have been substantial transformations of the modern public health systems. One of the major agents of change in these transformations, in Europe and, in particular, Spain, has been the conception of the patient as citizen.

In this area, Spain has developed important legislation that recognizes respect for patient autonomy and a right to health care. This legislation also defends a patient's right to information and the related requirement of informed consent. Additionally, the work of the Josep Laporte Library Foundation (Fundación Biblioteca Josep Laporte-FBJL), led by Dr. Albert Jovell, must be recognized for programs like the Spanish Patient Forum (Foro Español de Pacientes)[8] – which creates a network of more than 600 patient associations of diverse diagnoses in addition to relatives and volunteers – and the University of Patients (Universidad de Pacientes).[9] These organizations facilitate access to information and educate citizens and users of the public health system about different illnesses and services provided. The societal increase in utilizing the health care system and the provision of public health services is in part due to these organizations.

Under the direction of Dr. Albert Oriol Bosch, players at different levels of the public health care system have made a significant effort to critically examine the Spanish health care system, the current state of the health care professions, and the new role of the citizen as initiator of health care actions. These initiatives may serve as bridges to a healthier future (Oriol 2003).

Relevant to ethics, one must consider the contributions of Pablo Simón Lorda, an important figure in Spanish bioethics, who fights to ensure that the organization of the public health system is considered within the context of bioethics, with particular

[8] www.webpacientes.org.

[9] www.universidadpacientes.org.

attention paid to those values defining the system internally and differentiating it externally. He also tries to incorporate the behavior of *stakeholders* for the purpose of converting the organization into an institution of excellence (Simon 2005). He follows the path of the Chairs of the Department of Ethics at Valencia, Adela Cortina, and Jesús Conill (Conill 2002; Cortina 1986; Cortina and Conill 1998).

From the point of view of legislation, since the 1980s many norms and conditions have been incorporated into law, which affect issues of bioethical importance. Only the most important of these laws will be discussed below, and special attention will be paid to those regulations that reinforce patient rights (as users of the public health care system), as their effects pervade all levels of health care delivery and reflect the most progressive and liberal legislation in Europe.

- Transplants

On January 5, 2000, the Royal Decree 2070/1999 (dated December 30th) took effect. This law regulates the donation, removal, and transplantation of human organs, as well as the territorial coordination needed to carry out these activities. Law 30/1979 deals with organ removal and transplantation and continues to be in effect (cf. Terribas 2000).

- Assisted Reproductive Technologies

Law 14/2006 (dated May 26th) on Techniques of Assisted Human Reproduction is the most important law of this type. However, Royal Decree 411/1996 (dated March 1st) is also about the same legislation (Terribas 2003a).

- Research on Human Beings

Spain has adopted legislation regulating research on human beings, especially pertaining to the use of new medications and other health products. It was incorporated under Law 25/1990 on pharmaceuticals, and developed subsequently in the Royal Decree 223/2004 on clinical trials (dated February 6th). This decree adapts the original Spanish regulation to the corresponding directive of the European Union. Nevertheless, in the field of biomedical research, independent of the regulations on assisted reproductive techniques, the Bill on Biomedical Research must be mentioned because it is already in the advanced stages of parliamentary discussion.

- Patient Rights

In the last 15 years, Spain has widely developed legislation on the rights of patients and users of the public health care system. First to be enacted was the General Health Law (Ley General de Sanidad), which was later more rigorously defined by Law 41/2002 on information, patient autonomy, and clinical records (Terribas 2003b). It should be noted that there are autonomous governments in Spain with regulatory responsibilities that have also addressed these questions. The first autonomous government to tackle these issues was the Autonomous Government of Catalonia with Law 21/2000, which regulated advanced directives as a means of respecting patient autonomy (Terribas 2003c, 2004, 2006).

Relating to privacy and the protection of personal information, Law 15/1999 was enacted on December 13th and affects all areas pertaining to the confidentiality of information (Terribas 1999).

- Penal Code

Finally, the Penal Code must be considered, especially those aspects that are relevant to bioethical studies. Among them are:

- Abortion (Art. 144 to 146)
- Assisted suicide and euthanasia (Art. 143; cf. Abel et al. 2005; Armengol et al. 2006)
- Injuries to the fetus (Art. 157 i 158)
- Genetic manipulation (Art. 159 i ss.)
- Refusal of medical assistance (Art. 196)
- Breach of the patient–doctor privilege (Art. 199)
- European Agreement on Human Rights and Biomedicine (1997)

This agreement was ratified by the Spanish Parliament in 1999 and took effect in the year 2000. It addresses those regulations that are applicable within the European territory, in addition to those countries which have signed and ratified it – as is the case of Spain – and requires the adaptation of a country's internal regulations to the agreement. Included in its regulations are issues of informed consent, advanced directives, research on human subjects, and others. To date, the aforementioned Spanish legislation has been adapted to include all the principles of the agreement.

References

Abel F (2001) Bioética: Orígenes, presente y futuro. Institut Borja de Bioètica y Fundación Mapfre de Medicina, Madrid

Abel F, Terribas N, Busquets E, Camacho JA, Cambra FJ, Cardona X, Cusí V, Nello A, Salvat I, Torralba F (2005) Hacia una Posible Despenalización de la Eutanasia. Bioètica & Debat 39:1–7

Armengol R, Boladeras M, Broggi J, Busquets MA, Camps V, Espasa R, Hernández J, Morlans M, Pérez M, Royes A, Terribas N (2006) Informe sobre l'eutanàsia i l'ajuda al suïcidi. Prous Science, Barcelona

Barreau H (1989) Bioéthique et éthique de la vie. NRT Leuven: Hervé 111:194–216

Camps V (2005) La voluntad de vivir. Ariel, Barcelona

Conill J (2002) Ética y empresa sanitaria. In: Ferrer JJ, & Martínez JL (eds) Bioética: un diálogo plural. Homenaje a Javier Gafo, s.j. Universidad Pontificia Comillas, Madrid, pp 531–540

Cortina A (1986) Ética mínima. Introducción a la filosofía práctica, Tecnos, S.A., Madrid

Cortina A, Conill J (1998) Democracia participativa y sociedad civil: una ética empresarial. Siglo del Hombre (Serie Conversaciones), Bogotá

de Wachter M (2006) Revisiting the origins. EACME Newsletter, 15 April, Maastricht

de Wert G , Berghmans RPL, Boer GJ, Andersen S, Brambau B, Carvalho AS, Dierickx K, Elliston S, Nuñez P, Oswald W, Vicari M (2002) Ethical guidance on human embryonic and fetal tissue transplantation: A European overview. Med Health Care Philos 5.1, 79–90.

Gafo J (1979) El aborto y el comienzo de la vida humana. Sal Térrea, Santander

Gafo J (2003) Bioética teológica. UPC y Desclée de Broker, Madrid

Gracia D (1989) Fundamentos de bioética. Eudema, Fuenlabrada, Madrid

Gracia D (1991) Procedimientos de decisión en ética clínica. Eudema, Fuenlabrada, Madrid

Gracia D (2004) De la bioética clínica a la bioética global: treinta años de evolución. In: Selecciones de bioética. Instituto de Bioética – CENALBE, Bogotá, Colombia

Gracia D (2006) Contribución de las humanidades médicas a la formación del médico. In: Humanitas. Humanidades médicas. [Online] Available: http://www.fundacionmhm.org/revista.html
Lacadena JR (1995) Historia nobelada de la genética: Concepto y método. Discurso de ingreso como Académico de Número en la Real Academia de Farmacia, Real Academia de Farmacia, Madrid
Oriol A (2003) Libre blanc de les organizaciones sanitàries. Generalitat de Catalunya, Barcelona
Potter VR (1970) Bioethics: The science of survival. Perspect Biol Med 14:127–153
Potter VR (1971) Bioethics: Bridge to the future. Prentice Hall, New Jersey
Reich W (ed) (1995) Encyclopedia of Bioethics (rev. ed.), vols 5. Macmillan, New York
Rendtorff JD, Kemp P (eds) (2000). Basic ethical principles in European bioethics and biolaw, vols 2. Center for ethics and law, Copenhagen; Institut Borja de Bioètica, Barcelona
Simon P (ed) (2005) Ética de las organizaciones sanitarias. Nuevos modelos de calidad. Triacastela, Madrid
Terribas N (1999) Nueva ley de protección de datos personales. Labor Hospitalaria 32(257):217–231
Terribas N (2000) Nueva regulación sobre trasplante de órganos. Labor Hospitalaria 32(257):200–216
Terribas N (2003a) Destinos de los embriones sobrantes de TRHA. Bioètica & Debat 34:6–7
Terribas N (2003b) Derechos con rango de ley: pros y contras de la ley básica 41/2002. Bioètica & Debat 31:12–15
Terribas N (2003c) Las voluntades anticipadas y su especial consideración en el paciente geriátrico. Revista Española de Geriatría y Gerontología (monográfico de bioética) 38(suplemento 3), 53–64
Terribas N (2004) Las voluntades anticipadas y su problemática en la aplicación práctica, salud pública y derecho administrativo. Cuadernos de Derecho Judicial 5:267–296
Terribas N (2006) Un documento de voluntades anticipadas. Form Med Contin Aten Prim 13(7): 354–357
Viñas J (2004) Reptes de la cirurgia al Segle XXI. Reial Acadèmia de Medicina de Catalunya, Barcelona

Chapter 21
Bioethics in Venezuela: First Pathways

Ludwig Schmidt H.

21.1 Introduction

The task of retelling the recent history of Venezuelan bioethics and its establishment as a new way of thinking and an interdisciplinary concept is challenging because of the many details one must be careful not to forget.[1]

The beginning of bioethics in Venezuela occurred during the 1980s and was concentrated primarily within the setting of the health sciences. One of the primary figures of its establishment was Augusto León Cechini who published a book on medical ethics, taught at the Central University of Venezuela (UCV) and the Venezuelan Medical Federation, and was an authoritative member of the prestigious Academy of Medicine. During this time, there were also a number of scholars within ethics, medicine, and scientific research who were exchanging ideas at meetings or in informal conversation about international news or articles pertaining to bioethical issues. From these informal discussions grew more formalized activities; for example, during the 1990s, Alfredo Castillo, Isis Nezer de Landaeta, and Gabriel D'Empaire of UCV began to formalize discussions about health, law, and the environmental sciences. Others who came to be involved in these discussions included Professors Daniel Oliva, Ximena Páez, and Eliéxer Urdaneta of the University of the Andes (ULA); Professor Jacinto Robles y Yonis Sosa of the Pedagogic Experimental University Liberator, Maturín (UPEL); Eva Briceño of the National Commission of Scientific and Technological Research (CONICIT, now

L. Schmidt H.
Ph.D. Associate Professor of Bioethics at the UCAB -Universidad Catolica Andrés Bello, Faculdad Derecho, Caracas,VE
e-mail: lschmidt@ucab.edu.ve

[1] It is an interesting endeavor for me to prepare a part of the historical memory of bioethics in Venezuela. I say "part of" because often time things are discarded, perhaps by negligence, a desire to omit something, or by ignorance. In any telling of history there is always some subjectivity, but I will make a deliberate effort to be objective as possible in this essay. If I omit anything please inform me of my omission at lschmidt01@gmail.com.

L. Pessini et al. (eds.), *Ibero-American Bioethics: History and Perspectives*, Philosophy and Medicine 106, DOI 10.1007/978-1-4020-9350-0_21,

the National Fund of Science, Technology and Innovation [FONACIT]); Rafael Apitz of the Venezuelan Institute of Scientific Research (IVIC); and Rafael Bernad, Rafael Muñiz, and myself from the Andrés Bello Catholic University UCAB.[2] During these years, it was recognized that discussion criteria needed to be strengthened, especially the appropriate use of legal principles and case studies in decision making.

In 2000, the interdisciplinary field of bioethics, which integrates philosophy, theology, anthropology, psychology, and the social sciences, became a fashionable topic for discussion. As a result of its popularity, it began to lose some of its scientific rigor and was seen as something of a short-term trend. However, several experts managed to save its reputation by establishing it as an interdisciplinary approach to human knowledge.

These varying and sporadic events demonstrate the fact that the introduction of bioethics in Venezuela was the result of a number of spontaneous efforts and academic curiosity. This curiosity led to an invitation to a number of experts to visit Venezuelan universities for seminars and conferences.[3] As a result of these efforts, interest in bioethics began to grow and additional collaborators became engaged.

It should also be mentioned that there were some detractors who were not necessarily in opposition to the adoption of bioethics, but were not interested in collaborating and aiding in its diffusion. However, there were always highly motivated individuals to make up for their disinterest. In the several meetings held to promote bioethics – and in the meetings that continue to occur – professionals and students from varying disciplines were always in attendance.

When reflecting on the 1980s, the academic diffusion of bioethics was also accompanied by the creation of ethics committees within private and governmental institutions for the evaluation of research projects in the health sciences. Although most of the committees were ad hoc, they attempted to evaluate research projects based on their projected consequences and impact. Examples of institutions that developed such committees include CONICIT (now FONACIT) and the Polar Foundation (FP).

In selected hospitals, the medical societies established ethics committees, which sometimes considered topics in bioethics. In some research centers, experiments were evaluated according to broader criteria and in some cases professionals from outside disciplines were invited to participate in deliberations. Even with the development of these committees, bioethics still was not directly discussed, because it had not yet become an accepted concept. Discussion of establishing *bioethics* committees, with an interdisciplinary membership and approach, often times provoked extreme reactions. The primary objection was to the idea of introducing professionals outside of medicine to take part in the deliberation of *medical* cases. The situation was difficult because, although some doctors accepted bioethicists as well-suited experts, others were intimidated by the idea of having an outsider review their practice of medicine.[4] Fortunately, these prejudices have been minimized with time,

---

[2] I apologize for any name I haven't mentioned.

[3] Invited experts included: Javier Gafo Fernández (Pontifical University of Comillas, Madrid); Alfredo Llanos (Pontifical University Javeriana, Bogotá), Juan Ramón Lacadena (Pontifical University of Comillas, Madrid).

[4] This experience was naturally due to disciplinary zeal and the professional setting. However it often led to paternalistic arguments, absolutes, and resistance to interdisciplinary efforts. This occured not only in the medical setting, but also in biomedical and hospital engineering.

but they have not dissolved completely. A new generation of medical professionals has come to consider bioethicists peers with which they can discuss their experiences.

This rejection was not exclusive to the medical setting, but also occurred within the humanities (theology, philosophy, psychology, anthropology, and education), which resisted the idea of having specialists from the applied sciences introducing cases foreign to their professional setting. Additionally, the Vienna Circle had a significant influence on contemporary thought, causing universities to introduce humanistic thought into the curricula of scientific and technological programs, and vice versa, after the 1968 revolution.

In 1980, the usefulness of the interdisciplinary approach was still debated by some who asked, "Why do I have to study these matters? What use will these subjects be to my professional education?" Fortunately, this attitude has come to be diluted in both the sciences and the humanities, and bridges have begun to be formed among the varying disciplines to provide a multifaceted approach to problem-solving.

21.2 Human Rights

One of the primary means for the diffusion of bioethics in Venezuela was the media (i.e., press, radio, television), which, for every topic of bioethical significance, interviewed several bioethicists. Educational centers and scientific societies also contributed by inviting bioethicists to partake in seminars, forums, and studies.

Another important formative factor was the human genome and human rights debate, which encouraged the development of opinions about varying topics, such as abortion, euthanasia, patient care, and those issues related to the products of new technologies (e.g., regenerative medicine and stem cells, genetically modified organisms and transgenic food, pharmacogenetics and pharmacogenomics) as they were drawn into debate within the public forums. All of these topics were appropriate to and sought support within bioethics. Fifty years after the establishment of the Universal Declaration of Human Rights (United Nations 1948), international efforts increased in favor of this individual and social protection, prompted by the need to integrate the human genome into its purview.

The environment was also introduced as another topic of interest by the Declarations of the Earth Summit, Rio de Janeiro (United Nations 1992) and the Climate Change Conference, Bali (United Nations 2007). In addition, the Millennium Declaration (United Nations 2000) emphasized a joint commitment to the protection of the most vulnerable populations. Other declarations and resolutions were established during this time, but the aforementioned are those that were of primary interest to scholars in Venezuela.

The mass media provided coverage of these controversies and sought out the controversial positions held within the sciences. The universities also promoted public discussion forums to help individuals engage in these issues. However, the discussion often stopped at the level of public interest because there was no involvement at the governmental level. There was a distinct lack of an application of regulations, the drafting of new legislation, and juridical development.

The only governmental reaction occurred sporadically and usually as the result of a campaign or a demagogic event.

In Venezuela there are several advocacy groups and non-governmental organizations (NGOs) that promote the defense of life (both human life and nature), which are all pluralistic and natural, although some are distinctively religious, but have an ecumenical character, like the Forum Pro-Vida Venezuela (Pro-life Forum). All of these organizations seek to educate individuals and to warn them about potential threats to life and how to combat them. However, the quality of information they have is relative to the quality of the relevant studies being conducted and the evidence that is available.

At the national level, there were several meetings and forums developed for the discussion of patient rights, specifically in the context of health care institutions. A highly controversial issue within the debate was informed consent, which was the object of furious debate and even university theses.

The doctor–patient relationship was also addressed. Article 46 of the Constitution of the Bolivian Republic of Venezuela promotes a fair and balanced doctor–patient relationship by providing that:

> Every person has the right to respect for their physical, psychic and moral integrity … Every person deprived of freedom will be treated with the respect due to the dignity inherent to human being [and] no individual will be submitted without one's free consent to scientific experiments, or to medical or laboratorial examinations, except when one's life is in danger or in other circumstances as determined by law (Republica Bolivariana de Venezuela. Constitución 2000).

This article allowed for Venezuelan society to move away from a model of medical paternalism and to establish the autonomy of the patient (or one's legal representative if a surrogate is deemed necessary).

Standard activities in bioethics have persisted over the years, such as symposia, workshops, meetings, and discussions promoted by different groups, committees, or societies and concerning bioethical topics. However, the fruits of bioethical development are now beginning to be seen, and there is a renewed interest in promoting big events like those that occurred in 2001.

At present, the Centers for Scientific, Humanistic and Technological Development (CDCHT) and the national universities have established bioethics committees. In the work of these committees, bioethics is used to address the concerns relevant to research on human beings, human rights, animal rights, patenting parts of the genome, and more. The same type of standards is applied to environmental research, biological diversity, and food safety, all crucial topics because of the ecological imbalances they can generate.

Hospital bioethics committees are now trying to stay current with the ever-evolving knowledge of bioethics. For this purpose, the CENABI (National Center of Bioethics) prepares a monthly meeting to update its members on several study topics; the GTB (Interdisciplinary Bioethics Group) holds interdisciplinary meetings; the University of Clinical Hospitals (UCV) bioethics committee sponsors annual engagements; and the Week of Life is an annual ecumenical opportunity for organized communities to interact and consider several aspects of life. These events help to consolidate interdisciplinary efforts within the settings of health, education, scientific research, law, and the environment.

21.3 An Emergent Bioethical Thought

From the perspective of Van Rensselaer Potter's book, *Bioethics: A Bridge to the Future* (1971), "bioethics" calls on all human beings to understand, promote, and defend the survival of humanity and the earth.[5] Venezuela strives to actualize this call by founding bioethics as an interdisciplinary field (a bridge) meant to establish transversal axes of knowledge, allowing for individuals to interact with the life sciences[6] and to establish rational criteria between *techne* and praxis, guaranteeing the future of humanity. To achieve this call, one must take an approach that is broad, fair, rational, tolerant, and pluralistic.

While this concept is attractive, it remains complex and difficult to achieve due to a common resistance to change in a society that is divided between liberal and conservative perspectives, especially regarding professional activities. At the personal and public levels, one now sees a great deal of relativism and irreverence when faced with rules – at the personal level it is displayed in disciplinary sectarianism and in contemporary religious syncretism.

Venezuela has not been immune to post-modern thought, because it is deeply rooted in its conservative structures and has created a society riddled with ideological conflicts and false appearances. Professionals are not accustomed to taking a step back from a situation to consider it in detail so as to be able to make a well-informed decision. Instead, they argue over trivialities and end up making last-minute decisions for complex problems without appropriate reflection. This hastiness is symptomatic of a society lacking a rational structure within which one can effectively debate problems, instead of engaging in debates where understanding is based on prejudice and dialogue is not approached with the intention of reaching a plural, collective, and tolerant position.

The alternative perspective in Latin America and the Caribbean was the birth of bioethics taking place in the 1980s throughout the countries of Argentina, Colombia, Chile, Mexico, Brazil, and Venezuela. In this movement, different professionals sowed the seeds of the discipline, first in universities and medical centers, and later in research and development centers and secondary schools.

[5] Independently of controversies about whether Potter was the "father of bioethics," the meaning of *global* bioethics is his contribution. The fact that theologian Fritz Jahr used the term "bioethics" in 1927 for the first time, as Fernando Lolas informs us; or Albert R. Jonsen of the University of Washington, Seattle; or Henry Beecher, teacher of anesthesiology at Harvard Medical School; or the founder of the Kennedy Institute of Ethics, André Hellegers or the founders of the Hastings Center is irrelevant in the case of global bioethics.

[6] Both in the basic and applied sciences.

A figure of great influence was José Alberto Mainetti from Argentina, who founded the Institute of Medical Humanities in 1972 and the Latin-American School of Bioethics (ELABE) at the end of the 1980s, which is responsible for educating a majority of the current generation's bioethicists. Another influential figure was Fernando Sánchez Torres, who founded the Colombian Institute of Bioethical Studies (ICEB) in December 1985, which has served as a key center of bioethical thought.

Another significant development was the establishment of the Latin American and Caribbean Federation of Bioethics Institutions (FELAIBE) in 1991,[7] which has survived over the years and still functions in integrating the representatives of major bioethical associations throughout the region.

It must also be mentioned that the Pan-American Health Organization of the World Health Organization (PAHO-WHO) established the Regional Bioethics Program in 1994. In addition, the international graduate program of bioethics was also established by an agreement between the Regional Bioethics Program and the Complutense University of Madrid in partnership with the University of Chile. It also implemented the first itinerant graduate program in bioethics in 1996.[8] At present, it appears that the Latin American Sectional of the International Society of Bioethics (SIBI) and the Bioethics Network of Latin America and the Caribbean (UNESCO), which are responsible for educating the new generation of bioethicists, will also have a formative impact on the history of bioethics.

It is important to recognize that in the 1990s bioethics was already present throughout the entire continent. In the 1980s, bioethics was received with heavy influences from North America. However, over the course of a decade, it became more heavily influenced by European and Spanish bioethics. Finally, after another few years' time, a distinctively Latin American bioethics began to develop with a primarily social and global character (Leon 2004).

One can see that the development of bioethics in Latin America was in great part due to the international and united efforts throughout the region and the use of information and communication technologies, in addition to local, regional, and international meetings.

21.4 Stages of Development

In 1916, Venezuela promoted its own code of ethics in accord with the deontological tradition regulating the relations of doctors with each other, the public, and the state. Latin American medical ethics have traditionally been defined as naturalist,

[7] Its founders were José Alberto Mainetti (Argentina), Alfonso Llano (Colombia), and Pablo Pulido (Venezuela).

[8] The first was in Chile (1996–1998); the second, the Dominican Republic (1999–2001) and the third in Peru (2002–2004) specializing in clinical ethics and under the direction of Dr. Diego Gracia.

paternalistic, dogmatic, and authoritarian (Mainetti 1993). Currently, the same medical ethic is in place, but it is strengthened by bioethics. In the second half of the twentieth century, Venezuelan medical ethics, independently of French and North American influence, developed an ethic more compatible with its own local idiosyncrasies (Kranzberg 1985).

In Venezuela, the reforms of health science programs and other disciplines during the 1970s promoted radical changes due to the student revolution of 1968; the influence of bioengineering and biotechnology; and the new perspectives on professional responsibility brought about by codes of ethics and medical treaties. Once the relationship between technology and the humanities was promoted in medical schools during the 1980s, bioethics began to be taught as a situational ethics course with medical education programs.

It was not until the beginning of this decade that bioethics began to be considered an interdisciplinary approach to education, together with communication, research, teamwork, and citizenship. It is also challenging at this point to attempt to differentiate between bioethics and professional ethics, especially in health care facilities, because medical societies shape their ethics committees, and the facility's board of directors often asks advice from the bioethics committee. In other disciplines outside of the medical fields, bioethics will be developed from a more global perspective, with more of an emphasis on social matters instead of being so tightly linked to a profession and a professional ethic.

It is difficult to determine stages in the development of bioethics in Venezuela (Schmidt 2002), but two periods can be established, namely, the "First Steps" (1984–1995) (Leon 2004, p. 145) and its "Adolescence" (1996–2007) (Mainetti 1993). However, one should also be able to determine a third stage of "Maturation" in the near future.

21.4.1 "First Steps"

Bioethics in Venezuela began as medical ethics in 1975, when Augusto León published his book, *Medical Ethics*, which reinforced the existing disciplines of ethics, morals, and medical deontology.[9] His book served as a foundation for the emergence of a clinical ethics in medical schools and the establishment of a code of medical ethics and guidelines for practicing medicine (including nursing, pharmacology, and dentistry). However, during the mid-1980s, this initial vision began to be reoriented and redefined.

In this way, the universities were the primary actors in the dissemination of bioethics when they promoted it as a subject of study in their undergraduate and graduate courses in science, the health sciences, the political and juridical sciences, and the humanities.

[9] It should be mentioned that it was not until much later that Dr. León agreed to the use of the term "bioethics."

21.4.2 "Adolescence"

During the 1990s, bioethics was integrated into the disciplines of law, sociology, philosophy, theology, and engineering, allowing it to be considered an interdisciplinary method or approach. One of the reasons for this integration was the introduction of law and human rights into bioethical deliberation about the human genome and related topics (Wilkie 1994).

In addition, Argentina, Brazil, Colombia, Chile, Mexico, and Venezuela all created chairs, specialties, and graduate courses and programs in this new discipline. At the time, the content of these programs was centered on clinical bioethics as it was conceived in America and Europe. However, the current version of these programs takes an approach closer to that of a global bioethics.

In 1995, a policy was developed for the restructuring of the health sector; health law began to be developed that incorporated bioethical aspects. In 1997, the first legal project mentioned bioethics committees and the national bioethics committee. In 1998, the Minister Felix Oletta and his advisory team assembled the members of the National Bioethics Commission for their first meeting. Unfortunately, the initiative was discontinued subsequent to that meeting.

In the twenty-first century, Latin American and Caribbean bioethics have come to be associated with a social character concerned with addressing issues of justice, autonomy, and professional responsibility, in addition to protecting the environment and studying the consequences of scientific progress. In turn, there are debates about values and principles and consequences and aftermaths, which each country must face and address in accord with its own culture and social development.

21.5 Bioethics at the State Level

As an anecdotal note, in the year 2000, Van Rensselaer Potter wrote me an email asking me to congratulate the Constituent Assembly and the President of the Republic for having included the term "bioethics" in two articles of the Venezuelan Constitution, which was approved in December 1999 (Republica Bolivariana de Venezuela. Constitución 2000). The following are the articles in which the term appears.

> *Chapter VIII: Rights of Native Peoples*
> *Article 122*: Native peoples have the right to a health care system that takes into consideration their practices and cultures. The State shall recognize their traditional medicines and supplementary forms of therapy, subject to principles of bioethics.

> *Chapter IX: Environmental Rights*
> Article 127: It is the right and duty of each generation to protect and maintain the environment for its own benefit and that of the future world. Everyone has the right, individually and collectively, to enjoy a safe, healthful and ecologically balanced life and environment. The State shall protect the environment, biological and genetic diversity, ecological processes, national parks and natural monuments, and other areas of particular ecological importance.

> The genome of a living being shall not be patentable, and law relating to the principles of bioethics shall regulate the field. It is a fundamental duty of the State, with the active participation of society, to ensure that the populace develops in a pollution-free environment in which air, water, soil, coasts, climate, the ozone layer and living species receive special protection, in accordance with the law.

As one can see, protection began to be put in place for the native peoples whose rights had been infringed upon in a number of ways, and environmental rights began to be articulated with the proposal of the Organic Law of the Environment and Natural Resources, although it was not sufficient to prevent consistent violations.

In 2001, the government promoted the Organic Law of Science, Technology, and Innovation (Ley Orgánica de Ciencia, Tecnologia y Innovación [LOCTI]), which established in its articles that scientific and technological projects will be evaluated in light of the ethical principles established by the bioethics committees, which are also provided for by the law. This law marks the first time bioethics was given the status of an organic law. The articles relevant to bioethics are listed below.

> *Ethics, Righteousness, and Good Faith*
> *Article 6*: Public or private organizations, as well as legal and natural persons, must develop activities regulated by the present law according to principles of ethics, righteousness and good faith that must prevail in their acts in congruity with human rights.
>
> *Bioethical Principles*
> *Article 7*: The Government, by means of competent agencies, will oversee compliance with bioethical and environmental principles in the development of scientific and technological research, according to national regulations and international agreements signed by the Republic.
>
> *Commissions of Ethics, Bioethics and Biodiversity*
> *Article 8:* The Department of Science and Technology will promote the creation of interdisciplinary commissions of ethics, bioethics and biodiversity, which will define aspects of articles 6 and 7 of this law, by proposing codes of ethics, bioethics and environmental protection regarding scientific, technological and innovative practices.

Since 2001, the Minister of Science and Technology has taken part in the UNESCO meetings, presenting a report relevant to bioethics with a government representative (Freddy García) and an independent expert (Gabriel D'Empaire).

21.6 Bioethics Committees

In 1994, the first steps towards establishing the National Center of Bioethics (CENABI) at UCV's medical college took place and were consolidated in 1995. In 1996, the Interdisciplinary Bioethics Group (GTB) was created at the Andrés Bello Catholic University's (UCAB) College of the Humanities and Education, which is now the College of Law. In 1997, the Bioethics Commission of the National Council of Science and Technology (CONICIT, now the Commission of Bioethics and Biosafety of the National Council of Science and Technology [FONACIT]), was established.

In 1998, the Bioethics Committee of the Venezuelan Institute of Scientific Research was established, followed by the founding of the Association of Clinical Bioethics (ABIC) in 1999; the establishment of the Latin-American Institute of Bioethics and Human Rights at ULA in 2001; and the Venezuelan Society of Juridical Bioethics at UCV in 2005.

The Venezuelan Association of Catholic Doctors (AVEMECA), along with the Venezuelan Episcopal Conference of Venezuela, organized the Pro-Vida Forum and established a coordinating board for the Pro-Vida Program. During the meetings of the Interdisciplinary Bioethics Group, ministers from diverse religions (Jewish, Muslim, Protestant, Buddhist, and Catholic) attended, in addition to nationally recognized scientists, philosophers, and economists.

During these years, about 60 bioethics committees were created at the national level and in almost all hospitals of the third and fourth levels of health assistance, in addition to the main private clinics.[10] In 2007, the different Councils of Humanistic and Technological-Scientific Development (CDCHT) of the main universities consolidated bioethics committees.

Although bioethics education at the university level began almost a decade ago with a focus on clinical aspects, today it is primarily concerned with the global, social, and political aspects. This leads to specializations within bioethics; the first lines of research are defined as pertaining to malpractice, human reproduction, end-of-life issues, biotechnology, sanitary justice, the environment, biolaw, and biopolicy.

As mentioned in the Introduction, there were those who initially regarded bioethics as nothing more than an "academic trend." Nevertheless, over time, it has proved to be a serious academic discipline with the creation of spaces for bioethical discussion within universities, research centers, and other educational institutions. In addition, several events, such as the Bioethics Days of CENABI, the First Venezuelan Congress of Bioethics, the First Latin-American Congress of Bioethics at UCAB (February 2001), and the GTB's Interdisciplinary Reflection Days, have been promoted. Other events include the Ibero-American and Caribbean Congresses of Bioethics and Human Rights in Merida, the Days of the Scientific Societies, the Bioethics Seminars at UPEL, Maturín; the Universidad Gran Mariscal of Ayacucho (UGMA); the East University (UDO); and other events organized by the medical and legal associations in addition to the Society of Juridical Bioethics.

[10] About 60 Institutional Committees of Bioethics are taken into account, because some others are constituted but do not work as such. To be mentioned are: CB-Hospital Clínico Universitario de Caracas, CB-Maternidad Concepción Palacios, CB-Hospital de Niños J. M. de Los Ríos, CB-Hospital de Los Magallanes de Catia, CB-Policlínica Metropolitana, CB-Hospital de Vargas, CB-Hospital San Juan de Dios, CB-Hospital Militar, CB-Hospital Domingo Luciani, CB-Centro Médico Docente La Trinidad, CB-Hospital de Clínicas Caracas, CB-Instituto de Neurología y Neurociencias Aplicadas. Likewise, at the national level we mention: CB-Hospital General de Maracaibo, CB-Hospital de la Petrolera, Lagunillas, CB-Hospital de San Juan de Los Morros, CB-Hospital de Ciudad Bolívar, CB-IVIC, CB-UCV Malariología. Among them are some ad hoc or independent local research committees. But their primary function is of intermediation between the laboratory, research teams, and the National Institute of Hygiene, which gives the final approval.

Venezuela, like other Latin American countries, has come to establish educational events, professional gatherings, and formal publications on bioethics. At present, there are more than 1,000 professionals who have received a Master's degree in bioethics or have taken graduate or undergraduate courses. In addition, there are more than 100 bioethics teachers throughout the country. At the international level, Venezuela participates in a number of international institutions, takes part in various events, and has scholars publishing in the main journals on a global scale.

Recently, Venezuelan scholars presented at the Third South American Congress of History, which focused on professional education and bioethics in Latin American countries. The presentation from Venezuela was entitled "Bioethics as an Interdisciplinary Method of Teaching Health Sciences Graduate Courses in Venezuela."[11] The parallels in bioethics education among the different countries were interesting to observe, although countries such as Argentina, Brazil, Chile, and Colombia are more advanced.

21.7 International Participation

21.7.1 At the Institutional Level

Beginning in 1991, several Venezuelan institutions and scholars have become members of FELAIBE, the federation that integrates the main bioethics associations throughout the Latin American region. Similarly, some experts were invited to the International Council of Global Bioethics (ICGB), which was initially coordinated by Van Rensselaer Potter and is now by Hans F. Schweinsberg. Additionally, some experts have become members of the International Association of Bioethics or the Nuffield Council of Bioethics.

21.7.2 International Congresses

Since the 1990s, there has not been an international congress at which a Venezuelan was not presenting a paper or delivering a lecture, including the meetings of FELAIBE, SIBI, IAB, and Nuffield, among others.

In 2000, Venezuela organized the First Latin-American and Caribbean Congress on "Bioethics, Axiology and Human Rights" at ULA, Merida. Although it did not

[11] I made the presentation at the Third South American Congress of History, at the symposium "Past and Present Trends in Graduate Education in Health Sciences, Evaluation and Academic Accreditation in Latin America," Merida, July 19–21, 2007.

have a great impact, it drew a select group of international lecturers. In 2001 we also organized the First Latin-American Congress of Bioethics and the First Venezuelan Congress of Bioethics at the UCAB,[12] which had the participation of 35 international lecturers, 25 national scholars, and about 600 people from around the country in attendance. At this event, a FELAIBE meeting took place during which the Latin American *Journal of Bioethics* was established and has been published biannually since. It is currently in its 14th issue and is housed at the Nueva Granada Military University, Bogota. Currently, we are attempting to gain membership to the Bioethics Network of Latin America and the Caribbean of UNESCO.

21.8 Professional Education

Since 1990, a number of international experts have been invited to Venezuela. Salvador Bergel comes to ULA every year, Gilberto Cely visits the University of Carabobo, and Ramón Lucas has many chairs, among others. In addition, the United Nations University (UNU) Program on Biotechnology for Latin America and the Caribbean (BIOLAC) provided training for a group of Latin American experts at the First Ibero-American Congress of Bioethics and later at the International Seminar on Bioethics and the Genome at the Institute for Advanced Studies (IDEA), with the participation of Ramón Lacadena.

21.8.1 A Joint Request

A national commitment arose on February 9, 2001, at the First Ibero-American Congress of Bioethics and the First Venezuelan Congress of Bioethics, when the lecturers and more than 600 participants signed the Bioethics Declaration of Caracas, which read as follows:

> Taking into consideration the Universal Declaration of Human Rights of 1948, the American Convention on Human Rights of 1969, the Bioethics Convention of the Asturias on the Prohibition of Cloning Human Beings approved by the Committee of Ministers of the European Council in 1997, the Universal Declaration of the Human Genome and Human Rights of 1997, the Declaration of Manzanillo of 1996 (revised in 1998), the Letter of Panama of 2000, the Declaration of Bioethics of Gijón (World Congress of Bioethics) of 2000.
>
> We declare our firm adherence to the principles enunciated in these documents, our commitment to the defense of life and its quality, our commitment to the defense of dignity and human freedom and to respect global human rights, particularly of persons and peoples least favored in the current distribution of resources.
>
> And based on these convictions we ensure respect for the dignity and freedom of all human beings and every people and to their fundamental rights: civil, political, economic and

[12] Memoirs can be accessed at: http://www.ucab.edu.ve/eventos/bioetica/bioetica.pdf.

cultural, which includes respect for the rights of present and future generations and the entire community of living beings and their ecosystems. And so that this fundamental claim is translated into concrete achievements, we ask:

1. That bioethics education is promoted at all levels
2. That science and technology in all of its manifestations is in service to all of humanity, in particular persons, groups and peoples less favored in the current distribution of information, knowledge, resources and power, without discriminating against individuals because of gender, race or convictions
3. That information is provided at both the expert and lay levels about bioethical aspects of innovations and their scientific and technological use. Matters affecting the everyday life of citizens more must have priority. All persons must have the real possibility of expressing their opinion
4. That States favor the creation of National Bioethics Committees, which watch over the ethical dimension of the development and uses of science, technology and social services, in particular those concerning health. The above mentioned committees must be interdisciplinary, independent and pluralistic, so as to be representative of the knowledge necessary for analyzing bioethical problems and the traditional morals of each country
5. That the use of biosciences and their technologies takes into account the implications they have for the present, as well as future human generations, biodiversity and the environment
6. That every State recognizes and guarantees in an effective way the right of all citizens to quality health services
7. That our societies promote the most profound spirit of solidarity and social justice, and ensure equitable access to the services that guarantee an acceptable standard of living for all persons

Bioethics education has become a reality at all levels of primary and secondary education (basic, technical, and other) through the means of discussions, seminars, workshops, the development of teaching materials, and the direction of students who graduate into research work. At the national curriculum meetings, experiences and projects meant to insert bioethics into the curriculum as an interdisciplinary approach are presented.[13]

Several conferences have been organized by the Venezuelan Institute of Scientific Research of the IDEA,[14] at several of the main universities' research centers, some pharmaceutical companies, and among groups of Venezuelan scholars, for the purpose of creating the appropriate conditions for a dialogue aimed at understanding the role of ethics in the relationship between science and life. Seminars and workshops on bioethics and scientific and technological research have been promoted at the UCV, the UCAB, the UPEL, the UC, the ULA, the University of Zulia (LUZ), the Great Marshal University of Ayacucho (UGMA), the Rómulo Gallegos National Experimental University (UNERG), the Arturo Michelena University (UAM), Monteávila University (UM), and the Monsignor Rafael Arias Blanco Pedagogical Institute University (IUPMA), among others.

[13] Especially at the 4th and 5th, where I presented works on ethical education and the transversality of bioethics.

[14] These institutions governed by MCT have shaped bioethics committees or units that are centered primarily around biotechnological matters.

Since 2001, some bioethics committees have provided training in human rights and have joined with advocacy groups to ensure the protection of the environment and natural resources.

At present, thanks to UNESCO's Bioethics Network, several experts on research involving human beings are being trained, which will fill a gap in expertise within the country. The training takes place via the virtual Master's program of the Borjas Bioethics Institute at Ramón Llull University, Barcelona, coordinated by Francesc Abel and Núria Terribas, and the bioethics specialization at the Catholic University of Chile, coordinated by Francisco León.

In the past decade, between the bioethics committees and the universities, numerous professionals throughout the country have been educated at varying levels. For example, the CENABI, in partnership with the medical school of UCV, has promoted 20 professional development courses taken by approximately 500 professionals, in addition to several courses at the undergraduate and graduate levels in the colleges of health sciences (medicine, pharmacology, and dentistry) with the attendance of about 800 professionals.

The UCAB also offers annual undergraduate seminars (±350 professionals), the UPEL, Maturín, and the UGMA (±250 professionals), the UCSAR's Family Advising and Orientation Course (±250 professionals), UPEL, IUPMA, and others (±200 professionals).

There are other undergraduate and graduate courses at other Venezuelan colleges offering courses, such as ULA (±200 professionals), in addition to several medical, law, and sciences schools (e.g., Merida, Trujillo, St Kitts), such as the medical and law schools of LUZ (±200 professionals); the social sciences and medical colleges of UC (±120 professionals); the faculty of medicine of UNERG (San Juan de los Morros) (±200 professionals); and UAM (San Diego) (±120 professionals). Additional courses are also offered by USB (Baruta); UNEFM (Coro); UCLA's College of Medicine (Barquisimeto); UDO (Cumaná, Jusepín), UM (Caracas), and the Diocesan Seminars (Caracas, Valencia, Cumaná).

The creation of bioethics committees has been promoted in many institutions, primarily in the national reference hospitals, hospitals of the third and fourth levels, private clinics, and research and development centers at universities. The number of committees has grown to about 60 within Venezuela, and some of their locations are identified in Fig. 21.1 below. At present, some of the centers are trying to establish national chapters. The CENABI already has a chapter in the central region of Valencia, and one in Zulia is about to be established.

21.9 New Opportunities and Spaces for Reflection

Bioethics has already come to be understood as a possible venue for prudent future decision making regarding those life issues within which human beings, the environment, and science are all at stake. It encourages the valuation and promotion of life and human dignity as apodictic principles. However, changes in the curricula of the country's educational institutions do not happen overnight. They must occur

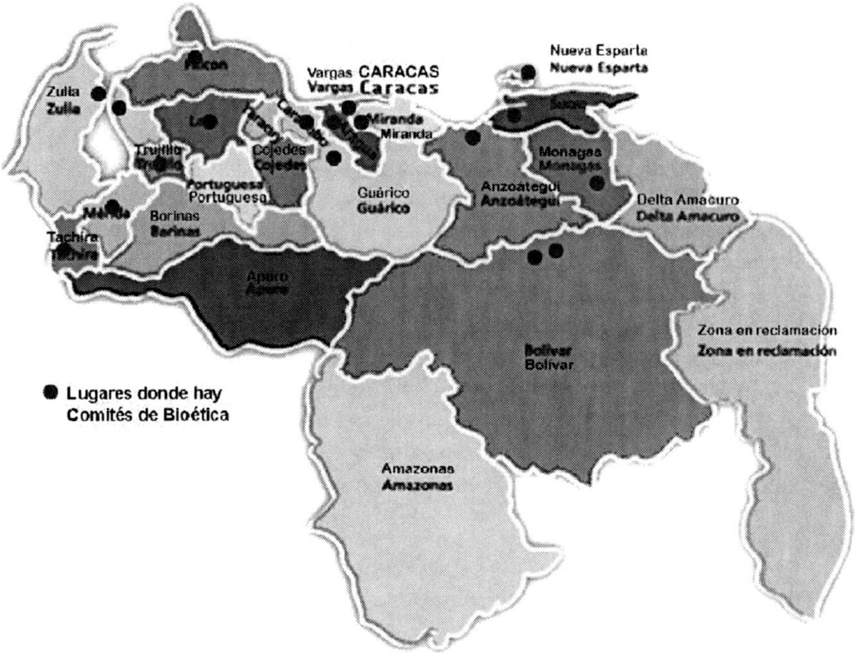

Fig. 21.1 Locations of Bioethics Committees in Venezuela

gradually as bioethics slowly begins to be seen as an interdisciplinary approach capable of integrating techne and praxis, where patient rights are taken into account, professional ethics are strengthened, the environment is respected, and scientific progress happens inside a principled and socio-political framework. Based on the experience of UNESCO, Venezuela has already integrated the primary concerns of international experts, as expressed in their report on the future of bioethics education, which do not differ from those of Latin America and the Caribbean.[15]

To sum up, it is necessary to take into consideration the attitudes and values that are part of human morals:

- Feelings of solidarity and justice
- Respect for others
- A sense of responsibility
- Regard for human work and its fruits
- The relation of attitudes and values to fundamental rights
- The defense of peace
- The protection of the environment
- The identity and cultural dignity of peoples (UNESCO 1981, pp. 26–27)

[15] In Latin American and Caribbean bioethics the focus is on social matters. That is, although it works from the techno-scientific level, it seeks justice, responsibility, and equality.

Other social, ethical, and moral values are used to evoke a broader vision of the world in young people. Education in the twenty-first century demands new trends and perspectives, and therefore it must go beyond the walls of the school and permeate the different dimensions of life (Botkin et al. 1980).

In this way, the voice of bioethics is sensitizing and dialogic and remains alert to any violations of life, especially before the developments of an unrestrained science (Russ 1994, pp. 107–108). Bioethics also serves to weave and interconnect life within the world by way of its interdisciplinary nature. It makes necessary the establishment of bridges throughout history.

On the other hand, interpretation is also needed. One must seek a vision that is both utopian and concrete in its nature. In this, we must also recognize a "respect for life" and a need for a certain "quality of life." This constitutes the primary challenge of discovering, assimilating, and reinterpreting the term "life" in accord with the bioethical reality of a life situated in the twenty-first century. Similarly, law, economics, politics, and other disciplines must create new spaces for reflection. Bioethics is currently located between anthropocentrism and cosmocentrism.

21.10 Conclusion

The interdisciplinary approach of bioethics has infused itself into the curriculum of university programs in medicine, political sciences, law, the humanities, and education. Bioethics allows us to rediscover being as a being-for-life and a being-for-encounter (Habermas 1996), an encounter with ourselves and with our world (other living beings and their environment).

At the same time, bioethics allows humans to develop a broader and more holistic vision of the interconnections of human life, the quality of life, scientific "truths," and the environment and the ecosystem. This serves to establish new limits and possibilities for every human being in one's particular context, aiming at the development of an interdisciplinary perspective on life, health, the environment, and science.

Bioethics considers the complexity of life and therefore requires a global effort sensitive to the socio-cultural context in which it develops. The interdisciplinary experience and one's vision of the world, science, and life develop within the epistemological framework proposed by bioethics. The complexity of life and its promotion continue to broaden, making the protection of human existence and the environment more difficult as one's context becomes ever more egoistic and unethical: there is increasing danger in the streets, and violence in general is relentless; tobacco, alcohol, and drug consumption continue to increase; young people are ever more frustrated about their futures; the world continues to be increasingly impoverished, social stratification increases and the hope of overcoming poverty becomes bleak; and there continues to be a need to reevaluate sex, marriage, family, and society.

The increasing influence of bioethics on the evaluation and supervision of research protocols requires additional coordination of efforts and better definitions as needed. Venezuela has been one of the first countries to conduct research for large, international laboratories. However, notwithstanding the quality of the results, there is a need to have the protocols and amendments evaluated by the home research team, the research ethics committees, the National Institute of Hygiene or the laboratories themselves. This is a problem that must be solved soon.

The expectation of increased knowledge of humans and the value of life, truth, and science has allowed for different experts to participate jointly in the reflections of bioethics. Educational institutions are always looking for curricula that will contribute to the evolution of the individual and that will allow one to acquire new knowledge from primary school to the university. Thus, we are trying to accomplish the first item of the Bioethics Declaration of Caracas (2001): "That bioethics education be promoted at all levels," in addition to life-long learning (UNESCO)[16] and continuous education (AUSJAL – Asociación de Universidades Confinadas a la Compañía de Jesús en América Latina 2000, 2001).

Bioethics demonstrates different tasks that are necessary to overcome some of the challenges of professional performance:

1. First of all, that we apply Cicero's maxim, "If you want to learn, teach." This challenge obliges professionals to acquire an aptitude both for learning and for teaching, since one learns while teaching. Similarly, they must encourage learning-by-doing.

   This constitutes a modality of self-education that accredits professionals in the exercise of their own profession. For example, it is not possible to practice within the health sciences without continued training in the innovations of the respective specialization, as biomedical knowledge doubles every two to four years.[17]
2. Second, it is urgent that one recognizes the value of life, especially within complex and critical situations, such as making end-of-life decisions or continuing to disturb environmental and ecological cycles.
3. Third and related to the second, one must be sensitive to the fact of how significant the consequences of an immediate and biased decision can be for health, the environment, biological diversity, climate, or the quality of water, soil, or air. Decisions must be carefully considered and evaluated, based on the consequences it could have.
4. The fourth challenge takes root in what Albert Einstein expressed when he said that study is not to be taken as a duty, but rather as an opportunity to enter into the wonderful universe of knowledge. This challenge can be linked to the first one, but one must recognize that human knowledge is never achieved in abundance,

[16] The works of UNESCO's International Commission on Education for the Twenty-First Century (1993) emphasize life-long learning as a key to entering the twenty-first century. This concept goes beyond its traditional articulation as education past the conclusion of one's formal education, and is meant to engender the educational society where everything is regarded as an occasion to learn and to develop one's capacities.

[17] I recommend reading the experiences of Pablo Polido, E-learning and Medical Education in Latin America. Meeting of Educational Technology (Caracas, UNIMET) November 5, 2004. Available at: http://www.ares.unimet.edu.ve/encuentroted/trabajos PDF/DrPabloPulido.ppt

if one is not exposed to the many opportunities that life has to offer to beings and their environments. One must be given a sense of human existence and its variegated contexts, and the need for one to seek truth and responsibility for oneself, others, and nature. It is impossible for education to be entirely neutral in its content, for it is littered with metaconcepts in which there are values and a need to oppose attitudes contrary to the promotion of life. There is also a need to emphasize that one generally treats these topics in a stereotyped way in the classroom, dismissing reality in its context.

5. From this stems the fifth challenge, the critical need to achieve the following factors for professional success: to improve the quality of expertise concerning the concept of life; to guarantee the continued evaluation and accreditation of educational institutions; offering the best development of clinical competence; to understand and to attend to the health needs of the population (Pulido 2004).
6. The sixth challenge concerns the social responsibility of bioethicists to their communities (Schmidt 2005). I denounce the complex Latin American and Caribbean educational reality in the words of the Mexican tenor, Plácido Domingo: "In most countries one is not interested in educating people, because when they learn to read they begin to be conscious of problems and begin to take [governments] to task; illiterate people say nothing." What I am interested in is the future I seek for my progeny, my friends, my compatriots, and other residents.

   Ethical responsibility is the integration of the subjective and objective realities. This occurs with the merging of subjects and action. There is an aspect of discovery revealed by action in the strict sense and its consequences. The ethical order is present, not as a visible reality, but as a reasoned appeal that asks for calmness, prudence, and balance. Hans Jonas names this order the principle of responsibility.

   Without question, medicine was the most ancient merger of science and art, done for the benefit of the patient, and essentially different from the technologies that destroy the environment. With medicine's clear goal of fighting illness through cure and the alleviation of pain, these methods have remained ethically unquestionable. However, today, with entirely new technological power, the advancements of techno-scientific progress can become the objects of doubt. Some of our current abilities make clear the criteria that arouse ethical doubt, especially, for example, those resources which can be used at the beginning and end of life. Our birth and our death touch the most essential questions of human life: the concept of *bonum humanum*, the meaning of life and death, the dignity of the person, and the integrity of the human image. These are real questions for philosophers. Here, a place where the individual paradigm has to tell the truth, the philosopher can promote the meeting of ethics with techniques (Jonas 1994).
7. The seventh challenge is based on complex thinking. Many people are concerned to find the fastest way to teach. As Seneca would say, "Lengthy is teaching by means of theories; brief and effective is teaching by means of examples." However, everything has a theoretical foundation that must be reached to understand the things we think we realize, the things that are approachable by means

of a diversity of disciplines, and a multiplicity of personal opinions, preconceptions, sentimentalities, and similar things. To return to Seneca: "Our defect is to learn more at school than in life". One of the problems is that what is taught is taken out of the context of the surrounding reality, where significant learning takes place. The problem is encapsulated in the reflection of Moisés W. Pérez: "A text said out of context is only a pretext."

Remembering the Bioethics Declaration of Caracas (2001), little by little educational programs must develop the interdisciplinary approach of bioethics. The curricula should strive for the development of significant learning, the promotion of cultural diversity, professional rationality, the revaluation of learning in terms of what is integral to a human being, and the adoption of new and adequate methods, modalities, and resources for teaching (Zabala 2000).

There have been many positive recommendations, but there are a few things that should be taken into account for the next stage of maturation:

First, we must not be selfish and follow the interdisciplinary nature of bioethics.

Second, we must consolidate and integrate the movement at a national level within the National Commission of Bioethics or the network we have been developing.

Third, it is mandatory to write and publish. It has been difficult trying to establish our first specialized journal in bioethics, and one must attempt to publish in the local journals of medicine, law, and philosophy, in addition to the international journals. Up until now, there have only been isolated efforts to do so. The truth is that publications can be increased, even though some bulletins already exist in Caracas, Merida, and Maracaibo. CENABI has a series of six volumes, one for every module of instruction that has already been updated for graduate courses.

Fourth, there needs to be a better effort in promoting more frequent national meetings. CENABI has held 10 annual Bioethics Days, the GTB has annual meetings, and the IAHULA has organized several events. However, in 2008, only the *Second* National Congress of Bioethics will be realized

Taking these challenges into consideration, if we overcome them, bioethics in Venezuela will move on to the maturation stage.

To finish, educational bioethics programs must promote a pluralistic and constructive dialogue that allows one the opportunity to reflect on life. From these reflections, one must make an effort to raise public awareness (ethical, social, and psychological) about human experience, an effort based on human dignity as a *sine qua non* condition and on the apodictic value of life in favor of human existence and mankind's cultural traditions and beliefs.

In this way, we will fulfill the Millenium Declaration (United Nations 2000) and the Universal Commitment to the Dignity of the Human Being (II World Conference on Bioethics 2002), the first commitment of which expresses the need for "Promoting and implementing the respect and protection of human dignity and the biosphere, such that they become universal and common habits exercised for peaceful living, the responsible exercise of freedom, liberty, and autonomy, which will be the legacy for future generations."

References

Academia Pontificia para la Vida the Pontifical Academy for Life. La naturaleza humana y el derecho a la vida. Available at: www.bioeticaweb.com/magisterio/PAV_nat_hum.htm

AUSJAL – Asociación de Universidades Confinadas a la Compañía de Jesús en América Latina (2000) Desafíos de América Latina y propuesta educativa. AUSJAL, Caracas

AUSJAL – Asociación de Universidades Confinadas a la Compañía de Jesús en América Latina (2001) Plan estratégico 2001–2005. AUSJAL, Caracas

Botkin JW, Elmandjara M, Malitza M (1980) Aprender, horizontes sin limites. Santillana, Madrid

Conclusion of First Ibero American Congress of Bioethics, Caracas, February 2-9, 2001. Updated and improved Caracas, July 27-August 1, 2008. Second Bioethics Declaration of Caracas (2008) http://www.debatecultural.net/Observatorio2/LudwigSchmidt.htm

Habermas J (1996) La lógica de las ciencias sociales. Tecnos, Madrid

II World Conference on Bioethics (2002) Universal commitment to the dignity of the human Being. Gijón, Spain. Available at: http://www.sibi.org/ingles/ddc/com.htm

Jonas H (1994) Ética, medicina e técnica. Vega-Passagens, Lisbon

Kranzberg M (1985) The information age: Evolution or revolution? In: Guile BR (ed) Information technologies and social transformation. National Academy of Engineering, Washington, DC

Leon FJ (2004) Diez años de bioética en América Latina: historia reciente y retroactiva. In: Lolas Stepke F (ed) Diálogo y cooperación en salud: diez años de la bioética en la OPS. Programa Regional de Bioética, Santiago de Chile

Mainetti JA (1993) Estudios bioéticos. Editorial Quirón, La Plata

Potter VR (1971) Bioethics: Bridge to the future. Prentice Hall, New Jersey

Pulido P (2004) E-learning y educación médica en la América Latina. In: Encuentro en Tecnología Educativa (Nov. 5). UNIMET, Caracas. Available at: http://ares.unimet.edu.ve/encuentroted/trabajos/trabajosPDF/DrPabloPulido.ppt

Republica Bolivariana de Venezuela. Constitución (2000) Gaceta Oficial Extraordinaria n. 5453 de la República Bolivariana de Venezuela, March 24

Russ J (1994) La pensée éthique contemporaine. Universitaires de France, Paris

Schmidt L (2002) La formación universitaria de la bioética al personal de salud en Venezuela. In: VI Congreso Nacional Latinoamericano y del Caribe de Bioética. Bioética en la calidad de la atención médica. En las memorias del Simposio Universidad y Salud en Latinoamérica (Oct. 27–30). Tuxtla-Gutiérrez, México

Schmidt L (2005) Global responsibility and bioethics: Humanization ways. In: Ethics and philosophy in the emergent medical technologies. Event sponsored by AECEM/EACME, the European Society for Philosophy of Medicine and Healthcare (ESPMH) and Institut Borja of Bioètica-University Ramon Llull, Barcelona; August 24–27

UNESCO (1981) Sobre el futuro de la educación: hacia el año 2000. Narcea, Madrid

United Nations (2007) Climate change conference. Bali. Available at: http://unfccc.int/meetings/cop_13/items/4049.php

United Nations (2000) Millennium declaration. Available at: http://www.un.org/millennium/declaration/ares552e.htm

United Nations (1992) Earth summit. Rio de Janeiro. Available at: http://www.un.org/geninfo/bp/enviro.html

United Nations (1948) Universal declaration of human rights. Available at: http://www.un.org/en/documents/udhr

Wilkie T (1994) El conocimiento peligroso: el Proyecto Genoma Humana y sus implicancias. Debate, Madrid

Zabala MA (2000) Diseño y desarrollo curricular. Nancea, Madrid

Bibliography

Adorno T (1975) Dialéctica negativa. Taurus, Madrid
Apel K (1991) Teoría de la verdad y ética del discurso. Paidós, Barcelona
Biagi S (1999) Impacto de los medios. Thomson, México
Boeri R (1993) Bioetica, pluralismo e principio di toleranza. Bioetica Riv Interdisc 1, p. 111
Carr W, Stephen K (1988) Teoría crítica de la enseñanza. MartínezRoca, Barcelona
Chadwick C (1987) Tecnología educacional para el docente. Paidós, Barcelona
De Corte E (1989) Toward a theory of learning from instruction: the case on cognitive skills. University of Leuven, Belgium
Eisner E (1979) Educational imagination. Macmillan, New York
Gadamer HG (1984) Verdad y método: fundamentos de una hermenéutica filosófica. Sígueme, Salamanca
Gracia D (1989) Fundamentos de bioética. Eudema Universidad, Madrid
Hegel G (1966) Fenomenología del espíritu. FCE, México
Howe L, Mary H (1977) Cómo personalizar la educación. Santillana, Madrid
Jonas H (1997) Técnica, medicina y ética. Paidós, Barcelona
Klaus D (1972) Técnicas de individualización e innovación en la enseñanza. Trillas, México
Kuhn TS (1978) La estructura de las revoluciones científicas. FCE, México
Lakatos I (1983) La metodología de los programas de investigación científica. Alianza, Madrid
MacIntyre A (1988) Historia de la ética. Paidós, Barcelona
Morin E (1981) El Método I: naturaleza de la naturaleza. Cátedra, Madrid
Morin E (1982) Para salir del siglo XX. Kayros, Barcelona
Novak J (1982) Teoría y práctica de la educación. Alianza, Madrid
Polanyi M (1966) El estudio del hombre. Paidós, Buenos Aires
Ricouer P (1969) Le conflit des interprétations. Seuil, París

Part III
Special Topics in Bioethics

Chapter 22
Bioethics and Religion in Latin America

Márcio Fabri dos Anjos

22.1 Introduction

The relationship between bioethics and religion is an intriguing subject that invites many questions. In this article, I want to discuss the intersection of religion and bioethics at this stage of its development in Latin America. As a Christian theologian, I tend to emphasize the contributions of religion to bioethics, but a critical examination reveals where they are at odds with each other. However, both are confronted with similar problems brought about by a broader cultural movement that demands the reinterpretation of the motivations of ethics and the grounds of religion. With this reinterpretation, a change simultaneously occurs in the social spaces affected by religion and ethics. Therefore, an appropriate starting place would be to discover the challenges common to both religion and bioethics and to determine how they can work together to solve these problems.

Bioethics, like ethics, has many currents and trends. In a specific way, the same occurs with religious diversity. In this article, I seek to find what type of bioethics is most appropriately applied in the Latin American context. When I speak of *religion*, I refer particularly to Christianity, in a Catholic theological reading, but remain open to the challenge of renewal that is common to the different religious confessions. I will also try to take into account the richness of religious traditions that precede Christianity.

22.2 "Bridges to the Future": Common Bridges

If we take into account Potter's (1971) concern regarding the survival of the future of humanity, bioethics finds in religion an approach that thinks about and considers life in relation to the future. Although significant differences become apparent

M.F. dos Anjos
Ph.D. Research and Professor of Bioethics at Saint Camillus University Center,
Centro Universitário São Camilo, Programa de Mestrado em Bioética, São Paulo, BR
Professor of Academia de Teologia Moral da Pontificia Universidade Lateranense, Roma
e-mail: mfabri@terra.com.br

L. Pessini et al. (eds.), *Ibero-American Bioethics: History and Perspectives*,
Philosophy and Medicine 106, DOI 10.1007/978-1-4020-9350-0_22,

when considering the possible outcomes of this approach, one cannot deny the importance of this fact. It becomes even more forceful when one acknowledges that religions participate actively in the cultural construction by which people understand life and the world, as well as its history and orientation towards the future. This is also the context wherein bioethics generates many questions and, while religion persists in this task, the cultural contexts cannot be ignored by bioethics.

From this perspective, Latin America has received from its aboriginal peoples an extremely rich cultural and religious inheritance. In this legacy, we find values that current bioethics starts to develop, especially concerning the significance of human beings in relation to the world and their relationship with the environment. For example, the Mayan and Aztec cultures, through ancient traditions, developed systems of understanding, including cultural and religious practices, in which human beings were integrated and became participants of a broader world. In the same way, many other Amerindian peoples persist today in supporting a more inclusive understanding of life. Their ethical conclusions become efficient for both caring for and protecting the environment and cultivating social relations favorable to life inside the culture. One cannot be so naïve as to ignore the asymmetries and inequalities in the cultures and religious systems of aboriginal peoples, but their systems remain deeply admirable for guaranteeing equity and cultivating reciprocity in relationships.

Today we are facing a radical cultural transformation. All references are put in question and aboriginal cultures and religious systems in particular are to a large extent surpassed by a hegemonic culture marked by science and technology. Still, it can be said that the wisdom of these institutions remains in the imagination. Bioethics, as a young discipline, has not yet been able to take full advantage of this wisdom. However, there are some indications of its capacity to critique the devastation of the environment and to posit an ethical requirement to take care of it.

The contribution of Christianity in Latin America takes an uncertain form, as it has been marked by a climate of conquest by the economic and political colonization which characterizes it. In this context, some scholars are not afraid to consider the Christian emergence on the Continent as a *spiritual conquest* (Suess 1992). This assessment has remained controversial in the 500 years since the arrival of Columbus to the Americas (1492). In this and other critiques of religious systems, we see something common to human organizations: an asymmetry between what is taught and what is practiced. Later we can revisit this topic to consider theological renewal in recent times.

Beyond the shadows, or even surrounded by them, Christianity has become an important influence for modern bioethics in the Latin American arena. By means of Christianity, the ethics of life inspired by a horizon beyond death is strengthened. The commandments of love and respect for life persist as a reference for relationships. And most of all the suffering image of the Christian Savior echoes in the suffering of the colonized people and aids in developing feelings of solidarity and compassion. Today, it would be deeply difficult to understand the reach of the concepts of *dignity* and *solidarity* in Latin America without an appeal to the religious conceptions that are part of their construction.

From a theoretical perspective, Christianity of a Catholic inspiration provides the manuals for Moral Theology which necessarily contain treatises related to the protection of life. Although they generally resemble European manuals and are basically restricted to the clergy, they nevertheless require ethical reflections of questions related to life. Thus, the arrival of modern bioethics in Latin America will find, particularly among the clergy, a theoretically informed ethical reflection on life, albeit a limited one. This same reflexive tradition allowed for the exploration of some dialogues between Pope Pius XII (1939–1958) and doctors and health professionals of his time, particularly pertaining to questions of euthanasia and dying. It equally allows for the understanding of figures such as the German theologian, Bernhard Häring, whose many writings were translated in Latin America and influenced the theological dialogue during the progress of Medicine in the 1960s and 1970s.

With these preliminaries and without intending to do a historical synthesis, I only want to recount how religion inside of cultural, political, and economic processes contributes to the formation of an *ethos* for modern bioethics in Latin America. In many ways, the "bridges for the future" that bioethics seeks to build have several points in common with religion which should be taken into account.

22.3 Bioethics: An Estrangement Between Reason and Religion?

The theoretical basis of bioethics brings into question its relations with religion. While religion follows faith, bioethics follows reason. This divergence suggests that bioethics would radically differentiate between a *lay* and a *religious* bioethics; they would have certain similarities and differences regarding their set of rules, but in their foundations they would always be *moral strangers*. This question appears crucial to the determination of their relationship. In fact, the question unfolds into two assumptions: that faith is really distant from reason and that the reason is really distant from spiritual motivations, or faith. But to what degree or in what measure, are these assumptions true?

It is true that Christianity, when recounting its experience of faith, has a long history of events which point to reason in belief and belief in reason. In its inception, due to the cultural context within which it was born, Christianity was marked by an emphasis for following the Master in its life practices and horizons of meanings. But it soon met Greek philosophical thought, from which the necessity of clarifying the reasons of faith took new routes. Although some philosophers, including H. Tristram Engelhardt, Jr. (2000) in particular, argue against this approach, Christianity, particularly in the West, begins to understand faith as having an intimate connection with philosophy. Among so many important thinkers, Saint Augustine (354–430) and Saint Thomas Aquinas (1225–1274) stand out. Augustine, reworking the inheritance of Greek thought, advocated for "a synthesis of a metaphysics of nature with a metaphysics of freedom, since liberty, by means of Christianity, is transformed into the very *matter* of philosophy" (Oliveira 2000, p. 73). Aquinas stands out due to his theological elaboration in seeking an understanding of the totality of beings, the world, and their relationship with the transcendent; he establishes a deep dialogue with thinkers in general, and particularly with Augustinian thought and Aristotelian philosophy (Oliveira 2000, pp. 75–104). Known for his well-worn phrases, Augustine (PL 33, 452 ad 3) said, already in the Fifth Century: "Far from us to think that faith stirs us up to refuse or to stop searching for reason, for we could not even believe if we were not rational." In our times, Pope Benedict XVI, in a speech addressed to the scientific community of the University of Regensburg, in Germany, made a clear statement "not to act according to reason, not to act according to *logos*, is contrary to the nature of God" (Benedict XVI, Pope 2006, p. 8).

History reveals the tensions that have manifested between reason and religion. These tensions are still persistent in preventing the Christian faith from having certain interactions with modern thought. But Christianity does not restrict itself to groups opposed to rationality for it develops itself significantly in another sense. Perhaps more comprehensively, the interaction between faith and reason is taken these days as a question that not only challenges religions, but also modern reason, as is demonstrated by, among other authors, Oliveira (2000). We will not discuss here the complex questions that the subject implies, but I want to suggest that faith and reason are not necessarily *moral strangers* except in those interactions that distinguish their respective discourses.

Christianity in Latin America participates in bioethics with a faith that seeks reasons. Liberation Theology (formulated in 1969) is a clear expression of this approach, as we will see below. Its perceptions and proposals appear to make significant contributions to some aspects of Latin American Bioethics, especially in its receptivity to social matters and persistent questions that defy Bioethics.

22.4 Religion and Bioethics in a Context of Persistent Inequities

Religion and Bioethics cannot be understood in the Latin American context without taking into account its history, which is marked by deep social inequities. We mentioned above the experience of colonialism. It is true that this cannot be reduced only to its negative aspects, but it is difficult to forget the scars of the deep social inequalities derived from it: the genocide to which the aboriginal peoples have been subjected; the exploitation of slave workers; and the voracity with which colonialism took the Continent to exploit its wealth. These are salient points in the history of Latin America which have established a heavy cultural inheritance, the effects of which are still felt today (Suess 1992; Chasteen 2001, 2005).

Thus, the Latin American culture with so much cordiality, joy, and celebration presents at the same time unlimited corruption and incredible social inequities that directly affect people's life conditions including health, housing, education, jobs, wages, and life expectancy. It is symptomatic of these circumstances that at least half of the Latin American population living below the poverty line are either of aboriginal or afro-descent. The Inter-American Development Bank concludes that "the poverty of socially excluded groups is permanent and not transitory" (Banco Interamericano de Desenvolvimento na América Latina 2005, p. 19). In one respect, we can say that Latin America is not properly conceived of as a continent of poverty, but more appropriately as a continent of deep inequities. The inequalities can also be located in international relations, as a product of a long history of dependence, international debts, and long drawn out promises of being "in development." The current emphasis on autonomy, in regard to societies that are debilitated in terms of citizenship, is, in the end, marked by a neo-liberalism that completely ignores individuals and legitimates inequalities. This contributes to the increase of violence and the resulting loss of confidence amongst the people and institutions.

The question is: how do liberation theology and bioethics function before and within such a reality? Liberation theology emphasizes, in religious experience, the question of coherence between the professed faith and the practices of social life. As such, it harshly criticizes a reality shaped by social and even religious injustices. Its action is understood in terms of a broader world process for understanding reality. We do not ask if Christian theology interacts with the sciences, and particularly with philosophy, but we do ask *which* philosophies and sciences are influential and construct the rational foundations of faith. Theology recognizes that one cannot understand the network of human history and social inequities only through *essentialist* philosophies. It instead considers those philosophies which may be more effective at exposing unjust structures that remain unacknowledged by other approaches; and is also capable of recognizing individualistic trends and perceiving the undeniable links between human inter-subjectivity and its social commitments.

It is easy to see that this function of theology also has much to do with the construction of the foundations of Bioethics, by assessing the correlation between its principles and reality. When the North American bioethical principles began to be criticized, I was asked to present this Latin American and theological conception to enrich the foundations of Bioethics (Anjos 1994, p. 130–147). But such contributions also emerge in the methodology for approaching specific subjects, as is seen in Pessini's writings on dysthanasia (Sorta-Bilajac et al. 2005) and euthanasia (Pessini 2004).

In this sense, Latin American theology, at least as a strengthening element, has contributed to the formation of Latin American bioethics. It has certainly helped to guarantee the ethical condemnation of injustices, with the corollary concern of revealing the processes by which one can expose the great inequalities deeply rooted in society. The Sixth World Congress of Bioethics sponsored by Brazil, in 2002, with the theme "Bioethics: power and injustice" (Garrafa and Pessini 2003), characterized this profile well.

22.5 Beyond Dogmatism

Although I do not aim to present here a synthesis of liberation theology, it is beneficial for bioethics to note that scientific dialogue has given theology a rereading of its very reference points and foundations. In Bible studies, for instance, theology assumes the history of the construction of texts as a basic and indispensable step to understanding the content of their message. Socio-cultural contexts are decisive for us to be able to evaluate the reach of terms employed and statements made. To sum up, *text, context, and message* are supposed to be three inseparable aspects to be considered in the theological exploration of Biblical references. This means that unfamiliarity with social–cultural contexts that are present in the elaboration of (verbal traditions and) texts leads to religious *fundamentalism*. On the other hand, in analyzing contexts, particularly those more deeply rooted in social–cultural systems and structures, the reach of faith proposals for life becomes clearer.

This process is also present in the understanding of *dogmas* of faith themselves. *Dogmas* stop being expressions of fundamentalism when one is aware of the social–cultural context of their formulation, particularly when we take into account the specific questions they were supposed to answer. Thus, one recognizes today, even officially, that an evolution in *dogmas* exists, and also recognizes the limits and the progressive character of human knowledge and its perceptions. These brief comments allow us to see how theology, as a rational moment of faith, allows for a close approach to the sciences for understanding the different processes of life. In its method, liberation theology consecrated as indispensable a moment called *analysis of reality*. This moment employs *social–analytical mediations*, that is, sciences with which one can adequately understand reality and make religious readings as a critique and proposal.

If we criticize dogmas in religion and theology, we can also ask whether there are dogmas in bioethics. It seems worthwhile to consider this question at least as a maieutic resource for some circumstances.

22.6 Bioethics and Theology on the Question of Transcendence

The question of transcendence is an extremely interesting point where bioethics and theology meet in the Latin American context. We can take here the concept of transcendence in a very broad sense that encompasses everything that goes beyond being, and includes questions of how human beings *survive* and self-actualize. I am not going to examine deeply the numerous theories that have searched for answers to these questions since Antiquity; however, I find it is important to point to the possibilities of mutual enrichment between the discourse of theology and bioethics in regard to the concept of transcendence.

It is well known that Christianity affirms that life only fully actualizes beyond history, in a definitive encounter with the Absolute. For those who do not have such a certainty or faith, this emphasis of life's actualization beyond death no doubt makes a dialogue difficult. Latin American theology makes an important step for promoting a dialogue precisely because it rescues the emphasis on human accomplishments inside history itself, in its processes of individual and social life. Even without losing sight of the horizon of life after death, it gives to religion a vigorous intra-historical transforming force that is just the reason for it being a theology *of liberation*. This is a productive space for it to come closer to bioethics. Let us examine some significant points of proximity in this sense.

Latin American theology aims to identify together with the sciences the challenge of human beings' survival, not only in their condition of finitude but also in the favorable or adverse situations of their social and environmental relations. It interprets this human condition as the great space of gestation of life itself, of *autopoiesis*, where human beings are at the same time creatures and creators. In this sense, the expression "to play God" should not be understood as a usurpation of divine power; on the contrary, the creative potentiality is certainly a human prerogative, one that theology itself sees as a *gift* given to human beings. From this comes not a prohibition but a challenge to act responsibly: what are we to do with so great a power? Still together with the sciences, theology examines the different human attempts to deal with this power throughout history and identifies different ways for dealing with that power. And so it comes across with great concentrations of power, oppression and destructive forms of violence. In the last analysis, there are ways for searching auto-affirmation, for guaranteeing this *autopoiesis*, of actualizing and surviving.

The specific contribution of Christian theology is very surprising (see Anjos 2003, p. 455–465), for it suggests that we understand the exercise of power in an eminently communicative and not concentrative sense. It goes against concentration of power and oppression. Here, vulnerability is not a field to be explored, but a challenge to the creative and potentiating spirit. The *other* we meet in relationships is not to be taken as a competitor, but to be searched for as a partner. Her lacks and sufferings are a provocative outcry. Survival, therefore, is not – according to this proposal – in exploiting or excluding the other, but in her respectful and unifying inclusion, grounded in mutual relationships and guided by love. Here is a key-concept that summarizes the set of its proposals: Jon Sobrino (1992), when considering oppressions and sufferings, enunciated it as the *principle of mercy*. It is obviously a principle that establishes a direction for all other attitudes and options that preside over action.

It is worth remarking that this theological perspective implies the image we make of God. The absolute is not mute, but communicative. It does not govern human history simply from outside, but enters it for manifesting itself inside it with its signs. It posits itself as a *spirit* that guides and livens up human potentialities and its fragile freedom in the construction of the ways of life. In this sense, a critique is in order for the transformation of the figure of Jesus Christ as legislator and conqueror; or many times, also as expiator of the disobediences of humanity before an angry God. In the counterproposal that is born from this critique, is first of all the image of a *master* who teaches by his practices and theory the ways the absolute *spirit* takes humanity in the construction of life.

Therefore, for a bioethical perspective it seems worth remarking that the theme of transcendence does not necessarily make religion the beyond or the distant and alien to historicity. Its relationship with history and even with daily life allows us to identify bioethics and religion in a confluence of perceptions and proposals. On the other hand, religion interrogates bioethics itself about its way of dealing with transcendence, about the spirit that presides over its criteria to evaluate and propose the exercise of autonomy and freedom.

22.7 Is There an Implicit Religion Within Bioethics?

When proposing this question, I am taking religion in a broad sense that precedes each and every specific religious institution. Considering that the conditioned human is situated in time, surrounded by deficiencies of all kinds and directed towards the desire of actualization, one can admit the necessity of human beings to go beyond themselves or at least beyond the situation in which they find themselves. There is in this a sort of *transcendence*. The Bible speaks of a *thirst* for God. The analogy of thirst is doubly interesting, because it first reminds one of the necessity we have of going outside of ourselves to seek feeding. Further, it also posits the question of what or who can really satisfy and actualize us.

This process includes dimensions of science and a type of faith. This is because human knowledge is limited and the challenge of living demands us to go beyond this knowledge and enter into the space of confident adhesion where scientific evidences are precarious. From that arises a question about what or whom we belive, either individually or collectively. With this integration of science and faith, we construct life projects, we deal with our desires, we create options, and we propose objectives for ourselves. I agree with Paul Tillich, who writes that "religion is unconditionally tied to the sense of life of the individual", and at the same time leads it to have expression in a "social group with symbols of thought and action" (Tillich 1988, p. 159).

Jean Bartoli (2005) conducted an interesting research project in the great city of São Paulo (Brazil) about the principles of life for executives, published in the editorials of a specialized magazine. The results show how principles, apparently lay and pragmatic, directed to enterprise professionals, involve religious components that go beyond a simple parallel. One sees that the ideals of perfection, proposed by those who lead the life of executives, impose a hierarchy of values, an ascetic route marked by acceptance and sacrifice, and even rituality similar to that found in conventional religions. Suggestively, the author titles his work with the question: "Is being an executive an ideal religion?"

Latin American theology develops an old tradition that consists in rendering in terms of *gods* the ideals that preside over human options, projects, and accomplishments. Rubem Alves observes that:

> … the same religious questions of the past are articulated now, altered, by secularized symbols. Names are metamorphosed. The same religious function persists. (...) If this is true, we will be forced to conclude not that our world secularized, but rather that gods and religious hopes had been given new names and new labels, and its priests and prophets, new clothes, new places and new jobs (Alves 1989, p. 13).

Among the relevant tasks this implies are the challenges of identifying the *gods*, their promises, and requirements, and also their capacities for fulfilling their promises.

Theology calls attention to the illusory side of promises that are attractive but will never be fulfilled; and names the *gods* of these deceptive promises *idols* (from the Greek word *éidolon*, meaning simulacra, imagination, ghost). This markedly religious language hides extremely practical questions that demand examination and reflection of the consistency of the senses and ideals that guide individual and social life. It has encouraged Latin American theology to unmask the sacrificialism with which some justify the great inequities in social systems which manifest in poverty, hunger, discrimination, and exclusion.

Bioethics as a rational discourse can conveniently take into account these inevitable vestiges of religion implicit in social systems. In addition, as sciences are not simply neutral, it would not be bad that in the field of bioethics we have the courage to argue about the *gods* that preside over our certainties and discourses.

22.8 Lay Bioethics and Religious Bioethics: The Challenge of Discourse

In one of the meetings where the preparations for the founding of the Brazilian Bioethics Society occurred, an interesting conversation took place which serves to introduce the theme of discourse between lay and religious bioethics. In the group's debates, the question of religion in bioethics arose, and someone was emphatic in saying, more or less, "As for me God does not exist. I do not see why we consider religion in Bioethics." In a cordial reaction, I simply stated: "Then, welcome to the club of theology." A little surprised, he continued: "What do you mean?" I explained that *theology* is a discourse about God, adding that to deny God's existence is a kind of theological discourse. Accepting the logic of the comment, he corrected himself: "Well! That is, I am an agnostic; I do not know God." But the second conclusion was: "If this is the case, welcome to the dialogue! Let's exchange knowledge about this in the field of Bioethics."

The polarization between a lay bioethics and a religious bioethics deserves particular attention, especially in the Latin American context. To talk about this requires considering first that Bioethics develops its reflection from a particular context that characterizes it. This is the function of the adjectives that at times qualify bioethics. Generally, they emphasize the type of references used by the subjects that elaborate it, and point to the area where reflection converges. This is a condition of human thought, a point from which they go seeking for the dimensions of universality. The dialogue between the different knowledge forms, sources, and contexts becomes a basic resource for the consolidation of concepts. In this sense, the distinction between lay and religious Bioethics would not be exclusive, but open to complementation.

However, one knows that live coals exist underneath these extinguished ashes. History shows a long hegemony of religious thought in the construction of senses and the interpretation of realities, with a deep influence in social organization. This hegemony did not bring with it only the power of religious thought, but also political power.

One knows how Leonardo Boff (1981) raised the question of power inside the religious community itself. The hegemony of religious power was broken by the eruption of modernity that attributes to the autonomy of reason the construction of the universe of significances that guide the senses of existence, thinking and acting of both societies and the individuals. Religion is now relegated to the private sphere.

In Latin America, this eruption appeared after some delay due to a large extent to the union between Church and State that persisted from colonial times to the Nineteenth Century. The numerous adjustments this transformation has required are still in progress in the Latin American Continent and present certain variations in the different regional experiences. Thus, it is understandable and fair that through the opposition between *lay* and *religious*, one posits in bioethical reflection the autonomy of reason before religious authoritarianism.

For this tension in the relationships to be overcome, theology must be in the bioethics of a pluralistic society, a "public theology," that is, a theology that presents itself as having its reasons overtly understood and discussed, and, consequently, that can also have a discourse open to counter-arguments. The discourse used inside communities of faith – where the weight of religious references and the authority of its leaders have another value – is not, for bioethics, an argumentative discourse. Even so, it can eventually clarify attitudes and behaviors. It is then necessary to recognize that not all theological discourses can participate in bioethics. However, in bioethics it is also indispensable to be able to distinguish, even if only a little, the different theological models, so that one does not identify all theological discourses as authoritarian. On the other hand, it seems equally indispensable to surpass scientific dogmatism, due to the fact that sciences are not neutral and do not constitute the only forms of human knowledge.

22.9 Bioethics and Religion: The Challenge of Their Places in Society

A deeper and more radical process exists that defies bioethics and religion. Gauchet (2003, apud Neutzling 2006, p. 59) observes that Christianity is *the religion of the exit from religion* precisely for having gradually allowed the political sphere to give up its religious legitimation and to find other models for legitimating itself. Historical Protestantism – as it is known – greatly contributed to this. Neutzling (2006, pp. 60–61) emphasizes the importance of the new directions followed by Roman Catholicism in the second half of the twentieth century and by liberation theology in their contact with modern culture.

This process ends the religious explanations and legitimations for the structures of social life. Hervieu-Léger (2003) speaks of a process of *exculturation* of Christianity (and religions in general) in post-modern society. Neutzling presents a synthesis of Hervieu-Léger's thought, saying that:

> For Hervieu-Léger, the logic of exculturation consists, thus, in the process for which religious significations collectively given to action in the world lose gradually all consistency for the

> actors themselves, who are inhaled, as it were, by action's economic and inexorably secular logic. This is not to say that these actors had necessarily lost as individuals all religious interest, but it does mean that the devices who allowed them to give a religious sense to their experience in the world – and, in the first place, to their professional experience – had lost their capacity of giving them a *collective signification*, perceived as such by them and by society (Neutzling 2006, p. 62).

Here there is an implosion of collective meanings previously guaranteed by religion. According to Blumenberg (apud Neutzling 2006, p. 59), this process causes the *senselessness* to be constructed with a *new* content. And the solution for this "new" content is in the last analysis looked for in the auto-affirmation of the individual (*Selbstbehauptung*), taken from then on as a reference for the construction of meanings (Blumenberg 1999).

This presents a radical challenge not only for religion but for bioethics. Bioethics, following the first intuition of Potter (1971, p. 1), is meant to be a guide for action in a pluralistic society which is able to utilize knowledge for the benefit of the society. What place does (bio)ethics really occupy in a pluralistic society? In many contexts, it is seen as an obstacle to the scientific race or as an evil to be tolerated due to the pressure of social groups.

To avoid falling into individualism, both Latin American theology and bioethics adopt *intersubjectivity* as a means to be able to dialogue, to be part of a network, to search and find the reasons that we have in common, to share meanings, and to actualize them in society. Here, a space is created where theology and bioethics can learn one from the other and work in partnership for the good of humanity.

References

Alves R (1989) O que é religião. Círculo do Livro, São Paulo

Anjos MF (1994) Bioethics in a liberationist Key. In: DuBose ER, Hamel R, O'Connell LJ (eds) A matter of principles? Ferment in U.S. bioethics. Trinity Press International, Valley Forge, PA, pp 130–147

Anjos MF (2003) Bioética em perspectiva de libertação. In: Garrafa V, Pessini L (eds) Bioética: poder e injustiça. SBB & Loyola & S.Camilo, São Paulo, pp 455–465

Augustine, A. Epistola XX Ad Consentium. In: Migne J-P. (ed) Patrologia Latina, ex Typis Destenay, Paris 1887, 452–462

Banco Interamericano de Desenvolvimento na América Latina (2005) Inclusão social e desenvolvimento econômico na América Latina. Campus, Rio de Janiero

Bartoli J (2005) Ser executivo: um ideal, uma religião?. Idéias & Letras, Aparecida

Benedict XVI, Pope (2006) Conferência em Regensburg. In: Vian GM (ed) Osservatore Romano (Ed. Português), 37, 38, 1.918, 23 de setembro de 2006, pp 8–9 (452–453) Tipografia Vaticana Editrice, Vaticano

Blumenberg H (1999) La légitimité des temps modernes. Gallimard, Paris

Boff L (1981) Igreja: carisma e poder. Vozes, Petrópolis

Chasteen JC, (2001) América Latina, uma história de sangue e fogo, 3rd edn. Editora Campus Rio de Janiero

Chasteen JC (2005) Born in blood and fire: A concise history of Latin America, 2nd edn. W.W. Norton, New York

Engelhardt HT Jr (2000) Foundations of Christian bioethics. Scrivener Press, Salem, MA

Garrafa V, Pessini L (eds) (2003) Bioética: poder e injustiça. Loyola, São Paulo
Gauchet M (2003) La condition historique. Stock, Paris
Hervieu-Léger D (2003) Catholicisme, la fin d'un monde. Bayard, Paris
Neutzling I (2006) Teologia e sociedade: relevância e funções. Algumas anotações. In: Freitas MC (ed) Teologia e sociedade: relevância e funções. Paulinas, São Paulo, pp 35–65
Oliveira MA (2000) Diálogos entre razão e fé. Paulinas, São Paulo
Pessini L (2004) Eutanásia: por que abreviar a vida?. Loyola, São Paulo
Potter VR (1971) Bioethics: Bridge to the future. Prentice-Hall, Englewood Cliffs, NJ
Sobrino J (1992) El principio-misericordia. Bajar de la cruz a los pueblos crucificados, Sal Terrae, Santander
Sorta-Bilajac I, Pessini L, Dobrila-Dintinjana R, Hozo I (2005) Dysthanasia: The (il)legitimacy of artificially postponed death. Medicinski arhiv 59(3):199–202
Suess P (1992) A conquista espiritual da América Espanhola: 200 documentos – século XVI. Vozes, São Paulo
Tillich P (1988) The spiritual situation in our technical society. Mercer University Press, Macon, Georgia

Chapter 23
Bioethics and Women in Latin America: A Biographical and Genealogical Essay

Debora Diniz and Dirce Guilhem

Bioethics consolidated in Brazil at the end of the 1990s. A similar phenomenon occurred in other Latin American countries, especially in Argentina, Chile, and Mexico, where the introduction of bioethics to academics was a notable occurrence (Diniz et al. 1999, pp. 244–248; Organización Panamericana de la Salud 2006; United Nations and Scientific and Cultural Organization 2006; Velasco-Suárez 2001). In this consolidation process, women assumed different roles: sometimes as academic protagonists and sometimes as interlocutors in the public sphere. This dual insertion is the trademark of women in Latin American bioethics and is part of the biography of this essay, a biographical and genealogical narrative of Latin American and especially Brazilian bioethics. The common thread of this narrative is our experience in this dual role as academic protagonists and as bioethical political speakers. Other women's reports about this process of the academic consolidation of bioethics in Latin America support the narrative; however, the authors assume total responsibility for the interpretation of the facts.[1]

D. Diniz
Ph.D. Anthropology, Professor of University of Brasilia (Universidade de Brasília) and Director of the non-governmental organization Anis - Institute of Bioethics, Human Rights and Genre. Member of the Board of Directors of the International Association of Bioethics
e-mail: d.diniz@anis.org.br

D. Guilhem
Ph.D. Professor in the Department of Health Sciences of University of Brasília (Universidade de Brasília), Brasília, Distrito Federal, BR
e-mail: guilhem@unb.br

[1] We analyzed two data bases of scientific papers in Latin America (Latin American and Caribbean Literature in the health sciences [Lilacs] and The Scientific Electronic Library Online [Scielo]) to get an overview of the state of the art in bioethics in the region. Forty-nine publications of women authors in bioethics were found. From these, key authors in Latin American bioethics were identified and in-depth open interviews were conducted with them in Argentina, Brazil, Chile, and Mexico.

L. Pessini et al. (eds.), *Ibero-American Bioethics: History and Perspectives*, Philosophy and Medicine 106, DOI 10.1007/978-1-4020-9350-0_23,

23.1 A Genealogical Overview

There is a growing feminization of academic activities in Latin America. Women are now the majority in most university disciplines; however, philosophy and theology are some of the exceptions in the humanities, and gradually, engineering is conceding to the entry of women. In medicine, despite the growing numbers of women physicians, the field continues to be marked by gender. Generally, women physicians are involved in caring activities and few are working in legal medicine, medical ethics, or even class politics (Diniz 2003, pp. 169–170). This social division of medical work helps one to understand women's participation in Latin American bioethics.

The genesis of Brazilian bioethics was similar to that of other countries in the region. As a general rule, the initial impulse came from two masculine fields: medical politics and Catholic theology (Corrêa 2003, pp. 1–6; Loyola 2002).[2] Medical entities, especially the Federal Council of Medicine, were in charge of the first initiatives to consolidate bioethics in Brazil. The journal, *Bioethics* (*Bioética*), for example, is the oldest journal specialized in bioethics to be published in the country and is under the editorial responsibility of the Federal Council of Medicine.[3] On the current editorial board, which is composed of 15 members, 80% are men, and most are physicians (Conselho Federal de Medicina 2006). A pioneering initiative for distance education in bioethics through television was also promoted by the Council at the end of the 1990s (Diniz and Guilhem 2002).[4] Moreover, the first graduate program in bioethics was sponsored by a Catholic university.[5] In the first decade of bioethics in Brazil, the interests of medicine, Catholic theology, and bioethics were quite similar, which facilitated the emergence of the field.

The closeness of bioethics to medicine, and more specifically to medical class politics, marked out two identities for Brazilian bioethics in the 1990s: it was a matter of interest for medicine and was in the hands of doctors dedicated to medical class politics and retired professors from other fields. For a short period of time, bioethics was understood as a sub-area of medical ethics and it was not by chance

[2] The concepts of field, field in dispute, and interests are from Pierre Bourdieu. See, for example, the author's ideas in the books *O poder simbólico* (Bourdieu 1989) and *A economia das trocas simbólicas* (Bourdieu 1989).

[3] *Bioethics* (*Bioética*) was first published in 1993. There is no peer-reviewed bioethics journal in Brazil with an international indexation. The national journals in bioethics are quite irregular and amateur. According to Braga, the amateur character of scientific communication in bioethics in Brazil – and to a certain degree in Latin America – is indicative of the field's weakness (Braga 2006).

[4] For two years, the Federal Council of Medicine produced a television program called "Bioethics, Science, and Citizenship" whose goal was to reach all Brazilian physicians. Debora Diniz was one of the people responsible for the program.

[5] *Centro Universitário São Camilo* (São Camilo University Center). Master's Course in Bioethics. The course began in August 2004 and is still the only one in the country (Centro Universitário São Camilo 2006).

that there was a migration from legal medicine and medical ethics to bioethics.[6] In addition, the introduction of bioethics in the universities was initially connected to graduate programs in legal medicine (Siqueira et al. 2002, pp. 85–95).

The initial understanding of bioethics as a matter of medical education and medical class politics still characterizes the field as is shown by (1) its strong emphasis on ethical reasoning to solve problems, which explains the fascination with checklist theories, as was the case with principlism; (2) understanding bioethics as a subject of interest for medical education and medical practice; and (3) a bioethical agenda defined by the daily lives of doctors. These factors were more prevalent in the first few years of bioethics, especially when medical groups were hegemonic in the field. Nonetheless, given the symbolic power of the medical profession in Brazilian society, the understanding of bioethics as a medical question, and not as an analytical or theoretical field pertaining to biomedicine and science, still persists (Diniz et al. 1999, pp. 244–248).

The relationship between bioethics and medicine was nevertheless important for consolidating the field. Bioethics rapidly rose to the symbolic level of an elite intellectual enterprise, the understanding of which was strengthened by the presence of Catholic theology. Different from the experience of other countries in Latin America, the theological groups that were interested in bioethics in Brazil were markedly open-minded for public debate. However, similar to physicians, the Catholic theologians also established an agenda according to their own interests, which gave rise to three other characteristics of the field: (1) the return of bioethics to applied ethics and the humanities; (2) a broadened thematic agenda meant to include new topics for Catholic theology, but still restrictive regarding dogmatic questions such as those related to biological reproduction; and (3) encouragement for establishing bioethics as an academic discipline, which resulted in the loss of the hegemony of the representatives of the medical class institutions as a legitimizing discourse in bioethics. The engagement and perseverance of theologians forced bioethics back to the humanities, despite the fact that some topics were restricted by Catholic dogma. Differently from central bioethics – which is mainly a philosophical field – Latin America bioethics began as a medical specialty and only later became a matter of philosophical interest (Andre 2002, pp. 14–77; Garrafa et al. 1999, pp. 35–42). In the beginning, theology was responsible for maintaining the theoretical connection to the humanities.

Although the connection between medicine and Catholic theology initially served to empower bioethics, this strategic partnership has gradually been dissolving. The entry of women into bioethics was crucial for the reinterpretation of this initial trilogy – bioethics, Catholic theology, and medicine. In addition, during the first years of Latin American bioethics, women introduced feminism as an alternative analytical and political tool for understanding moral conflicts.[7]

[6] In reality, this understanding of bioethics as a specialty of medical ethics is still hegemonic among doctors who are dedicated to medical politics. Recently, the journal *Bioethics* changed its title to *Bioethics: A Journal of Bioethics and Medical Ethics*.

[7] It is possible to recognize the presence of some women in the genesis of bioethics who were not feminists. However, they were not women protagonists nor were they interlocutors for bioethics who remained in the field during the last decade.

23.2 Between Doctors and Theologians: Feminist Women

There is a false assumption that being an active woman in bioethics means being a feminist specialized in biological and social reproduction, or at least a researcher on care and vulnerability. This false assumption facilitates the gender distribution of bioethical expertise: issues related to the feminine, such as reproduction and sexuality, are women's issues in bioethics. In fact, there was a convergence of interests as the first women in bioethics were truly specialized in these topics, but this is not the rule for all women in Latin American bioethics (Corrêa 2000, pp. 863–870; Corrêa 2001; Diniz and Velez 1998, pp. 255–263; Diniz and Guilhem 1999, pp. 181–188; Diniz and Guilhem 2000, pp. 237–244; Diniz and Gomes 2006, pp. 55–67;Diniz and Velez 2006, pp. 111–130; Guilhem 2002, pp. 161–171; Luna 1995, pp. 93–100; Oliveira 1997, pp. 166–77; Rotania 1998, 2000; Sommer 1998; Valdebenito et al. 2006, pp. 145–150).

This false generalization also caused the strategic rearrangement of the field provoked by the entry of women (especially feminists). Taking for granted that abortion, reproductive technologies, and homosexuality were feminist topics solved a series of political challenges for the pioneers of bioethics: both for the doctors, since they were topics of heightened moral disagreement, and for the Catholic theologians, because reproductive issues had limited space for reasonable discussion or the contestation of dogma. The first Brazilian publications in bioethics with women authors were evidence of how this new distribution of the field served the different interests involved (Costa et al. 1998; Pessini and Barchifontaine 1996; Sorokin 2002). As a general rule, books were compiled in which women wrote analytical chapters on biological and social reproduction, while men authored the theoretical discussions.

The entry of women in bioethics caused a political restructuring of the field in Brazil: (1) Catholic theologians took the job of making bioethics an academic career and of dealing with challenging yet less controversial questions, such as population aging and issues concerning the end of life (Anjos 2005, pp. 325–225; Barchifontaine 2004; Pessini and Bertachini 2005, pp. 495–509); (2) doctors fought against the distancing of bioethics from medical ethics and attempted to maintain political control of the field in the face of the juridical invasion (Grisard 2002, pp. 97–114); (3) feminists assumed the role of academic protagonists for feminist epistemology and became the public interlocutors of bioethics, introducing a new identity of Latin American bioethics as a tool for advocacy and social criticism (Diniz and Velez 1998, pp. 255–263; Oliveira and Mota 2001, pp. 151–180). This political rearrangement does not mean that Catholic theologians or physicians were silenced regarding the issues of abortion or reproductive technologies.[8]

[8] The anencephaly case in Brazil is an example of the redistribution of the responsibilities in the field. The Catholic theologians in the forefront of the public debate are not specialists in bioethics. The anencephaly case involved the official representatives of the Catholic Church in Brazil and not the Catholic intellectuals from the bioethics community.

The redistribution of responsibilities in the field occurred inside the emergent community of specialists in bioethics, where the organization of these sub-areas can be more easily identified.[9]

The distinct boundaries between the different groups described are not as clear in practice due to the "under construction" character of Latin American bioethics. It is not the case that only these groups exist, especially if one considers the growth of bioethics in juridical communities. In Brazil, there have been feminists in bioethics who were also active participants in medical class politics, in addition to cases of feminist theologians who were key authors in the emergence of bioethics (Gebara 2000, 2004; Oliveira 2001, pp. 99–112; Oliveira et al. 2001, pp. 483–511; Oliveira 2003, pp. 349–358). While one can recognize differences among these groups, the identity of bioethics as a developing field requires the analysis of these different perspectives in the region.

23.3 Between Academic Protagonists and Public Speakers

Bioethics is a new discipline at the intersection of academic knowledge and political action. Due to its status as a developing field, epistemological disputes are intense, especially in those countries where academic institutionalization has been recent. In Latin America, there are two different arenas of dispute, and in both the role of women has been expressive.

In the academic arena, the protagonism of women can be expressed in two ways. The first movement occurred at the universities: women were at the forefront of the efforts to establish bioethics in the universities. As part of the self-fulfilling prophecy, women bioethicists have ended up in those areas dedicated to the study of biological and social reproduction. In Brazil, the State University of Rio de Janiero was the first public university to establish and hire a bioethics position in 1999, specifically for the position of "Biological and Social Reproduction, Medicalization and Bioethics." The second bioethics position was at the Catholic University of Brasilia for the "Bioethics, Vulnerability, and Ethics in Research with Human Beings" position in 2000.[10] The first doctoral dissertation in bioethics to be defended in Latin America was titled "New Reproductive Technologies and Genetics, Ethics, and Feminism: the Celebration of Fear" and was defended in 1998 (Rotania 1998). In 2002, the Pan American Health Organization instituted the "Manuel Velasco-Suárez Bioethics Award," which sought to award young Latin

[9] The Brazilian Society of Bioethics is one of these forums. The Latin American Forum of Ethics Committees for Research in Health (*Foro Latinoamericano de Comités de Ética en Investigación en Salud* – Flaceis) is another example at the regional level.

[10] In the first post, Marlena Corrêa was approved and Debora Diniz was one of the evaluators on the jury. In the second post, Debora Diniz was the approved candidate. The posts represent an important benchmark for the field since the academic community is recognizing the emergence of a new specialization.

American researchers in bioethics. The award has been given four times to date, and each time has been awarded to a woman.[11]

The other aspect of the academic protagonism of women in bioethics brings Brazil closer to other countries in the region, especially Argentina, Chile, and Colombia. Due to the scarcity of local bioethical literature, the first decade of bioethics was characterized by an intense exchange of ideas within the region, as well as between the region and central bioethics, especially the United States. In the case of the United States, bioethics had not only already been consolidated in the universities and in public debates, but the feminist perspectives of bioethics were already part of the field. The regional distribution of knowledge associated with the flourishing of critical feminist theories made feminist bioethics grow rapidly in Latin America, especially in countries with structured graduate programs (particularly in Argentina, Brazil, and Mexico).

The exchange of ideas occurred primarily by means of the bioethics associations that emerged in the 1990s. International meetings were rich encounters for the formation of alliances and partnerships. Since its foundation in 1992, the International Network of Feminist Approaches to Bioethics (FAB) has actively participated in the principal international bioethics association, the International Association of Bioethics (IAB). In 1996, FAB organized the first satellite meeting of the IAB congress and, since then, has been the most active network with the largest number of participants (Feminist Approaches to Bioethics 2006). FAB entered Latin America at the same time that the network itself was forming, with Alejandra Rotania as the first country representative in 1996.[12] The FAB has also had country representatives in Argentina, Brazil, Chile, Colombia, and Mexico. In addition, Brazil hosted one of its world meetings in 2002.

The participation of Latin American researchers in FAB was a decisive step for the self-fulfilling prophecy of women as specialists in reproductive issues. FAB is a network of academics dedicated to the study of such topics as reproduction, ethics, and bioethics, from the theoretical perspective of feminism. As an epistemological tool for the humanities, feminism emerged in the 1960s with the fields of ethics and moral philosophy most directly challenged by feminists' critical perspectives (Harding 2006; Haraway 1991; Haraway et al. 2006). Feminist contributions quickly became a part of Brazilian bioethics, because they represented a resistance to the dominance of Tom Beauchamp and James Childress principlist theory, which had taken hold during the first years of bioethics in the region (Beauchamp and Childress 2008; Diniz and Guilhem 2000; Wolf 1996). Moreover, the participation of women researchers at FAB and IAB broadened the region's bioethical horizons by strengthening the theological perspective of bioethics as a field in the humanities, especially in social ethics.

[11] The first award, in 2002, went to Debora Diniz from Brazil with the project "Genetic information and justice: a bioethical challenge"; the second went to Rosa Angelina Pace from Argentina with the project "Organ transplants and the teachings of bioethics"; the third went to María Graciela Ortúzar from Argentina with the project "International justice, the right to health, intellectual property, and the human genome"; and the fourth, in 2000, went to Patricia Sorokin from Argentina with the project "Treatment of personal data in the genomic investigation: bioethical, legal, and social aspects" (Pan American Health and Education Foundation 2006).

[12] Latin America already had some country representatives. Debora Diniz (Brazil), Susana Sommer (Argentina) and Ana Cristina Gonzalez Veléz (Colombia) were members of the board.

Nevertheless, one of the main challenges was to overcome resistance to the category of "feminist" bioethics (Diniz 2009). The Latin American feminist movement had had a history of social conquests, especially in controversies over political and social rights. Nevertheless, the social movements were mainly political ones, and the place for action remained in civil society and government. The inclusion of feminist perspectives within the university was not considered a high priority. It was not until the emergence of feminist epistemology that feminist bioethics in Latin America was accepted into the universities.

In the 1980s and 1990s, some women's groups in the universities found a way to avoid the stigma of "feminism". They managed to avoid this label by defining themselves not as "feminist researchers," but as "gender specialists" (Diniz and Foltran 2004, pp. 245–253). The substitution of "gender" for "feminism" facilitated the emergence of new areas of research interest in women's studies programs, and avoided the stigma associated with feminism as a political movement instead of as a valid academic perspective. This was possibly a decision made for academic survival shared by several Latin American women researchers, especially those working in confessional universities (Diniz 2006, pp. 71–104). However, the entry of feminist bioethics in Latin America coincided with a moment of recognizing the epistemological boundaries between feminism and gender, which made easier the self-identification of the young bioethicists as feminists.

There are important differences between feminist and gender perspectives in science (Wolf 1996). Feminism is committed to a political criticism of the so-called "gender neutrality" in science and takes charge of re-describing academic discourse in terms that favor the interests of subordinate groups. For this reason, the category of vulnerability is seductive for feminist bioethicists: it represents the fragility of some groups, and at the same time it demands protection and care for the oppressed (Guilhem 2005). Unlike gender studies, feminist perspectives are committed to an intervention in the world and its inequalities. This theoretical and methodological perspective of feminist bioethics has attracted some of the young Latin American bioethicists.

Feminist perspectives on bioethics strengthened the political dialogue that had already been started by women's movements in Latin America. Feminist bioethics became a new argumentative tool, especially because of the growing secularization of societies in the region. Unlike central bioethics, which emerged in societies with secular constitutions, Latin American countries have a different legal reality where there are cases of multiculturalism challenging secular legislation. In this context, the topics discussed by feminist bioethicists are the ones that demand the most negotiation in public debate.

The emergence of a regional feminist bioethical research agenda was a result of this double insertion of women – as academic protagonists and as public interlocutors.[13] Some topics, abortion for instance, have always been issues of

[13] A privileged space to analyze this double insertion of women in Brazilian bioethics would be the history of participation in research ethics committees and in the National Commission of Ethics in Research (Brasil et al. 1996, 1998). Women participated decisively since the formation of the multidisciplinary workgroup that was instituted to elaborate Resolution 196/96.

international bioethical debate, but the Latin American reality has demanded a re-description of these international perspectives. Different from the American or French debates on abortion, where the bioethical agenda includes new perspectives about the fetus' status without banning abortion as a woman's right, in Latin America the main issue is to guarantee a deep acceptance of a secular State in the promotion of bioethics. The consequence of such different political configurations among societies for Latin America was the emergence of a critical perspective regarding international bioethics.

23.4 Women and New Challenges

The fact that bioethics is an emerging field encourages the attempts of different groups, languages, and argumentative strategies to be recognized by the bioethics community. The reality is that the emerging character of bioethics does not allow for unlimited possibilities for argumentative expression. The initiative of bioethics to define itself as an academic discipline is growing, and therefore the permanent effort of women in bioethics is to guarantee the inclusion of feminism as an analytical tool. Today, a large proportion of the graduate programs in health or in the humanities have courses in bioethics in their curricula that include international and regional feminist references. This is an indication of how deeply the field has been challenged by feminist perspectives.

In this effort to both maintain and widen the field's boundaries, one of the main contributions of Latin American women has been the conquest of different argumentative forums: women in bioethics are not confined to the university or to peer dialogues. Initiatives such as the Brazilian and Mexican video and documentary production in bioethics are examples of this effort to broaden the horizon of academic protagonism and of public dialogue to make the understanding of bioethical arguments more democratic (Catholics for a Free Choice 2005; Diniz and Brum 2005). Another example of this diversity of languages is the insertion of bioethicists in research institutions, universities, social movements, and non-governmental organizations, a phenomenon that has been observed among all the more active feminist researchers in Latin American bioethics.

However, few women participate in Latin American bioethics. This unequal expression of gender is a consequence of the genesis of the field and its closeness to the knowledge of medicine and theology which restricted the participation of women. Another explanation is that it is not common for a woman to dedicate herself exclusively to bioethics work in the region: the figure of the professional bioethicist has not yet been established. The first generation of bioethicists from Latin American universities is still being formed.[14] Considering the expansion of the field in the region and the increasing professionalization of women, a fast gender transformation in the field is to be expected.

---

[14] One should understand a specialist in bioethics to be the young researchers with doctorates in bioethics or who defended dissertations in bioethics.

Acknowledgments The authors thank Cristiano Guedes, Fabiana Paranhos, and Sergio Costa for their comments. Translation: Julie Ciancio.

References

Andre J (2002) Bioethics as something new. Bioethics as a territory: An allegory. The language of bioethics. Bioethics as practice. In: Andre J (ed) Bioethics as practice. The University of North Carolina Press, NC, pp 14–77

Anjos MF (2005) O corpo no espelho da dignidade e da vulnerabilidade. O Mundo da Saúde 29(3):325–335

Barchifontaine CP (2004) Bioética e início da vida: alguns desafios. Idéias e Letras, São Paulo

Beauchamp T, Childress J (2008) Principles of biomedical ethics, 6th edn. Oxford University Press, Oxford

Bourdieu P (1989) A gênese dos conceitos de habitus e campo. In: Bourdieu P (ed) O poder simbólico. Bertrand Brasil, Rio de Janeiro, pp 59–73

Bourdieu P (2003) Campo do poder, campo intelectual e habitus de classe. In: Bourdieu P (ed) A economia das trocas simbólicas, 5th edn. Perspectiva, São Paulo, pp 183–202

Braga KS (2006) A comunicação científica e a bioética brasileira, UnB/Departamento de Ciência da Informação e Documentação. [Projeto de Doutorado – Programa de Pós-Graduação em Ciência da Informação], Brasília

Brasil, Ministério da Saúde, Conselho Nacional de Saúde (1996) Normas regulamentadoras sobre pesquisas envolvendo seres humanos. CNS, Brasil

Brasil, Ministério da Saúde, Conselho Nacional de Saúde (1998) Como funciona a Conep. Cadernos de Ética em Pesquisa, 1, 8. [Online] Available: http://conselho.saude.gov.br/docs/doc_ref_eticapesq/cadernos de etica 1.pdf

Catholics for a Free Choice (2005) No estás sola. Catholics for a free choice [Documentário], Washington, DC

Centro Universitário São Camilo (2006) Cursos de pós-graduação [Online] Available: http://www.saocamilo-sp.br

Conselho Federal de Medicina (2006) Revista Bioética [Online] Available: http://www.portalmedico.org.br/revista/bio13v1/index.htm

Corrêa M (2000) Novas tecnologias reprodutivas: doação de ovulos. O que pode ser novo nesse campo? Cadernos de Saúde Pública 16(3):863–870

Corrêa M (2001) Novas tecnologias reprodutivas. Limites da biologia ou biologia sem limites? Ed UERJ, Rio de Janeiro

Corrêa M (2003) Perspectivas da bioética no Brasil. Polêmica 8:1–6

Costa SIF, Oselka G, Garrafa V (1998) Iniciação à bioética. Conselho Federal de Medicina, Brasília

Diniz D (2003) Editorial – Educação médica: também, uma questão de gênero. Revista de Educação Médica 23(7):169–170

Diniz D (2006) Quando a Verdade é posta em Dúvida. In: Diniz D, Buglione S, Rios RR (eds) Entre a dúvida e o dogma: liberdade de cátedra e universidades confessionais. LetrasLivres, Brasília; Livraria do Advogado, Porto Alegre, pp 71–104

Diniz D (2009) O desafio da bioética feminista no Brasil. In press

Diniz D, Brum E (2005) Uma história severina. ImagensLivres [Documentário], Brasília

Diniz D, Foltran P (2004) Gênero e feminismo no Brasil: uma análise da Revista Estudos Feministas. Revista Estudos Feministas 12, n. espec., 245–253

Diniz D, Gomes R (2006) Infertilidad e infecundidad: acesso a nuevas tecnologías reproductivas. In: Cáceres C, Careaga G, Frasca T, Pecheny M (eds) Sexualidad, estigma y derechos humanos: desafios para el acesso a la salud en América Latina. FASPA/UPCH, Lima, pp 55–67

Diniz D, Guilhem D (1999) Bioética feminista: o resgate político do conceito de vulnerabilidade. Bioética 7(2):181–188
Diniz D, Guilhem D (2000) Feminismo, bioética e vulnerabilidade. Revista Estudos Feministas 8(1):237–244
Diniz D, Guilhem D (2002) O que é bioética. Brasiliense, São Paulo
Diniz D, Guilhem D, Garrafa V (1999) Bioethics in Brazil. Bioethics 13(2):244–248
Diniz D, Velez ACG (1998) Bioética feminista: a emergência da diferença. Revista Estudos Feministas 6(2):255–263
Diniz D, Velez ACG (2006) Aborto y razón pública: el desafío de la anencefalia en Brasil. In: Checa S (ed) Realidades y coyunturas del aborto. Paidós, Buenos Aires, pp 111–130
Feminist Approaches to Bioethics (2006) Newsletter [Online] Available: http://www.fabnet.org
Garrafa V, Diniz D, Guilhem D (1999) Bioethical language and its dialects and idiolects. Cadernos de saúde pública 15(Suppl. 1):35–42
Gebara I (2000) Rompendo o silêncio. Vozes, Petrópolis
Gebara I (2004) Novas relações de gênero são possíveis [Online] Available: http://latinoamericana.org/2004/textos/portugues/Gebara.htm
Grisard N (2002) Ética médica e bioética: a disciplina que falta na graduação médica. Bioética 10(1):97–114
Guilhem D (2002) Bioética feminista e o conceito de vulnerabilidade nas pesquisas biomédicas envolvendo seres humanos. In: Sorokin P (ed) Bioética: entre utopías y desarraigos. Libro homenaje a la Prof. Dra. Gladys J. Mackinson. Editora Ad Hoc, Buenos Aires, pp 161–171
Guilhem D (2005) Escravas do risco: bioética, mulheres e aids. Editora UnB/Finatec, Brasília
Haraway D (1991) Simians, cyborgs, and women: The reinvention of nature. Routledge, New York
Haraway D, Shelley M, Perkins G, Moore CL, Merril J (2006) Unfamilial bonds: Technological fiction and the reimagination of gender. ProQuest/UMI, Ann Arbor
Harding S (2006) Science and social inequality: Feminist and postcolonial issues (race and gender in science). University of Illinois Press, Chicago/Champain
Loyola M (2002) Pierre Bourdieu entrevistado por Maria Andréa Loyola. EdUERJ, Rio de Janeiro
Luna F (1995) Razones internas y la discusión acerca del aborto. Mora [Universidad de Buenos Aires], 1.1, 93–100
Oliveira F (1997) Filhos da tecnologia: questões éticas da procriação assistida. Mundo da Saúde 21(3):166–177
Oliveira F (2001) As novas tecnologias reprodutivas conceptivas a serviço da materializaçäo de desejos sexistas, racistas e eugênicos? Bioética 9(2):99–112
Oliveira F (2003) Feminismo, raça/etnia, pobreza e bioética: a busca da justiça de gênero, anti-racista e de classe. In: Garrafa V, Pessini L (eds) Bioética: poder e injustiça. Loyola, São Paulo, pp 349–358
Oliveira F, Ferraz TC, Ferreira LCO (2001) Idéias feministas sobre bioética. Revista Estudos Feministas 9(2):483–511
Oliveira F, Mota JAC (2001) Bioética e as mulheres. In: Rede Nacional Feminista de Saúde e Direitos Reprodutivos, Saúde da mulher e direitos reprodutivos: dossiês. Rede Saúde, São Paulo, pp 151–180
Organización Panamericana de la Salud (2006) Unidad de bioética [Online] Available: http://www.bioetica.ops-oms.org/E/ehome.htm
Pan American Health and Education Foundation (2006) Premio Manuel Velasco-Suárez [Online] Available: http://www.pahef.org/awards/bioethics
Pessini L, Barchifontaine CP (1996) Fundamentos de bioética. Loyola, São Paulo
Pessini L, Bertachini L (2005) Novas perspectivas em cuidados paliativos: ética, geriatria, gerontologia, comunicação e espiritualidade. O Mundo da Saúde 29(4):491–509
Rotania A (1998) Novas tecnologias reprodutivas e genéticas, ética e feminismo: a celebração do temor. UFRJ/ Instituto Alberto Luiz Coimbra de Pós-Graduação e Pesquisa de Engenharia – COPPE. [Tese de Doutorado – Programa de Pós-Graduação em Engenharia], Rio de Janeiro

Rotania A (2000) Formas atuais de intervenção no corpo das mulheres: um questionamento. Caderno da SempreViva – Mulheres, Corpo e Saúde, p 13 [Online] Available: http://www.boell-latinoamerica.org
Siqueira JE, Sakai MH, Eisele RL (2002) O Ensino da ética no curso de medicina: a experiência da Universidade Estadual de Londrina (UEL). Bioética 10(1):85–95
Sommer S (1998) Genética, clonación y bioética: cómo afecta la ciencia nuestras vidas?. Biblos, Buenos Aires
Sorokin P (ed) (2002) Bioética: entre utopias y desarraigos. Libro homenaje a la Prof. Dra. Gladys J. Mackinson. Editoria Ad Hoc, Buenos Aires
United Nations Educational, Scientific and Cultural Organization (2006) UNESCO Chairs [Online] Available: http://portal.unesco.org/education/es/ev.php-URL_ID=2557&URL_DO=DO_TOPIC&URL_SECTION=201.html
Valdebenito C, Lama A, Lolas F (2006) Relación mujer y biotecnología: aproximación al impacto de la bioética. Acta Bioética 12(2):145–150
Velasco-Suárez M (2001) IX Aniversario de la Comisión Nacional de Bioética, Ciudad de México [Online] Available: http://www.salud.gob.mx/unidades/dgcs/sala_noticias/discursos/2001-04-05-IX-ANIVER-BIOETICA.htm
Wolf S (1996) Feminism & bioethics: Beyond reproduction. Oxford University Press, Oxford

Chapter 24
The Environment and Bioethics: A Brazilian Perspective

José Roque Junges and Lucilda Selli

24.1 Introduction

The increasing awareness and concern caused by global warming has led to the inclusion of environmental issues in international politics and global agreements. Awareness of a global environmental crisis has encouraged a search for planetary answers, because no nation is capable of solving ecological challenges independently. The promotion of global agreements by a community of individual nations acting as a whole under the aegis of the United Nations (UN) is required.

The role of certain countries in solving the environmental crisis is necessarily more significant due to their being more responsible for its causes or having the resources to contribute more significantly to a solution. Brazil – owning the world's largest tropical forest, possessing vast freshwater resources, and responsible for the planet's most significant biodiverstiy – is certainly one of the latter. This natural wealth increases its responsibility and political leverage in the international debate on climatic changes. Given its resources, Brazil needs to accept its share of internal responsibility for defending the environment and addressing the issues of an unjust distribution of wealth and the environmental burden thereof.

Brazil's environmentalist call – as well as the country's longstanding social injustices – makes it an ideal candidate to propose discussions, at international forums pertaining to the close relationship between environmental protection and social justice. The country possesses one of the most advanced legal systems regarding environmental protection, but its legal culture remains notorious for failing

J.R. Junges
Ph.D. Professor of Bioethics in the post-graduate courses at the Universidade Vale do Rio dos Sinos, São Leopoldo, Rio Grande do Sul, BR
e-mail: roquejunges@hotmail.com

L. Selli
Universidade Vale do Rio dos Sinos, Programa de Pós-Graduação em Saúde Coletiva,
Died in May, 25, 2009

L. Pessini et al. (eds.), *Ibero-American Bioethics: History and Perspectives*,
Philosophy and Medicine 106, DOI 10.1007/978-1-4020-9350-0_24,

to endorse the laws it creates, or causing more corruption in the course of their application. This results in increased indifference to environmental protection and its social ramifications, as well as the occurrence of ecological crimes without reaction from the authorities due to a lack of political will and the absence of effective means with which to act. On the other hand, Brazil has developed alternative energy sources, including hydroelectrical power plants and the use of sugar cane ethanol, which can help reduce carbon emissions.

The United Nations Conference on Environment and Development (UNCED, or the "Earth Summit," held in Rio de Janeiro, Brazil, in 1992) has given rise to ecological awareness in Brazil by originating opportunities for debate as well as initiatives for action. During this time, the inception of bioethics at the national level was witnessed for the first time in Brazil, although it was initially detached from ecological concerns and favored a clinical approach. At present, ecological concerns are becoming more prevalent in Brazilian bioethical debate, as can be seen in the organization of an environmentally themed congress of the Brazilian Society of Bioethics in 2005. In addition, Brazilian representatives participated in the debates held in Paris to promote the inclusion of the environmental protection clause in the drafting of the Universal Declaration on Bioethics and Human Rights, later issued by UNESCO.

According to Potter (1971) and Naess (1989), cosmetic solutions are insufficient if they do not reach the root of the environmental crisis. Technical solutions are important, but a genuine response should be both ethical and cultural. The dimensions of the crisis ask for a deepened ecology. Casuistry and isolated efforts will not suffice. The solution should be ecosystemic, with a hermeneutic perspective, which interprets cultural assumptions and dynamics so as to provide an in-depth explanation of the deterioration of the environment and its social effects.

Human action always employs a pragmatic dimension, to the extent that it attempts to respond to immediate needs by utilizing common-sense morality and paying close attention to the circumstances of a particular case. Environmental management is based on this perspective. However, environmental action, of greater ethical significance, has a symbolic dimension that expresses cultural dynamics and makes apparent those effects that can only be seen in the long run. The expressivity of action demands an interpretation that may shed light upon assumptions and identify those values at stake. Therefore, ecological bioethics cannot be reduced to casuistry, and should include a hermeneutic perspective, as will be discussed in this article (Junges 2005).

24.2 Natural and Cultural Biodiversity

An environment is more propitious to the reproduction of life if it contains a diversity of living beings with a developed set of interdependencies. Environmental protection that does not respect biodiversity does not exist. Brazil, due to its paramount biodiversity, has greater ethical and political responsibilities concerning international agreements related to this topic, such as the Convention on Biological Diversity, issued during the 1992 UNCED.

The abundance of natural resources, understood as a means to promote the country's economic progress, has long been an obstacle to environmental awareness and political decision making aimed at preserving biodiversity. Measures of protection have resulted from the condemnation of biopiracy and the assumption that biodiversity may have economic relevance. However, this is a narrow and utilitarian view, because it reduces biodiversity to its economic dimension. The primary importance of biodiversity lies in its role of promoting the biological sustainability of ecosystems. From this perspective, we must overcome its reductionist interpretation as merely providing the natural resources needed for economic progress.

The Convention on Biological Diversity defined biodiversity as "the variability among living organisms from all sources, including, inter alia, terrestrial, marine, and other aquatic ecosystems, and the ecological complexes of which they are part: this includes diversity within species, between species and of ecosystems." Biodiversity refers to the integration of a diversity of species, genetics, and ecology, although it is not a mere catalogue of genes, species, and environments. It is the set of interactive dynamics between those different levels. Through genetic diversity, different species may adapt to changes in the environment as diversity evolves over time and is a response to change. Interaction between biological systems and ecological conditions explains the evolution and the diversification of a species and the fact that different ecosystems house different flora and fauna. Thus, the notion of biodiversity is a modern variant of the theory of evolution, including discoveries resulting from the study of molecular biology and ecology.

Biodiversity plays an essential role in the regulation of natural ecosystems and, at the global level, the biosphere. A reduction in diversity affects the adaptation of living beings to disturbances. Therefore, biodiversity has a basic ecological function in the process of regulating bio-geo-chemical cycles and, consequently, the survival of humanity (Lévêque 1999).

The debate over the preservation of biodiversity revolves around the relationship between human beings and nature. Biodiversity cannot only be understood from the point of view of nature, but must also be considered from a cultural perspective. Cultural models affect biodiversity as much as cultural diversity, making them mutually dependent. The reduction of biological diversity is proportional to the reduction of cultural diversity. Given this, we need to act as a liaison between ecological and socio-cultural systems by studying which methods of preserving biodiversity are compatible with sustainable forms of socio-economic development.

Apart from biological aspects, Brazil also has great cultural diversity, in the different ways that Brazilians relate to nature and their many different local interactions with ecosystems. The great regional diversity is reflected in the cultural sprouting of different types of cattle agriculture, the many different ways of handling and cultivating natural resources, varied alimentary and medical systems, and distinct cultural customs, which contribute to Brazil's rich socio-cultural variety. The human variances of Brazil, in addition to its cultural diversity, have created many different modes of human contextualization within natural ecosystems.

This rich cultural diversity is currently undergoing gradual homogenization due to the introduction of capitalism, the globalization of agribusiness, and the consequent loss of traditional knowledge about how to adequately handle nature within such an ecosystem. Great expanses of land with soy bean, sugar cane, and eucalyptus plantations are uniformly found in any region of Brazil, regardless of their interdependency with the environment.

On the other hand, preliminary experiments in preserving the traditional communitarian handling of agrarian biodiversity are now being performed. For example, the Study Group of Agro-Biodiversity (NEAB10, Núcleo de Estudos em Agrobiodiversidade), comprised of researchers and students from the genetic and plant resources and agro-ecosystems graduate program at the Federal University of Santa Catarina (Universidade Federal de Santa Catarina-UFSC) in Florianópolis, promotes continuing education in the community and research based on nuclear family agriculture via the handling and use of agro-biodiversity. The group promotes nutritional self-sufficiency and the autonomy of local communities through agricultural production and socio-economic development, which is based on four principles: the reappraisal of traditional and scientific knowledge in a participative context; the use of production strategies based on the structures and sustainability of family-based agriculture; the use of participative and integrated methods of research and education; and the promotion, handling, and use of local germplasms to preserve agro-biodiversity (Boef et al. 2007).

Native Brazilian culture once influenced the country's development through its harmonic practices of relating to nature; however, those practices have gradually been lost, due to a new way of relating to natural resources based on the rules of a globalized market, which rejects the holistic vision of a traditional peasant. The traditional vision of locating oneself within a set of interdependencies in nature provides one with a sense of ecological sensitivity from which one can perceive the dynamics of the surrounding ecosystem. Although traditional culture lacks scientific knowledge of biodiversity, peasants intuit their role due to the systemic vision inherent in their knowledge of nature.

What, then, is the importance of preserving biodiversity? First of all, biodiversity is important for ecological reasons (Lévêque 1999). It is indispensable to the evolutionary processes of life; the regulation of the biosphere's physical and chemical balances; ground fertility and the regulation of hydrological cycles; the absorption and decomposition of pollutants; and the cleansing of water. Secondly, it is important for ethical and patrimonial reasons. Human beings have a duty to refrain from exterminating other life forms and to preserve their ecological heritage for future generations, because natural ecosystems help individuals understand the evolution and survival of humankind. Finally, biodiversity is also important for economic reasons. It provides food products, raw materials, and medicines important to human health, in addition to constituting the basis for all agrarian production and the development of biotechnologies.

In understanding these reasons, it is possible to point out two ethical problems related to biodiversity that have environmental and economic implications for Brazil: biopiracy and the monopoly and homogenization of genetically modified seeds. The term "biopiracy" means the appropriation of biogenetic resources or knowledge of traditional communities by individuals or institutions that strive to obtain exclusive control, without authorization from the State or the community and without the fair and equitable distribution of the benefits obtained from the acquisition and appropriation of such resources.

The interest of multinational companies in biotechnology and Amazonian biodiversity is widely known. Access to these resources is gained in an unethical and predatory manner, motivated by pure economic interests, and with direct effects for the local communities by disrespecting their traditional culture and knowledge, and harming their sustainability.

Biopiracy has been made easier by globalization and has increased the possibility of international patenting. There have been recent examples of multinational companies demanding exclusive rights to Amazonian plants. The Convention on Biodiversity has been used as a precedent for fighting against these practices because it supports the preservation of biological diversity, sustainable economic exploitation, and the fair and equitable sharing of obtained benefits, in addition to ensuring each country's sovereignty over its genetic patrimony.

Another frequently debated issue in Brazil is the planting and marketing of genetically modified seeds (Scholze 2002). The new Biosafety Law allows their use, but it has not settled the debate entirely. Popular movements, such as the Movement of the Ones Without Land (Movimento dos Sem-Terra – MST) and the Peasant Way (Via Campesina), have promoted actions against the use of genetically modified seeds. Consumer associations also fight for the labeling of genetically modified food products and the right of consumers to decide independently whether or not to make use of such products.

The central debate revolves around the consequences of planting genetically modified organisms for the environment and human health. There is a strong evidence that genetically modified foods may cause allergies, but more detailed and verifiable studies on their long-term effects are still lacking. This is a common problem for impact studies, since effects may only arise after long periods of time. The side effects of genetically modified agricultural products still cannot be properly assessed due to their novelty; this includes effects on human health in addition to the grand effects it may have on nature, in terms of changes in genetic and environmental levels, which will take even more substantial periods of time to discover. Due to these uncertainties, it is wise to impose the principle of precaution as an ethical minimum in this process.

At present, the primary focus is on the unethical economic monopoly of multinational companies on genetically modified organisms, which gives them the upper hand when dealing with farmers. Exclusive rights over the seeds are secured by the genetic deactivation of the seeds' germination to prevent farmers from producing their own seeds. This limits the farmers' autonomy and puts them in a position of complete dependence on the multinational companies.

Agricultural production does not cater to the needs of communities, but rather to globalized economic interests, moved by the commodities of agribusiness. It produces grains for export, feed for the animals of meat production, and renewable energy for transportation. The promotion of sustainable agriculture and sustainable development should take priority; the agricultural industries are related to the production of automobiles and meat for human consumption, which are the main causes of environmental problems because of the vast areas they require.

24.3 Sustainable Development

The report of the World Commission on Environment and Development, Our Common Future, issued in 1987, has proposed the concept of sustainable development (Sachs 2002, 2004; Da Veiga 2005) as a way of combining the use of natural resources for economic development with sustainability of the environment. It has defined as sustainable all development that satisfies the needs of current generations without compromising those of future generations. This concept was accepted in 1992 by the Conference of the United Nations. Due to the vagueness of this definition of development, it has since been identified with the classic economic vision that measures progress through the per capita income and the national GIP – a decision which has determined the understanding of sustainability itself (Nobre and Amazonas 2002).

If development were to be understood in terms of its human and social sense, as quality of life, sustainability would also be assessed by other standards. This was the intention of the UN when it created the Human Development Index (HDI), which attempted to overcome the previously held economical and monetarist vision of development.

To define sustainability in relation to the needs of future generations is to be unaware of the geometric progression of the needs of human beings and the corresponding economic progress, which causes the deterioration of the level of biodiversity necessary for the preservation of the ecosystem, hampering the reproduction of its resources for future generations. On the other hand, Amartya Sen contends that to understand human beings only in terms of needs amounts to an impoverished idea of humanity (Sen 2000). Consequently, sustainability cannot be strictly defined by mere human needs, but rather in terms of the environmental complexity of life reproduction within an ecosystem (Leff 2003).

Until recently, economists were uninterested in environmental topics because natural resources were considered free and abundant properties that need not be estimated for price – which prevented natural resources from being recognized as objects of value. Natural goods such as rivers, forests, and regional climates were not valued because they were not assigned a price. They existed in abundance. Since natural resources did not have prices, their depreciation was not recorded in the budget as that of buildings, facilities, or equipment would have been.

In light of this, some economists have started to consider the environment and its depreciation or preservation in budgetary calculations, using as a criterion "he who pollutes must pay for the damage." This approach regards the preservation of the environment as a profit, because "saving the planet can be an income-producing business." This solution seems opportune in a situation of environmental emergency; yet, it is insufficient and dangerous, in the long run.

The attribution of market values to common and interdependent natural properties utilizes the very cause of environmental degradation and unjust wealth distribution as its own solution. This proposal must be corrected and extended from an ecocentric and social perspective, by adopting an interactional and ecosystemic understanding of the environment, including the natural and social ecosystem.

The developmental ideology of economic progress has long been a strong influence upon the social imagination of Brazil, which stands to imagine itself as a developing country, rich in natural resources. The criteria for measuring progress have always been reduced to economic indexes, and although Brazil has always had high indexes of economic growth, it has never truly experienced a qualitative social jump. The country still maintains one of the most unjust income distribution indexes in the world. The Brazilian economist Celso Furlado has transformed this dominant ideology into a myth through skillful analysis (Furtado 1974).

In Brazil, growth has been promoted at the cost of its abundance of natural resources and has depended on a neglect of its environmental implications through the predatory use of nature to do so. It has been based on archaic socio-economic structures that operate through loopholes in the political mechanisms of the distribution of generated wealth. Consequently, it is difficult to understand the environmental question in Brazil if this socio-economic process is being ignored. Thus, the question of developmental sustainability is necessarily complex, because it requires the consideration of both environmental and social factors. This is the thesis of the environmental justice group.

24.4 Environmental Justice

The environmental justice movement was born in the United States and was inspired by the marches in defense of African Americans' rights. It was found that the highest levels of industrial pollution and toxic residues were detected in regions inhabited by populations of African and Latin descent. Polluting chemical companies used the vulnerability and low levels of awareness and organization of these groups to their advantage. They were able to establish their plants in these regions, releasing toxic residues and unsanitary dejections into water courses and landfills, without having to fight against any organized opposition of the population. This practice of extending the environmental burden to the black population was called environmental racism. The discovery gave rise to increased organization and denunciation by the population, which fought against the social acceptance of the unjust degradation of their environment and demanded egalitarian measures in environmental policy. This movement established an ethical principle which prevented vulnerable populations from having to bear a disproportionate burden of the negative environmental consequences of commercial transactions, industrial or municipal activities, or the performance of public policy for federal, state, local, and tribal programs (Bullard 2004).

Inspired by the socio-environmental movement of African Americans, the Brazilian Network of Environmental Justice was established in 2001, with its founding manifesto issued during the World Social Forum of Porto Alegre, in 2002. It defined "environmental injustice" as the mechanism by which economically unequal societies place the heaviest burden of environmental damage over the low income populations, the socially discriminated groups, the traditional ethnic peoples, the working class neighborhoods, and the marginalized and vulnerable populations (Freitas and Porto 2006).

The movement of environmental justice is involved in socio-environmental conflicts created by the local changes brought about by industrial, agricultural, and mining processes. These processes cause pollution, which affects the life and health of the surrounding populations. In central countries, environmental laws do not accept productive structures that may cause harm to the environment. Consequently, those structures are exported to peripheral countries that lack the strict legislation for protecting the environment. The externalization of environmental damage, which is made possible by a globalized economy, is not considered as a factor in cost analysis. Ecological economics calls this process "social metabolism," a visible process in Europe, where countries import six times more than what they export and still accrue a much greater profit even if production does not occur within their territory, due to the knowledge added in the pricing of the product. Human and ecological degradation are not considered in the final cost calculation; for those run on the account of the peripheral countries (Freitas and Porto 2006).

To be unaware of the collateral effect of these macroeconomic processes on the environment would be to embezzle the phenomenon of environmental degradation in peripheral countries. The underdeveloped countries are made responsible for the environmental degradation in their territories, forgetting that it is an externalization of environmental damages by the rich countries. The degradation, apart from destroying ecosystems and their biodiversity, affects the health of the populations, destroying the natural environment and cultural basis for the social reproduction of life.

Environmental wounds are disclosed by the use of the land for the monocultures of the exporting agribusiness, spreading green deserts of soy, sugar cane, and eucalyptus along with the exploitation of seasonal workers in subhuman conditions; the mineral exploitation that generates pollution and risks for the ecosystems and surrounding populations; the production of hydroelectrical energy through the construction of dams, exterminating biomes and banishing small agriculturists from their lands; the social conflicts that arise involving access to urban land for housing; and the localization of industrial pollution and toxic residues in the proximity of poor neighborhoods (Freitas and Porto 2006).

The environmental question cannot be answered without taking into consideration the proportional relation between environment and health, which is made clear by the reflection of environmental degradation in the health of humans, as the environment configures the conditions for the reproduction of life. To understand this relation, it is necessary to employ an ecological perspective of human health.

24.5 Health and the Environment

The relation between health and the environment has always been a human concern, as is demonstrated by its being responsible for the understanding of illness as a consequence of miasmas from the environment – an essentially environmental explanation of disease.

The progress of microbiology has substantially changed this conception. Causes were no longer found to be poisonous gases, but rather microbes that invaded the body of the patient. The environment remained important, because it was seen as a reservoir for hosts and vectors of pathologies. The cause was no longer vague, as miasmas were, but was identified as the contagion of a microbe. Medical ecology studies the relations of the physical and biological factors with the illness and the interrelation between the environment and the vectors of pathologies (De Ávila-Pires 2000).

The bacterial revolution brought great benefits; however, it had the negative side effect of the retrogression of the social vision of medicine. The diseases of the new civilization, of non-microbial origin, brought back the importance of the environment as an ecosystem of natural, social, political, and cultural interdependencies, influencing health and illness. Thus, an ecosystemic understanding of health has become prominent, propagated by Brazilian public health officers (Sabroza and Leal 1992; Minayo and Miranda 2002).

According to this conception, the focus on the environment includes a deeper concern for health (rather than disease), combining the binomial "health environment" with concepts of ecological sustainability, quality of life, social justice, democracy, and human rights. Thus, the environment in its broad definition is integrated into the understanding of health itself. Before, the surroundings of a human being were merely an external condition for the spread of disease, reduced to a mere physical aspect. Today, the vision of disease and health itself does not consider only specific factors, but the interaction between them. This conception demands a more complex approach to the presence of risks in the environment.

The ecosystemic model combines three simultaneous reflections: health, the environment, and, as a mediator between the two, the conditions, situations, and life styles of specific population groups. It means combining health and environment, interlacing the ecological sustainability of the natural environment with the socio-economic development of human surroundings and the quality of life. Sustainability and development are basic for quality of life, as those concepts are understood by Minayo, as "a process of construction of new subjectivities through the participation in change projects, from a perspective of sustainable development and joint responsibility with future generations. Although there are attempts to quantify indicators ... the definition of quality of life is eminently qualitative," since it combines, "at the same time, a feeling of well-being, the vision of the finitude of the resources to achieve it, and a willingness to solitarily, through the widening of possibilities, present and future" (Minayo 2002, p. 174). Thus, the ecosystemic approach to health, seen as quality of life, "is like an umbrella, sheltering our desires of happiness, our parameters of human rights, our efforts to widen the boundaries of social rights and the conditions of being healthy and promoting health" (Minayo 2002, p. 174).

Another way of considering the relation between environment and health is the theory of social reproduction proposed by the Argentinean public health scholar, Juan Samaja (2000, 2004), who has had a strong influence in Brazil. To him, the object of health sciences is "the encounters and transactions among the various spaces of value assignment and regulation of the problems posed by social reproduction to all spheres of human sociability: namely, the biosocial, socio-cultural, socio-economic and political–ecological spheres" (Samaja 2000, pp. 95–96).

Health, as an object, includes the conceptions and practices of health officials in the spheres of bio-communal activity (biological and environmental reproduction), communal-cultural activity (reproduction of awareness and behavior), social activity (associative and economic reproduction), and the state (ecological–political reproduction). This focus on health in the social reproduction of life conditions exceeds the subject of medicine, and includes ecological, anthropological, sociological, legal, economic, and environmentalist epidemiology. For Samaja, life conditions determine health situations. Therefore, health situations must be studied from the perspective of the conditions of the reproduction of life. This means that, if health is the complete state of physical, psychic, mental, and social well-being, then "it is inseparable from the conditions of life, and can only be defined as the contrail over the processes of reproduction of social life. This means, health is the regular order itself of this reproductive movement" (Samaja 2000, p. 100). Environment is identified as the life conditions that make the social reproduction of health possible.

The integral concept of the promotion of health, spilling over the borders of its simple understanding as prevention, was explained by the Ottawa Charter for Health in 1996. It defines the promotion of health as providing the means for the population to improve their sanitary situation, exerting greater control over it. The conditions and requirements for health are: peace, education, housing, feeding, income, a steady ecosystem, social justice, and fairness. Strategies to promote health include the establishment of healthful public policies, a favorable environment, the strengthening of communitarian actions, the development of personal abilities, and the reorientation of the health services (Buss 2003).

This broad and integral understanding is the result of many worldwide conferences for the promotion of health. This movement is based on the analysis of the contradictory proposals formulated in cities, because their sanitary conditions are the biggest challenges for the promotion of health. Therefore, the idea of healthy cities was created in order to combine health and environment, making cities politically responsible for the creation of the structural and communitarian conditions for a healthful urban environment (Organização Pan-Americana da Saúde, 2002; Andrade and Barreto 2002).

24.6 Conclusion

Brazilian environmental bioethics points to an increasing awareness of the country's responsibility for the preservation of its rich biodiversity. On the other hand, it is characterized by strong social connotations, due to the unjust distribution of national wealth. In Brazil, the binomial of nature and society has historically and culturally been adjusted until the moment of its economic insertion in the global market. Nature was then transformed into natural resources for exporting and industrializing. The quick process of modern acculturation, without the necessary time for a creative assimilation, created socio-cultural disintegration. Human spaces also went through a fast cultural change due to urbanization, which detached society from nature and watered down social relations.

The concern for human ecology springs from the necessary integration between the natural and the cultural, always present in the relation between humans and nature. The configuring of ecosystems and human communities occurred up until the industrialization and urbanization of modern times when this harmonic interaction was severed. That is why it makes no sense to oppose human beings and living beings, or communities and living ecosystems, as is seen in the conflicts between anthropocentric and bio-centric tendencies. The harmonious relation within an eco-centered perspective must be ethical, so that humans are understood to be a central link of the interdependencies within any ecosystem, based on an empathic interrelation with living beings.

References

Andrade LOM, Barreto CHC (2002) Promoção da saúde e cidades/municípios saudáveis: propostas de articulação entre saúde e meio ambiente. In: Minayo MC, Miranda AC (eds) Saúde e ambiente sustentável: estreitando nós. Fiocruz Abrasco, Rio de Janeiro, pp 151–171

Boef WS, Thijssen MH, Ogliari JB, Sthapit BR (eds) (2007) Biodiversidade e agricultores. Fortalecendo o Manejo Comunitário, L&PM, Porto Alegre

Bullard R (2004) Enfrentando o racismo ambiental no século XXI. In: Acselrad H, Herculano S, Pádua JA (eds) Justiça ambiental e cidadania. Relume Dumará, Rio de Janeiro, pp 41–66

Buss RM (2003) Uma introdução ao conceito de promoção da saúde. In: Czeresnia D, Freitas CM (eds) Promoção da saúde: conceitos, reflexões, tendências. Ed. Fiocruz, Rio de Janeiro, pp 1538

Da Veiga JE (2005) Desenvolvimento sustentável: o desafio do século XXI. Ed. Garamond, Rio de Janeiro

De Ávila-Pires FD (2000) Princípios de ecologia médica. Ed. Da UFSC, Florianópolis

Freitas CM, Porto MF (2006) Saúde, ambiente e sustentabilidade. Ed. Fiocruz, Rio de Janeiro

Furtado C (1974) O mito do desenvolvimento econômico. Ed. Paz e Terra, Rio de Janeiro

Junges JR (2005) Bioética como Casuística e como Hermenêutica. Revista Brasileira de Bioética 1:28–44

Leff E (ed) (2003) A complexidade ambiental. Cortez Editora/Blumenau, Edifurb, São Paulo

Lévêque C (1999) A Biodiversidade. EDUSC, Bauru

Minayo MCS (2002) Enfoque Ecossistêmico de Saúde e Qualidade de Vida. In: Minayo MCS, Miranda AC (eds) Saúde e ambiente sustentável: estreitando nós. Fiocruz -Abrasco, Rio de Janeiro, p 174

Minayo MCS, Miranda AC (eds) (2002) Saúde e ambiente sustentável: estreitando nós. Fiocruz-Abrasco, Rio de Janeiro

Naess A (1989) Ecology. Outline of an ecosophy. Cambridge University Press, Cambridge, Community and Lifestyle

Nobre M, Amazonas M (eds) (2002) Desenvolvimento sustentável. A institucionalização de um conceito. Ed. Ibama, Brasília

Organização Pan-Americana da Saúde (2002), Municípios e Comunidades saudáveis: guia dos prefeitos para promover a qualidade de vida. Disponível em http:www.opas.org.br/sistema/arquivos/Mun_SAUD.pdf

Potter VR (1971) Bioethics, bridge to the future. Prentice Hall, Englewood Cliffs

Sabroza PC, Leal MC (eds) (1992) Saúde, ambiente e desenvolvimento sustentável: uma análise interdisciplinar. Hucitec-Abtrasco, São Paulo and Rio de Janeiro

Sachs I (2002) Caminhos para o desenvolvimento sustentável. Ed.Garamond, Rio de Janeiro

Sachs I (2004) Desenvolvimento: includente, sustentável e sustentado. Ed. Garamond, Rio de Janeiro

Samaja J (2000) A reprodução social e a saúde: elementos teóricos e metodológicos sobre a questão das "relações" entre saúde e condições de vida. Casa da Saúde, Salvador (BA)
Samaja J (2004) Epistemología de la salud: reproducción social, subjetividad y transdisciplina. Lugar Editorial, Buenos Aires
Scholze HC (2002) Patentes, transgênicos e clonagem. Implicações jurídicas e bioéticas. Ed, UnB, Brasília
Sen A (2000) Desenvolvimento como liberdade. Companhia de Letras, São Paulo

Chapter 25
Human Vulnerability

José Eduardo de Siqueira and Marco Segre

25.1 Vulnerability in the Singular

The concept of "human vulnerability" at first makes one think of the miserable, the socially marginalized, the elderly, children, and the ill. This is a valid reflection, because we are accustomed to seeing people through the lens of our own values, whereas misery and scarcities of all types, as well as diseases, are objective elements preliminarily restrictive of what has conventionally been denominated "quality of life."

The perspective on "quality of life" promoted in this essay is in accord with the view of Flavio Carvalho Ferraz articulated in his paper, "The Concept of Health," published in the *Brazilian Public Health Magazine* (*Revista Brasileira de Saúde Pública*) (Segre and Ferraz 1997) – which holds that subjectivity is a determinant condition upon which being or not being well is valued. However, one must approach this issue with the understanding that the unprotected, according to socio-medical criteria, do not necessarily feel more vulnerable than any other whose quality of life is considered normal.

Through the lens of health policy, it becomes evident that the social–medical view must prevail. Despite the dominance of this view in approaching the vulnerability of the human condition, especially within the context of bioethics, it is important to consider an alternative approach to vulnerability: a more generic component of the human species that is deeper, subjective to each person, and, perhaps, paradoxically, more real.

J.E. de Siqueira
Ph.D. Physician. Researcher and Professor at Universidade Estadual de Londrina, Department of Clinical Medicine, Londrina, Paraná, Brazil

M. Segre
Ph.D. Physician. Researcher and Professor at Department of Forensic Medicine, Medical Ethics and Social and Work Medicine, University of São Paulo, Brazil
e-mail: msegre@uol.com.br

L. Pessini et al. (eds.), *Ibero-American Bioethics: History and Perspectives*, Philosophy and Medicine 106, DOI 10.1007/978-1-4020-9350-0_25,

Luiz Tenário de Oliveira, a psychoanalyst from São Paulo, finds that with the weakening of traditional values in contemporary society – including family bonds, nationality, and religion – one has a more acute perception of oneself as subject to the immanent conditions of vulnerability. The term "subject" has purposely been employed to better characterize one's condition as less susceptible to external injunctions and, therefore, freer and better able to realize one's unfamiliarity with one's own existence, origin, and destiny. One also perceives oneself as more confident and self-assured, while at the same time being more fragile and vulnerable.

Each individual can only rely on his own reality – an exclusive consequence of one's particular way of thinking, feeling, and "seeing" the world – and one can only live in one's own present, as any effort to actualize the past in the present remains useless. In other words, the yearning to feel safe or to revive a lost belief or feeling is fruitless, unless new experiences can modify one's feelings. To better illustrate one's desire to return to the past, consider it similar to an attempt to abort an airplane during its takeoff, the disastrous consequences of which are well known.

Atheists teach that God is a creation of human beings. Whether one believes in His existence or not, and this is an affective issue, no matter how much one tries to rationalize one's belief, God was created to explain and justify our existence.

One need not reference psychoanalytic theory to realize that the subjective essence of vulnerability is loneliness. The perception of an affective bond from within the womb is crucial to human beings. The feeling of being loved, beyond all rationality, supports life. An attempt to escape the feeling of being unloved can lead to endless cogitation, which expends significant emotional energy without constructive results, and can also lead to externalization and dependencies (e.g., drugs, compulsions, etc.). Man, alone, has an unbearable burden of suffering. The anguish that arises from the absence of rational explanations for one's existential questions subsides or disappears when one's lack of affection is satisfied. What I am, where I come from, and where I am going are all replaced by "I am" when the *subject* feels affectively balanced.

In this brief essay, due to the authors' lack of complete theoretical knowledge of psychoanalysis, the task of thoroughly investigating the role of loneliness in perceiving human vulnerability will be impossible; however, consideration of the anguish experienced by the lonely when confronted with death will be its main focus. From the point of view of the authors, it is the thought of complete identity loss, of a sleeping state with no return, that makes the idea of death unbearable. One dies unappealingly alone. One disguises this monster with illusions: of eternally postponing death; of understanding it within a utilitarian calculus (how one's death could benefit others); or of appealing to religion and/or an afterlife (where one will be reacquainted with lost loved ones or rewarded for a lifetime of good deeds). Additionally, the delusion of suicidal or homicidal escapes allows one to believe that the unbearable anguish of an expected death will be avoided.

The primary approach for considering human vulnerability, more specifically man's vulnerability when confronting death, will be within the context of bioethics in this essay. In other essays, the authors have argued that the concept of apriorism (understanding distinctions like *good* and *evil*, virtue and sin, and heaven and hell as absolute principles) does not have a place in bioethics. As a result, they contend that there must be a condition serving as a common factor to every ethical reflection. They state:

> Under the vast umbrella of praised hierarchies of values, which we propose to shelter and respect within bioethics, there are inevitable presuppositions.... No matter how much the different ethical positions diverge, each praised for its own understanding of life, from different people and/or cultures, there is a perception that ethical uniformity is unattainable and undesirable, and any uniformity appears impossible without a condition present in the human being. This condition is about the capacity to comprehend your fellow man, to get in tune with him, to realize his individuality, to be able to feel solidarity. We no longer speak of love and respect aprioristically, although they are, from our point of view, decisive components in the structuring of ethics. However, let us be careful not to base our doctrine, immediately, on a vision used by religion.... We see ourselves defending a theory pervaded by belief and the appreciation of feelings, therefore, by religiosity, but with the intention of allowing for other understandings of its use outside of an obedience to dictates, be they from religion or any other codified moral system, nevertheless, not denying them value (Segre and Cohen 2002; Segre 2006).

The ability to experience alterity is inherent in all people, regardless of where or when one has lived. It is also said to exist in other animal species, at least at specific stages of life, which justifies our distain of any attempt to defend ethnocentricity as resulting from just instincts (Lévinas 2005).

Referring back to the bioethical analysis of human vulnerability when facing death, more specifically within the context of a professional health care relationship – a relationship where the participant's life is expected to be abbreviated – one will see that the affective-solidarity amalgam is indispensable to attenuating the pain of an individual whose moment of self-loss is perceived to be drawing near. These conditions are readily adapted to the health care relationships one may have with the elderly. As a result, proposals for the care of the elderly will be made, keeping in mind that the elderly maintain their own interests.

The conception of the "existential flame wavering" with the years is often false. It is a label often applied to the elderly as a way of justifying one's interfering with how an elder meets one's needs. While it is obvious that physical limitations often impede an elderly individual's ability to meet certain needs, it is far from realistic to assert that the elderly must be aided in meeting all of their goals.

The point to be made is that the restrictions on the elderly are more often imposed by external rather than internal constraints, due to the stigma of being old in a contemporary society that no longer associates age with wisdom. Recently, the field of mental health has more readily acknowledged the damage caused by isolation, especially in mental institutions. In light of this realization, one should approach relationships with the elderly in a manner that reinforces the values of equality, understanding, and solidarity.

This essay began with reference to the *Animus Vivendi*, or *Moriendi*, of human beings, which is close to the statement "one dies when one wants to." The predominant view of Western bioethics, at this time, is moving strongly toward the appreciation of one's quality of life. It is possible that these values may change over time in the interest of the collective good. It is commonly said of European countries that the decreased birth rate brings about the inversion of the age pyramid.

The perspective from which one approaches bioethics is influenced by one's background and personal convictions. At present, at least in theory, one of the most important goals of bioethics is to respect the preservation and quality of life. It has been shown that loneliness is a decisive condition for vulnerability. One dies alone, and, as a very real consequence of vulnerability, it can also be interpreted: "when one is alone, one dies."

The presence of an affective bond can serve as a breath of life. This point is reinforced in a selection from the book, *Is There Human Solidarity?* (*Arte di Crescere*):

> We would all say yes, even though it is not a constant. Do we believe that it is an autonomous feeling developed in man due to a spontaneous identification with his fellow creature, in joy and pain, sharing his reaction to existential phenomena? We would like to think so, in the attempt to convince ourselves that we really are "good," even though we harbor feelings of hatred, envy, etc. Psychology, supported by Freud's psychoanalysis, demonstrates that human feelings are varied and changeable, leading us to hear their voices according to the situation, one's nature, conditioning, or other factors. Feelings germinate in the child, and become accentuated throughout his life, according to his individuality. It is about what is "good" or "bad," according to changeable affective perceptions.

It is impossible to distinguish the innate from the acquired features of human nature. Can one learn solidarity? Certainly, even a person's constitution, including one's genetic structure, is of great importance. He can be just as good as his father, even if his kindness results from emulation rather than genetics. (Segre 2007).

One may also consider the effect of religion or morality on one's behavior, when one's kindness may be the result of fear of punishment instead of the performance of an innate kindness. This cannot be true solidarity, since it cannot be externally induced but must naturally emerge from one's psyche.

There is a perspective in bioethics that rejects the idea of having such duties to others and instead adopts the principles of autonomy and beneficence (Beauchamp and Childress 2008) as the most humane. This perspective is differentiated from an "ethics of care," which gives a primary role to the affective bond. The "ethics of care" approach was established by two women, Carol Gilligan, a psychologist, and Annette Bauer, a philosopher, who did not intend to establish a system of principles, but, instead, to stimulate human solidarity. One could also call this approach an "ethics of the heart," which appears closest to a feeling of solidarity (Gilligan 1998).

25.2 Vulnerability in the Plural

What makes the contemporary human being a member of a species which is dominated by overlapping existential crises, making one a stranger to oneself, a rebel actor, increasingly more complex and aggressive? No matter where one looks, people are dissatisfied and apprehensive in their daily lives. Paradoxically, in a century marked by extraordinary technological breakthroughs and the most pronounced expression of individual liberties, the manifestation of human vulnerability is most blatant. The initial promise of complete happiness, engendered by the material abundance and unfettered individual liberties of the twentieth century, is no longer apparent.

This dream resulted in a nightmare. We became the lowest and most disposable species of a greedy market, open to manipulation by big financial conglomerates promoting the continuous deregulation of social institutions. The consequence has been the establishment of a society of unhappy people, who, in their unrestricted consumption, have sought to ease their anguish and insecurities.

The word *crisis*, derived from the Greek *krisis*, originally meant that one would examine a situation and reach a decision when faced with a moral dilemma. Curiously, in modernity, another meaning has been adopted of having no way out when faced with a difficult decision. There are those, however, who would prefer to define yet another meaning for *crisis*, one which reveals a hidden challenge of *creating*. This reading has been advocated for by scholars of varying capacities. Such thinkers include, the polemic Italian sociologist, Domenico De Masi, who understands the future as belonging to those who free themselves from traditional ideas of work as obligation and, instead, conceive of a life where professional labor is minimized and more time is given to leisure, allowing for free time to be filled with "creative leisure"(De Masi 2000).

Happiness has also been promoted by authors of the successful self-help literature. Rowland, for instance, promises in his books the easy achievement of absolute happiness, a path to a life of self-fulfillment. In the introduction to one of his works, he states: "What you are about to read in this book will surprise and free you in a way you have never dreamt possible before (...). I am going to show you how you can obtain happiness and joy in ecstasy and full existence, as well as obtaining the material possessions, intrapersonal relations and other opportunities you desire" (Rowland 1995).

In the writings of both the sophisticated De Masi and the superficial Rowland, one is meant to orientate oneself through the invulnerability of the absolute power of the human mind as a means to achieving one's personal goals. It is clear in these works that although the authors travel through fascinating territory, the reliance on mental powers makes it easy for one to lose direction. Although the achievement of complete happiness is described as an "easy" task, the author warns that the responsibility falls solely on the reader and any failure must be accepted as an indication of incompetence.

Phrases such as "your own mind will dictate your destiny," "you will truly become the creator of your own life," or "you cannot change that which cannot be changed," sound like mantras to the passive readers who devour this literature, even though the phrases are discordant with each other.

The separation of the social from the internal dynamics of the Freudian psyche makes it difficult to interpret the impact of the cultural–historical condition. The perception of the social as an external objective and indifferent to individual behavior began being questioned in the 1960s through the reflections of different authors. These authors had carried out deep analyses of complex social situations and the respective individual and/or group responses to the indignation and disgust which had influenced the accomplishment of changes in the conduct of institutional powers regarded, up to this point, as hegemonic.

The atom, symbolic of the individual, may be considered an icon of the twentieth century. Similarly, one may consider a net, symbolic of the social, as the new icon for the twenty-first century. The atom, revolving around its own axis, is the greatest expression of individuality, whereas the net, devoid of a nucleus, an orbit or certainty, is the ideal model of all manifestations of intelligence and human feelings. It represents the interdependencies of the social, economic, and environmental variables. All means of communication, from the family microcosms to the cosmos, from small tribal decisions to the imperatives of a global participative democracy, are included.

While the atom represents an isolated and solitary unit, the net is composed of channels which promote a complex reality through the permanent communication of multiple social actors. Non-governmental organizations are exemplars of those institutions that adopt a net model for the purpose of performing social transformations while remaining entirely independent of formally established institutional powers (Kelly 1998). Unlike the Soviet Union's school of psychology, which promoted the social as essential and irreplaceable through the use of behaviorism and Pavlovian reflexology, the concept of a network is not incompatible with nor does it invalidate human subjectivity. An inadequate dependency relationship allows the social to become the determinant cause while rendering human subjectivity a mere effect.

For the Soviets, it was Vygotsky who recovered the complex and systemic view of the individual psyche situated within a social universe. He used scientific argumentation to defend the thesis that the social is not something external to the individual, but instead represents the production of feelings associated with objective conditions that transcend the space and time of the individual. That is to say, it is essential to determine the parameters of one's environment, the comprehension of which will naturally be incorporated into an individual's subjectivity. For Vygotsky, atomistic subjectivity gives way to an approach, not necessarily focused on the dynamics of intrasubjectivity, but capable of recognizing one's interaction with the environment and social conditions (Vygotsky 1993). Vygotsky's theory refers to the dialectic between the individual and the environment, as described by Ortega y Gasset, when answering the question of whether one can represent another without relying on the inseparable reality between the individual and one's biographical circumstances (a thesis rescued by Edgar Morin in his theory of complex thoughts [Morin 2005]).

Furthermore, market rules are chosen to establish the superiority of the whole over its parts (which Amartya Sen has identified as the most deceiving motto in post-modern reflection), allowing individuals to disengage themselves from any responsibility of tending to community matters. The alleged virtues of the market's regulating mechanisms are so blatant and obligatory that any attempt at justification can immediately be disregarded. Society has become subordinate to the market's dictatorship. Sen argues that while many attempt to defend capitalism as a scientifically based economy that must succumb to the demands of the market, the fact remains that it takes no interest in defending social democracy over the liberty of foreign capital, which, in recent history, has been shown to significantly increase social inequalities with the most perverse disregard of citizenship in the history of mankind (Sen 1999).

The underestimation of the value of human dignity associated with chronic problems, such as hunger, misery, insalubrity, and unemployment, has encouraged the development of violence at all levels of society, both domestically and globally.

To compound the injury, hegemonic powers have waged war against poor countries and have paradoxically and pretentiously defended their actions as an attempt to promote democratic ideals.

Such an indisposition generated a wealth of scholarship seeking a reconstruction of society in accord with the ideals of solidarity and peace. Authors, such as Adela Cortina, advocate for the recovery of a Kantian universalist model and the discursive ethics of Jürgen Habermas to define the minima of global justice. Cortina emphasizes that such minima will not emerge from the liberal political tradition and, therefore, must be arrived at through the establishment of an inclusive discussion among the leaders of global society. She also warns that an unequal, non-communal world without liberties cannot establish the minimum conditions for harmonic survival. Solidarity, as a moral value, cannot pertain to a particular group; it must be universal. It is opposed to individualism, nepotism, and a lack of community. Once universal solidarity has been achieved by permeating the boundaries of groups and countries, it will encompass all human beings and nourish itself with peace by welcoming inhabitants of underdeveloped regions and maintaining respect for the environment. Once this has been achieved, the unsustainability of a possessive, individualistic market economy will become evident (Cortina 2001).

Alternatively, some Latin American authors, including Garrafa, Porto, and Schramm from Brazil, suggest more forceful political actions by institutions to bring about a more effective means of social inclusion. In 2002, Garrafa advocated for an intervention bioethics, marking a theoretical landmark, at the opening ceremony of the Sixth World Congress of Bioethics hosted by the International Association of Bioethics in Brasília (Garrafa and Porto 2003). Similarly, Porto supported the prioritization of policies and methods of decision making that privilege the largest number of people for the longest possible period of time and may also result in better life conditions, especially those of the most vulnerable (Porto and Garrafa 2006). Schramm suggests a bioethics of protection that seeks to assist in the resolution of a category of moral conflicts particular to Latin America and will simultaneously serve as a tool that is both intelligible and effective (Schramm 2006).

What appears undeniable is the fact that bioethics, as an applied ethics, cannot adopt a purely reflexive attitude when addressing moral problems; it must, instead, actively seek concrete proposals for change. Leopoldo e Silva articulates this position by affirming that "the attempt to simply explain and comprehend inequities … is profoundly unethical…It is necessary to know the reality in which the ethical judgment will be performed; trying to make this judgment translate into a mere justification of what exists is to renounce ethics" (Leopoldo e Silva 1998).

One cannot divorce the individual from the social within subjectivity; in other words, one cannot conceive of any complex social process without integrating both of these organizational levels of the human personality. Within this analytical perspective of human problems belonging to a network system, the social subjectivity concept understands the behavior of an individual or a social group as an inseparable part of a wide subjectivation generated at different levels and moments of social organization.

Even though bioethics holds in high esteem a social contructivist approach in accord with Habermas' dialogic theory, it also acknowledges the warnings of

Michel Foucault about the asymmetrical discursive practices that exist in the communication of real communities. From a Foucaultian perspective, liberating dialogue ceases to exist once the discretionary imposition of the power of the strongest becomes an objective. It appears undeniable that living in a real community is to experience, on a daily basis, the authoritative actions of some over others, and, according to Foucault, trying to imagine a human society without such asymmetrical power dynamics is a dangerous and unproductive abstraction (Foucault 1984).

To better understand this warning, we must refrain from the verification of the violence imposed by totalitarian regimes, such as Hitler's fascism and Stalin's communism, marked by the imperative denial of the Other while supporting diverging ideological positions from the one officially imposed. These political regimes perpetrated the cruelest and most extensive genocides recorded in recent history.

Furthermore, the global market economy has generated a new form of violence affecting marginalized countries in the form of extreme poverty, miserable life conditions, a lack of minimal access to education and health care, and, based on these conditions, an outright denial of any social rights. This large contingent of marginalized populations has not even been granted the first generation of citizenship rights. A lack of resources, the State's legitimacy crisis, and the growth of institutional emptiness contributable to organized crime have only increased the existential imbalance of a people overwhelmed by fear who have lost their personal identity due to a lack of social support. At the start of a new millennium, humankind exists in a state of perplexity similar to that experienced at the end of the First World War. In the words of Ralph Linton: "This book was written at a time of confusion and uncertainty. It is still too early to say whether the western world will ever recover from the self-inflicted wounds of the World War, or [if it will be] the beginning of a second and presumably more efficient suicide attempt. There have been times of darkness. Therefore, there is no reason to rest assured that the darkness will not return again" (Linton 1970).

It is clear that there are a number of differences between modern warfare and the armed conflicts of the past; however, the twenty-first century began with the terrorist attacks of September 11th, announcing a new period of darkness. The new globalized world is shaken by the novelty of terrorism and organized crime and begins to seek new regulations for the recognition of citizenship. One finds oneself inserted into a world of increasing complexity as technological advancements are rapidly achieved, and the condition of what some economists have called "impoverished enrichment" allows for a small number of elites to maintain a large percentage of the wealth with the better part of the population existing in conditions of misery.

Sophisticated security alarms available in gated communities are fooled by armed criminals who receive orders from convicts, devoid of their freedom, serving their time in "maximum security prisons." Never before has humankind relied on so many material resources in the possession of so few, denying to so many the most fundamental human rights. We have come to realize the nightmare foreshadowed in Josué de Castro's book, *The Famine Geography* (1946), which predicted big cities inhabited by a large contingent of sleeping people, those who could not sleep due to hunger, and those who would not sleep due to a fear of the legions of famished (Castro 2005).

Undoubtedly, there are those individuals who are isolated and introverted, who practice an exacerbated individualism, dominated by fear and incredulous of utopias and the intervention of State power. Having deemed life in the community unfeasible, one seeks refuge in the fantasy of individualism. Their identity, which should be built on the richness of cultural diversity, is replaced by the unreasonable logic of the self. As Allan Bloom illustrates: "The uncertain future and lack of a binding past means that the soul of the youth finds itself in a similar state to the first men: spiritually naked, disconnected, apart, with no inherited or unconditioned relations with anybody or anything. They can be whatever they wish, but have no particular reason to be anybody in particular" (Bloom 1989).

As a consequence of the true *I*, the tyranny of the *other* begins to be seen as a strange element to be manipulated, raped, and excluded from the community of equals. The physical destruction of the other has become increasingly common in big urban centers. Hetero-destruction was what motivated Freud to reflect on destruction as the pulsation of death. When questioned by Einstein in the late 1930s about the reason for war, which had decimated entire communities in Europe, Freud referred back to his thesis in which destruction and death constituted a form of exteriorization, explained by one's impulse for the death of the other as a replacement for one's wish for self-death and by the pleasure of being powerful enough to impose suffering on another (Freud 1981).

A representative case of insane cruelty was recorded by the murder of the native Brazilian Pataxó Indian leader, Galdino Jesus dos Santos. Invited to represent his community at the FUNAI's meeting, Galdino, without a place to sleep, fell asleep on a bus stop bench in Brasilia. While he was asleep, five middle-class young men soaked his body in alcohol and set fire to him. He was checked into a hospital with third-degree burns all over his body and died the next day. One of the murderous young men, in a testimony published in the April 21, 1997, issue of the newspaper *Correio Brasiliense*, justified his aggression as follows: "We were only kidding! We didn't know he was a native Indian, we thought he was some beggar."

Motivated by this crime, Endo, a member of the UNESCO Cultural Sector, resumed a study in Brasilia surveying middle-class young men. The results of the study showed that young men believed that humiliating transvestites, prostitutes, and homosexuals was a less reprehensible behavior than defacing public buildings or destroying phone booths and traffic signs. Over 20% of the interviewees believed it was unjustifiable to punish an individual for harassing an individual who had publicly displayed unconventional conduct (Endo 2005).

The Galdino case allows one to understand the discrimination and refusal to live with one another, as well as the vulnerability caused by conditions of social misery. It also forces one to confront the fallacy of global citizenship, because society exercises a policy of social exclusion when it is convenient. In the testimony of the murderous young men from Brasilia, they made a distinction between its being a crime if they had known he was a native Brazilian Indian and being otherwise justified if he were just "some beggar." One can see that begging has become intolerable in a developed society such as Brazil and, as a result, beggars are regarded as scum or as an element of trash that must be removed from social life. This illustrates that, for the beggar, the right to be different amongst equals is not respected. One lowers the status of the beggar to that of a stray animal and therefore respects the principle of treating equals as equals only by regarding the beggar as a class of animal, which is the social role they have created for him. The more tragic realization is that by not acknowledging his status as a human being, endowed with moral value, one may then physically eliminate him at random, through the arbitrary and perverse actions of young men who will undoubtedly find shelter in the society that conceived them. The right to life becomes reserved for those who are included by society's standards. To complete the analysis, the passivity of society when faced with a horrific event can be considered, as conventionally described by Hannah Arendt, the "banalization of evil."

Bioethics urges one to step outside of one's comfortable life and to take control of life's theatre, to create a new plot that will acknowledge the full citizenship of all human beings, especially the most vulnerable ones.

25.3 Seeking a Conclusion

The essential issue, which the historical study of humankind reveals, is the complexity of life and destiny, whether individual or social. Over 20 centuries, humankind still appears to have failed to realize the intrinsic value of humans. In 1783, when Kant manifested his belief in human rationality as "a man's abandoning of his minority [which would be] the incapacity of making use of his [own] understanding without the guidance of another individual," he inaugurated a new proposal for humanity (Kant 1985).

After two centuries, one now sees the Kantian ideal of one's full autonomy being reduced to what has conventionally been called an "ethics of realization." This approach understands the individual as a unique source of measurement, and one's priority becomes the disengaged personal fulfillment of any social commitment. Contemporary thinkers propose the substitution of the "self" for the "connect," a person guided by reflexive and critical consciousness who seeks the other's recognition through "implicated pluralism" (Castiñeira 1995). Lévinas aims for transcendence to the Other in an imperative relationship dominated by *alterity* (brotherhood). It is not achieved by privileging the Kantian universe, but simply by the "here and now" of community life, linking transcendence to the commonplace of reason and practice.

The relationship with the other is accomplished "face-to-face," and the feeling of fraternity is no longer generated from the nature of beings, but is revealed through the epiphany of the Other's face. The mission of every human being would not simply be "being," but "being for." The "one to another" model breaks the hegemony of the egoist being and proposes the construction of a society humanized by fraternity (Lévinas 1993).

Therefore, the question that has persisted throughout the centuries of humanity's history remains as to whether the ideal man conceived of by Lévinas, who exists for the Other, will subsist in an increasingly materialistic, competitive, and individualistic society. On the other hand, for the first time in history, the twenty-first century demands of every human being the elaboration of reasonable and prudent solutions to exceedingly complex moral issues. These decisions can only be reached if individuals from different moralities are able to partake in deliberation. The desire to establish new landmarks for an ethics of solidarity and responsibility emerges, because the ethical models found in an individualistic society are incapable of reaching such a resolution. Therefore, the primary task of global development should be the recognition and reinforcement of humanity in the face of market idolatry, the resultant ethical emptiness, and the abandonment of community. It has never been so urgent to recreate a universal ethics of solidarity. At a moment when economic globalization pervades all national borders, humankind lives with unbearable unemployment rates, hunger, and misery, in addition to the most consistent and egregious violations of the principles of human dignity (Herrero 2001).

References

Beauchamp T, Childress J (2008) Principles of biomedical ethics, 6th edn. Oxford University Press, New York

Bloom A (1989) O declínio da cultu ra ocidental. Best Seller, São Paulo

Castiñeira A (1995) Hábitos del corazón, comunidad civil y pluralismo implicado, Rev. Sal Terrae 83(1):3–18

Castro J (2005) Geografia da fome. Civilização Brasileira, São Paulo

Cortina A (2001) Ciudadanos del mundo. Alianza Editorial, Madrid

De Masi D (2000) O ócio criativo. Sextante, Rio de Janeiro

Endo P (2005) Sobre a violência: Freud, Hannah Arendt e o caso do índio Galdino. In: Zugueib Neto J (ed) Identidade e crises sociais na contemporaneidade. Editora UFPR, Curitiba

Freud S (1981) Más allá del princípio del placer. Biblioteca Nueva, Madrid

Foucault M (1984) Microfísica do poder. Graal, Rio de Janeiro

Garrafa V, Porto D (2003) Intervention bioethics: A proposal for peripheral countries in a context of power and injustice. Bioethics 17:399–416

Gilligan C (1998) In a different voice: Psychological theory and women's development. Harvard University, Cambridge, MA

Herrero FJ (2001) Ética do discurso. In: Oliveira MA (ed) Correntes Contemporâneas da Ética. Vozes, Petrópolis

Kant I (1985) Immanuel Kant: Textos Seletos. Vozes, Petrópolis

Kelly K (1998) New rules for the new economy: Radical strategies for a connected world. Penguin Books, London

Leopoldo e Silva F (1998) Da ética filosófica à ética em saúde. In: Costa S, Garrafa V, Oselka G (eds) Introdução à Bioética. Conselho Federal de Medicina, Brasília

Lévinas E (2005) Entre nós: ensaias sabre a alteridade. Vozes, Petrópolis

Lévinas E (1993) Humanismo do outro homem. Vozes, Petrópolis

Linton R (1970) O homem: uma introdução à antropologia. Martins Fontes, São Paulo

Morin E (2005) O método 6: ética. Sulina, Porto Alegre

Porto D, Garrafa V (2006) Bioética de intervenção: considerações sobre a economia de mercado. Bioética 13(1):111–123

Rowland MD (1995) Absolute happiness: The way to a life of complete fulfillment. Hay House Inc., Carlsbad, CA

Schramm FR (2006) Bioética sem universalidade? Justificação de uma bioética latino-americana e caribenha de proteção. In: Garrafa V, Kottow M, Saada A (eds) Bases conceituais da bioética: enfoque latino-americano. Gaia, São Paulo

Segre M, Ferraz N (1997) O conceito de saúde. Revista Brasileira de Saúde Pública 31(5):538–542

Segre M, Cohen C (2002) Bioética, 3rd edn. EDUSP, São Paulo

Segre M (2006) A questão ética e a saúde humana. Atheneu, São Paulo

Segre M (2007) L'Arte de invecchiare, bioética e terza etá. Patron Editore, Milano

Sen A (1999) A development as freedom. Alfred Knopf, New York

Vygotsky LS (1993) The collected works of L.S. Vygotsky. Plenum Press, New York

Chapter 26
Ethics of Research Involving Human Subjects: The Brazilian Experience

William Saad Hossne and Corina Bontempo Duca de Freitas

26.1 Introduction

Human experimentation cannot be analyzed in isolation because many forces shape social interaction – man's quest for knowledge and mastery, his willingness to risk human life, and his readiness to delegate authority and to rely on professional judgment (Katz 1972). It was man's capacity for seeking justice that made ethics committees possible, while at the same time it was man's capacity for deceiving people that made ethics committees necessary (Ramsey 1982, p. 533). As Raul Hilberg wrote in *The Destruction of the European Jews*, "If the world was so shocked at what it discovered to be the extremes to which experimental medicine would go, it has yet to condemn the method or find the means to control it" (Hilberg 2003). From our point of view, the right choice is to control experimentation on human beings.

By all means, this type of control is not an easy task. Considerations of the doctor–patient relationship, such as confidentiality and consent, are complicated

W.S. Hossne
Physician and researcher, Emeritus Professor of State University of São Paulo - UNESP, Botucatu Campus, Medical School, Member of the National Commission of Ethics in Research - CONEP, Member of the International Committee of Bioethics - UNESCO, Coordinator of the Master Course in Bioethics of University Center São Camilo, São Paulo - Centro Universitário São Camilo, Programa de Mestrado em Bioética, São Paulo, BR
e-mail: whossne@saocamilo-sp.br

C.B. Duca de Freitas
MD. Ph.D. Evaluation of Health Programs and Services, Pediatrician and Public Health Doctor at Teaching and Research Foundation in Health Science Secretaria de Estado de Saúde Pública do Distrito Federal, Fundação de Ensino e Pesquisa em Ciências da Saúde-FEPECS, Brasília, Distrito Federal, BR
e-mail: corinabdf@hotmail.com

L. Pessini et al. (eds.), *Ibero-American Bioethics: History and Perspectives*, Philosophy and Medicine 106, DOI 10.1007/978-1-4020-9350-0_26,

by special issues in this context, such as the interest of society in medical advancements and the uncertainty of experimental treatments. An important question becomes: how can we ensure that the risks of scientific advancement never outweigh the value of human life? The dangers of performing or not performing research have to be weighed on the same scale and the only way to accomplish this is to continually monitor research ethics by any means available.

Historically, the doctor–patient relationship has been based on trust. However, this relationship has also been one-sided, requiring the patient to relinquish one's right to an opinion, while trusting completely in that of one's doctor. As Jay Katz has put it, there was a silent world between doctor and patient. Nowadays, there is a growing need for honest communication between physicians and their patients, which requires informed consent to be more than just a judicial attempt. Doctors and patients must understand trust as an interrelationship based on mutual communication.

In human experimentation, it is not enough to offer an explanation to a potential subject and then to distribute a consent form. The decision-making process takes time, because self-determination is a process of self-reflection and reflection with others (Katz 1984, pp. 121–129). The quality of the consent one obtains varies in relation to the similarity of social positions between the doctor and the patient. In fact, informed consent is meaningless unless the patient has the appropriate level of education and medical knowledge to understand the terms of the research project. Most sick individuals are not in a position to argue with their physicians and are "coerced by disease, by pain, by fear of death, and often by ignorance" (Katz 1984, p. 2). It is important to realize that this is the situation of the great majority of sick people in Brazil. In addition, the distinction between therapy and experimentation is often blurred in such a way that it is difficult to make a precise judgment about the appropriate medical procedure.

Data can be provided to confirm this statement. It is well known that the implementation of the Brazilian Public Universal Health Care System (Sistema Único de Saúde - SUS) around 1990 was followed by a significant expansion of private insurance coverage. However, it is troublesome to know that in 1998 only 7.2% of the population had health insurance, while the health expenditures of this group represented 52.5% of the health expenditures of the whole population (Kilsztajn et al. 2002, pp. 258–262). In 2005, 19.9% of the population had private insurance coverage and public universal health care system (SUS) expenditures were around 3.7% of the Gross Internal Product (DATASUS 2006).

These data explain why some pharmaceutical companies choose to perform their research studies in Brazil. It is relatively easy for companies to find volunteers who are "treatment virgins," meaning that they have never received drugs to combat their diseases. In addition, many Brazilians are desperately seeking medical treatment and therefore may accept any form of experimental medicine, provided it is free. Brazil is a large country (8,514,876 km^2) with an estimated population in 2007 of around 190,000,000 inhabitants with an unfair income distribution associated with varying levels of education.

What used to be called "human experimentation" is now referred to in the more technical terms of "clinical studies" or "clinical trials." "Clinical studies" refer to the class of scientific approaches that evaluate disease prevention, diagnostic techniques, and treatments, while "clinical trials" refer to the subset of clinical studies that evaluate investigational medicines in phases I, II, and III (Spilker 1991). In addition to these terms, research on human beings also involves the understanding and use of cohort studies, retrospective studies, cross-sectional studies, different types of questionnaires and inquiries, and control groups.

In Brazil, all research participants are aware when the treatment they receive is part of a research study. The question becomes whether they really had a choice to participate in research to begin with. The only real protection subjects may have depends on the ethical behavior of investigators and their peers. This ethical protection of participants is the primary responsibility of research ethics committees concerning the involvement of human subjects in Brazil.

26.2 Guidelines for Ethical Research in Brazil

26.2.1 Motivation

During the 1980s, the ethical requirements of and procedures for medical research involving human subjects were debated all over the world. Some of the relevant efforts included: the revision of the World Medical Association's Declaration of Helsinki at the Twenty-Ninth World Medical Assembly in Tokyo, Japan (1975); the publication of the International Ethical Guidelines for Biomedical Research in 1982 by the Council for International Organizations of Medical Sciences (CIOMS); and the publication of many rules and regulations applicable to research involving human subjects by the World Health Organization (WHO) and the Department of Health and Human Services of the United States of America.

In Brazil, a demand for the revision of the Brazilian constitution arose as a result of all the political changes that were occurring. Consequently, a revised constitution with the clear expression of human rights was promulgated in 1988 (Constituição da República Federativa do Brasil). Following these changes, a new code of medical ethics was addressed, taking medical research into account (Código de Ética Médica 1988). Additionally, a book on experimentation with human beings was published (Vieira and Hossne 1987). All of these factors catalyzed a reaction among physicians regarding the lack of governmental regulations pertaining to research involving human beings, in particular, biomedical research. As a result, in 1988, the Brazilian Council of Health (CNS), subordinate to the Brazilian Institute of Health (MS), approved the first guidelines for medical research under the Resolution CNS 1/88. Unfortunately, many mistakes were made and the resolution was ineffective.

In 1995, a revision to the resolution was proposed and the Brazilian Council of Health (CNS) established a working group, whose president was William Saad Hossne, to elaborate new guidelines for research on human beings in Brazil. The team was an interdisciplinary assembly of 15 people from a variety of fields, including medicine, philosophy, religion, sociology, law, government, the pharmaceutical industry, and some representatives from voluntary health agencies that focused on various illnesses and handicap conditions. All members of the team were chosen by the CNS and were sufficiently qualified through experience and expertise to promote respect for their advice in safeguarding the rights and welfare of participants in research.

It was first decided that the guidelines should be established within a free and independent system, which meant that it would not be subordinated to professional boards or governmental agencies and would require the creation of an advisory panel for counseling and advising. Additionally, the code was not to include statements with strong wording like "must" or "forbidden" or even some weaker terms such as "ought" or "should." Instead, it was meant to indicate how the requirements of ethical principles could be met when research on human beings was being carried out. The team then identified, based on data from The Brazilian Institute of Health and the Brazilian Institute of Education, approximately 30,000 people and institutions that could be of help in the process of elaborating guidelines. A copy of Resolution CNS 1/88 was sent to each identified individual or institution, with a cover letter asking for any comments, suggestions, or tips. Resolution CNS 1/88 was also published in some of the leading scientific journals. Responses were received from 119 institutions with a significant number of associated individuals, marking a significant contribution. The team then analyzed and discussed the responses they had received in conjunction with the examination of 18 different international codes and guidelines. In addition, seminars, meetings, lectures, and multiple document revisions took place.

An early draft soon emerged and was presented at the First Brazilian Congress of Bioethics. The Brazilian Society of Bioethics had already been established two years prior by Dr. William Saad Hossne. Suggestions from the conference were accepted, corrections were made, and, finally, after working for 10 months on the revisions of Resolution CNS 1/88, the team sent a written proposal to the Brazilian Council of Health (CNS). The new guidelines were established under Resolution CNS-196/96 in October 1996 and therefore marked the date when Brazil officially adopted guidelines for research on human beings approved by the Brazilian Council of Health (CNS) and Brazilian Institute of Health (MS). The revised guidelines are now well known throughout the country and investigators acknowledge and comply with them - National Health Council (Brasil 2000).

Resolution CNS-196/96 was a significant advance and demonstrated a notable difference between the initial regulations set forth and those which Brazil had come to establish. The resolution provided for the creation of the National Commission for Research Ethics (CONEP) (2000), which is responsible for evaluating the ethical concerns of all research involving human subjects when there is a risk of harm. It should be noted that many individuals understand the word "risk" to imply dreadful consequences (Vieira and Hossne 1987). However, CONEP defines risk as the possibility of physical, psychological, social, economic, or legal harm. Resolution CNS-196/96 also provided for the creation of institutional research ethics committees (CEP) at those institutions where research on human beings was being carried out. These committees will be discussed in further detail below.

It is interesting to note that Resolution CNS-196/96 also provided guiding principles regarding the responsibilities and obligations of all parties involved in an investigation with human participants. However, it is not a code. Part one of the Resolution CNS-196/96 links its recommendations with Brazilian laws and was written by lawyers and jurists. Hence, it makes clear to an investigator when a departure from the guidelines can be prosecuted. But the major intention of Resolution CNS-196/96 is to allow the reader to become aware of human experimentation and its consequences from the vantage point of various fields.

26.2.2 Research Ethics Committees (CEP)

In Brazil, these committees usually exist at academic institutions and medical facilities and are most commonly applicable to studies in the fields of medicine, dentistry, nursing, psychology, and other health sciences. Some CEPs also exist in the social and human areas. All committees are subordinated to the National Commission for Ethics on Research (CONEP), which is subject to the Brazilian Institute of Health (MS). Any research involving human subjects has to be approved by a CEP before it begins.

Each CEP must have at least seven members who demonstrate sensitivity to the rights and welfare of human subjects and have different background profiles, including gender, field of interest, and profession. Not more than half of the members can be of the same profession. In addition, CEPs must have members of suitable professional competence to review specific research activities. At least one member must serve as a representative for the patients attended to by the health care system of the committee's institution. Since special attention must be paid to those investigations involving vulnerable populations, such as indigenous peoples, children, prisoners, the elderly, or persons with diminished capacities, an ad hoc advisor who is familiar with a particular vulnerable population is allowed to assist in revising relevant protocols.

A CEP must review proposed protocols within a reasonable time period (usually one month) and must present its assessment in writing, substantiating one of the following decisions:

(a) Approved
(b) Modifications required prior to approval
(c) Disapproved

The CEP may also request additional information and may require alterations or adjustments to the consent form if they improve the protection of the rights, safety, or well-being of subjects. An institution, and when appropriate a CEP, must keep records of all members, identified by name with addresses and phone numbers included, in addition to maintaining copies of all research protocols reviewed and the relevant meeting minutes to document attendance.

When submitting a research protocol to a CEP, an investigator must send a copy of the project, the consent form, a description of the recruitment procedures, the financial plan, the curriculum vitae of all investigators, and the available safety information. The investigator also must inform the institution where the research will take place and provide a detailed description of the facilities to be used. To ensure a fair judgment, members of a CEP should consider the qualifications of investigators for the proposed research by asking for the curriculum vitae of all investigators and any other documents that, in the judgment of the CEP, are relevant.

However, the most important aim of a protocol review is to ensure safeguards for research subjects once they have enrolled in a project. Voluntary participation by prospective subjects is always required. Participants who are competent to make decisions are required to sign a consent form, while those who are not competent must have a suitable proxy to act on their behalf (surrogate decision maker). It is preferable that one's consent to participate in an experiment is truly informed and free from coercion. Therefore, an important task of all members of a CEP is to examine and evaluate whether a consent form is comprehendible to subjects. A major concern is the ability of patients to understand the consent form and freely, that means by their own decision, choose between participation and non-participation in a research project. All means should be exhausted to avoid "the engineering of consent" (Levine 1986, p. 39).

In addition to a valid consent form, the scientific merit of a research project must also be assessed. Accordingly, a CEP must have the professional competence necessary to review specific research activities and must be able to determine the acceptability of any proposed investigation in terms of institutional regulations and standards of professional conduct and practice. For this reason, a CEP shall include members with expertise in the scientific areas it regularly reviews and may invite ad hoc referees to assist in areas of specialization that the committee lacks. Effective monitoring of research protocols requires the simultaneous assessment of scientific and ethical soundness in the protocols.

In 2005, around 17,000 protocols involving 700,000 human subjects were reviewed by 475 committees with approximately 7,000 committee members distributed throughout Brazil. At the present time, there are 551 research ethics committees with a total of 8,107 committee members. The background breakdown for these committee members includes more or less 32% professionals in social sciences or law, 30% physicians, 23% health professionals but not physicians, 10% from mathematical fields, and 5% biologists.

Brazilian guidelines forbid the practice of paying research participants. However, the investigator is required to cover any additional expenses a participant accrues as a result of participation in research. Some committees in Brazil represent non-profit organizations and their recruitment for research participants may not include the use of advertisements.

While the guidelines are fairly well established, they still allow for changes and advances. The guidelines approved by the Brazilian Council of Health (CNS) were written with the biomedical and laboratory sciences in mind. CEPs are most often used for the review of studies in the fields of medicine, dentistry, nursing, psychology, and other health sciences. However, the methodologies of the social sciences, such as psychology, do present some concerns, because they can rely more heavily on qualitative research methods. In general, one should be guided by the principle that harm must be minimized and informed consent must be maximized in any research protocol.

26.2.3 National Commission for Research Ethics (CONEP)

This commission has the final authority to determine whether a particular research protocol can be performed. In addition, CONEP is responsible for maintaining the ethical conduct of investigators at the highest professional level, educating investigators about relevant ethical standards, and endeavoring to protect research participants against harmful conduct by investigators. CONEP has an advisory function regarding those ethical questions that are relevant to research involving human participants.

Protocols should be reviewed by CONEP within two months. During 2005, 1,253 protocols involving around 50,000 human subjects were reviewed by CONEP and an on-line database recording those research protocols that have been approved is available. Entries may be listed by the project title, the institution where the investigation will be performed, or by the name of the primary investigator.

Most investigations (around 90%) carried out in Brazil are approved solely by a CEP. However, in special research areas, such as new drugs and vaccines, diagnostic testing, human reproduction, investigations on indigenous people, human genetics, biosafety, new procedures in general, and international research projects, a review by CONEP in addition to the regular review by an institutional CEP is required. A CEP may also defer to CONEP when there are uncertainties in a given protocol.

In order to ensure the protection of research subjects and to guide the judgment of research projects in special areas, CONEP established rules and provisions pertaining to:

- Investigations of new drugs, medicines, vaccines, and diagnostic tests – Resolution 251/1997
- Investigations with international cooperation – Resolution 292/1999
- Investigations on human reproduction – Resolution 303/2000
- Investigations on indigenous peoples – Resolution 304/2000
- Investigations on human genetics – Resolution 340/2004
- Investigations on multicenter research – Resolution 346/2005
- Investigations involved stored or storing biological material – Resolution 347/2005

CONEP now has 13 members: three physicians, two dentists, a lawyer, a social worker, a psychologist, a pharmacist, a biologist, a theologian, a nurse, and a patient representative. Members were chosen by the CNS from those nominees indicated by CEPs spread all over the country. Profiles of the designated nominees were submitted and analyzed (Freitas 2006, p. 67). The results showed that nominees had high academic qualifications and almost all had taken courses on research methods or bioethics, with about two-thirds of these courses being of short duration. In 2005, both males and females were equally represented.

The awareness of investigators pertaining to the evaluative system and guidelines employed by CONEP in reviewing protocols was also analyzed (Freitas 2006, pp. 103–112). Major concerns included how to find patient representatives for participation in a research committee and how best to reinforce their role; how to monitor projects, how to prepare a member appropriately for a CEP; and how to improve communication among different CEPs. A self-evaluation of CEP members also found that approximately 90% believed they were able to do the work, were satisfied with what they were doing, and valued the responsibility and cooperation demonstrated among committee members.

However, there is still cause for concern. A survey of Brazilian scientific journals found that most of the submission instructions for authors fail to include a policy regarding the ethical components of any research findings published, and when they are present, requirements vary significantly among journals (Sardenberg et al. 1999, p. 289; Sardenberg et al. 2002, pp. 15–18).

26.3 Final Considerations

It is a challenge to establish an investigator-subject decision-making process that involves a genuinely mutual effort. It is also difficult to make investigators realize that the protection of subjects depends heavily on their ethical behavior. However, Brazilian guidelines are intended to make investigators consider the need for a sound and ethical protocol in addition to recognizing those critical issues that investigators and participants must confront related to informed consent. In this way, the Brazilian guidelines are not a normative code.

This problem remains because, for a normative ethics to be established, students and professionals must become more familiarized with the field. The introduction of ethics into professional schools would require either introducing it into the curriculum during the first year, which would often lead to the mere memorization of facts by students, or introducing it in the latter years of study, which, alternatively, runs the risk of students being unreceptive to philosophy because they only want to learn and practice their professional skills. Despite these challenges, a change must be made. A decision not to act will likely bring about as many problems as a decision to act. Therefore, not to act is to only adding to the current problem.

The observable efforts currently being made include: the existence of a body of literature on the subject written in Portuguese; bioethics journals being edited in Brazil; several attempts to introduce bioethics at the undergraduate, graduate, and post-graduate level; and the existence of a first graduate course in bioethics at the University of São Camilo.

Over the last decade there has been an increasing interest in research ethics in Brazil and it continues to grow. CONEP and all of the CEPs have changed investigators' behavior and should be credited for making this difference. However, there is still much to do in order to give the public a basic understanding of health care research and its requirements: not only regarding the money spent on it, but also regarding their participation as subjects. Brazilian investigators are now more aware that scientific investigation requires social controls as well as all other professional activities. So, the seed is sown and we hope that from this seed a plant will flourish.

References

Brasil (2000) Ministério da Saúde. Conselho Nacional de Saúde. Disponível em: http://conselho.saude.gov.br/Web_comissoes/conep/arquivos/resolucoes/resolucoes.htm. Accessed 5/20/2009

Código de Ética Médica (1988) Cf http://www.m.org.br. Accessed 2/22/09

DATASUS (2006) http://tabnet.datasus.gov.br/cgi/idb2006/matriz.htm. Accessed 2/26/09

Freitas CBD (2006) O sistema de avaliação da ética em pesquisa no Brasil: estudo dos conhecimentos e práticas de lideranças de Comitês de Ética em Pesquisa. PhD dissertation, São Paulo

Hilberg R (2003) The destruction of the European Jews [1961]. Yale University Press, New Haven, CT

Katz J (1972) Experimentation with human beings. Russell Sage Foundation, New York. Part One

Katz J (1984) The silent world of doctor and patient. Free Press, New York, pp 121–129

Kilsztajn S, Camara MB, Carmo MSN (2002) Gasto privado com saúde por classes de renda. Rev Assoc Med Bras 48(3):258–262

Levine RJ (1986) Ethics and regulation of clinical research, 2nd edn. Urban & Schwarzenberg, Baltimore

National Commission for Research Ethics (CONEP) (2000) Rules on Research Involving Human Subjects (Res. CNS 196/96 and others). National Health Council, Brasília

Ramsey P (1982) Consent as a Canon of Loyalty. In: Beauchamp TL, Walters LR (ed) Contemporary issues in bioethics. Wadsworth Publishing, Belmont, pp 430–433

Sardenberg T, Müller SS, Pereira FIR, de Oliveira RÃ, Hossne WS (1999) Analysis of ethical aspects on human experimentation included in the instructions for authors in 139 Brazilian scientific journals. Rev Assoc Med Bras 45(4):295–302

Sardenberg T, Müller SS, Pereira FIR, de Oliveira RÃ, Hossne WS (2002) Análise dos aspectos éticos da pesquisa em seres humanos contidos nas instruções aos autores de 38 revistas de ortopedia e traumatologia. Acta ortop bras 10(2):5–18

Spilker B (1991) Guide to clinical trials. Raven Press, New York

Vieira S, Hossne WS (1987) Experimentação com seres humanos. Moderna, São Paulo

Constituição da República Federativa do Brasil (1988). http://www.planalto.gov.br/ccivil_03/Constituicao/principal.htm. Accessed 03/05/09

Part IV
The Future of Ibero-American Bioethics

Chapter 27
A Prospective Examination for Discovering Challenges from the Hispano-American Historical Context

Hubert Lepargneur

27.1 Introduction: Defining the Historical Context

The beginning of bioethics in Hispano-America and Brazil requires an understanding of the particular life conditions of that subcontinent, which have been expounded in Diego Gracia's reflections. Despite recent advances, most individuals still live under or near the poverty line, making one's fundamental concern socio-economic survival: something that precedes any discussion of bioethics pertaining to issues like ad hoc committees so common in the Northern hemisphere.

Due to the limited context of this essay, a detailed discussion of these socio-economic conditions cannot be undertaken. As a foundation for the present discussion, historical lessons will be extracted and used as a basis from which one can make future projections. The prevention of past misfortunes and missteps will influence the projected path, and attention to the continued effects of these historical blunders will be given. The aim in moving forward is to pay heed to the lessons of the past while reviving an idealistic perspective with which to approach the future.

27.2 The Universalist Perspective of Bioethics Returns Relativized but Strong Enough

Idealisms, utopias, and supposedly universal religions provide glimpses of the ideal of a more humanitarian and collaborative humankind, which goes beyond the globalization of communication and finances and is better reconciled with its own constitutive diversity. Located within this multi-secular history, bioethics begins an important stage, after almost half a century of progressive preparation and anticipation. Christians have a word to symbolize the supreme unit of completely reconciled humankind: *pleroma*. However, this concept is only intelligible within the Christian

H. Lepargneur
Professor do Programa de Mestrado em Bioética do Centro Universitário São Camilo. Seminário Camiliano, São Paulo, BR
e-mail: pessini@saocamilo-sp.br

L. Pessini et al. (eds.), *Ibero-American Bioethics: History and Perspectives*, Philosophy and Medicine 106, DOI 10.1007/978-1-4020-9350-0_27,

faith. After a long journey, bioethics is now in an exceptionally relevant phase. It was born as a universal perspective, motivated by a need to improve life on our planet; however, it assumed conditions and a capacity for good will beyond that which could be guaranteed within each nation. A number of disappointments proved that this idealized concept was neither as accessible or generalized as it was intended to be. The time has therefore arrived for its reconsideration through scientific, political, cultural, and religious perspectives.

While this account of the various routes taken by Latin American bioethicists, starting from 1970, cannot be exhaustive, it remains a far-reaching and serious approach. The documents presented aim to contribute to the research and informational exchanges and collaborations of the near future. An understanding of the historical routes taken will also lead one to appreciate the work required to preserve the future of humankind.

The polarity of a universal ethics active in bioethics is not a surprise, even if this seems a distant and utopian ideal, because bioethics incorporates all cultures. Although unattainable outside of limited sectors, this ideal demands the constant efforts of well-meaning communities to be successful. A concept of shared morality is employed in relation to the idea of a universal human nature, which develops a common good that promotes a natural right to be constructed, investigated, stimulated, and updated.

History, both past and recent, presents concerns, especially when – regarding, for instance, the Israeli–Palestinian conflict – no theoretical or practical consensus has been reached pertaining to serious issues such as reaching a cease-fire to allow for establishing the conditions for an enduring peace. Consider the obstinacy of the Hamas party, now dominant in Palestinian ideology, which refuses to respect the three demands which would make possible a peace treaty: (1) accepting the existence of Israel as an independent nation; (2) abolishing terrorism and violence; and (3) respecting political and legal agreements signed by representatives of the two countries. Can one sail in deeper waters if rocks so settled prevent the first reliable moves? Love is a great force and justly celebrated, but obstinacy fueled by hatred has usually not recognized its real historical strength. Maybe history would register fewer wars if mentalities or psychologies were different. A contribution from bioethics is required for human beings to attain the ideal of understanding and peace.

In a 2006 declaration, the writer Salman Rushdie pointed out:

> We witness today a proliferation of irreconcilable world views that battle for the same space. We observe a conflict that opposes less cultures or religions than dissimilar perceptions of reality. We live in a fractured world. I am not a believer; between reason and religious faith, I always choose reason. However, neither believers nor atheists can be satisfied with a view of humans as only rational beings. We are also dreamers, which opens us to another dimension. How to integrate the idea that something exists that is beyond meat and blood? (Rushdie 2006).

Dissimilarities, of course, are not absent from Latin America. Bioethics demands us to go beyond the strictly physiological aspects of human beings to exercise the symbolic capacity of human words and thought, with the purpose of reflecting on the transcendental experience that leads a few towards religious lights. Even humanistic projects fail to take into account all beneficial connections, as Xico Graziano reminds us when he states that "the environmental sensitivity of the so-called social movements is next to zero" (Graziano 2007).

Bolivia appears to emphasize the importance of heterogeneity in a national or Latin American bioethics. A problem arises when considering the ambiguities of the expression "health," or "good life," since not all definitions of these concepts share the same elements. For example, what is better: an intensely happy but short life, or a long but mediocre life? Do we prefer to smoke, with the accompanying risks, and die young, or do we value a long ascetic life? Another point, on which all will not agree, is the degree of acceptable interventionism ("hard bioethics") useful for the national or international common good. The fact is, conceptions of the common good diverge and affect the institutionalization of bioethics. What do we think, for instance, about the increasing European prohibitions of smoking in public places? Is it conceivable to prohibit cocaine use in Bolivia or poppy production in Thailand or Afghanistan?

Beginning in 1994, the Pan-American Health Organization (PAHO), the Chilean government, and the University of Chile created a "Regional Bioethics Program," focusing in principle on all of Latin America and the Caribbean, and aiming to sponsor several activities and publications. The Chilean Society of Bioethics preceded the registry of the first bioethics committee in Chilean hospitals, occurring at the beginning of the decade, but only later did it begin to function. In addition, Chilean Catholic institutions had an early interest in bioethics that encouraged a conservative approach (for better or worse: protection of the family and opposition to abortion, but also a clear opposition to reproductive technologies and embryonic stem-cell research). The National Commission of Bioethics in Chile was established after much debate and opposition, and its authority remains very limited and its work wanting. North American principlism was received in Chile before other countries, but the impediment of an extreme conservatism remained uncompensated for by the irruption of great market forces. The behavior of medical elites and the slower evolution of the people's mentalities were recognizably different. Ultimately, each Latin American nation was socially and culturally fragmented by economic resources, despite substantial humanitarian efforts.

The appeal and receptivity to a universal ethics in bioethics is no surprise, because it has been justly encouraged by the works and movements initiated by Hans Küng. A universal ethics relates all cultures and therefore demands intense and constant efforts from all the communities involved in the interchange. It would be an achievement to be able to coordinate the Latin American countries in a way similar to that achieved by the European Union. A similar coordination is what this work seeks to support, but at the same time wishes to acknowledge the World Health Organization and other organizations currently working in Latin America for the value of their contributions.

The counter-forces at work historically have not prevented the production of bioethical works, especially by Hispano-American and Portuguese groups, which have aimed at advancing a science and an art to benefit, as far as possible, all human beings. These works were inspired by conditions of hardship and therefore have come at a cost. For this reason, we appreciate the preliminary work done by many researchers and bioethicists, knowing that some day, after many and discreet stages, a new progress for humankind will arise. One of the characteristics which distinguishes human beings from other animals is an ability to accumulate and transfer knowledge and know-how across generations. Significant advances have happened almost by chance, under the pressure of unforeseen and unavoidable circumstances. In the future, similar circumstances will inevitably arise; however, it is important to respond to and understand them in a way that will challenge individuals to create more perceptive and effective solutions.

27.3 Complimentarity and Parallelism Among the Identified Bioethics Nuclei

The bioethics of each nation or region reflects the culture of its own context without denying common objectives. In general, each community has a unique contribution to make but also has room to accommodate those of other cultures. No authority is able to accommodate all of the nuances of a complex situation involving many cultures. Such pluralism is frequently taken into account by the members of a bioethics committee, but disadvantaged countries are not always capable of establishing an appropriately qualified and diversified team. Many doctors prefer only to consult their peers in the medical profession, due to their distrust of the potential "aberrations" that could arise from an outside perspective.

One cannot overemphasize the vital need for the participation of individuals from the different religions and cultures representative of the region, as well as therapists and doctors who have different specializations and practices. The representation of patients is admittedly very rare and difficult to establish in practice; and yet, the patients are the ones who have the most intimate knowledge of their situation and have the most at stake in improving their condition. While it is acknowledged that the greater the number of participants, the more difficult it is to reach unanimous decisions, sometimes a certain degree of convergence is enough to justify certain decisions.

Practice seems to show that disagreement between doctors and jurists is frequent. The divergence of beliefs among religious individuals and agnostic scientists is another location of strong disagreement. The conflict of beliefs also becomes more pronounced as particular religious fundamentalisms proliferate, as is shown by the expansion of Islamic influences. Religion imposes dogmas whose grounds are "supernatural" revelations that believers cannot challenge. Scientists do not have access to the apodictic value of these dogmas and, instead, ground their beliefs in mathematics and the observation of concrete facts through verification by experience and experimentation. It should be noted that, except for some domains of declining scientism, science is much less certain of its "definitive" position than the believer of religious dogmas. However, scientists who do have a faith are reluctant to admit to its influence on their scientific pursuits, because it may affect the interpretation of data offered by history and nature. Some issues of interest here are abortion, IVF, embryo manipulation, euthanasia, and assisted suicide.

Complementary approaches must prevent or correct threats of myopia in bioethical treatment or biogenetic experiments that would exceed genetic or morphologic characteristics of human nature. Advancements in bioethical research follow the developments of democracy and to an extent rely on them: democratic cultures take more readily to the theory and practice of bioethics. Many contemporary discoveries are the product of research teams who cooperate and integrate their findings to produce new knowledge. It is rare for a single individual to accomplish such discoveries on his own; however, a few scientists have received the Nobel Prize for such discoveries. In this way, the practice of bioethics encourages the convergence of individual or collective findings for the benefit of human integrity. This does not confuse biomedical sciences with philosophy or religion, because some cultural concept of the deeper nature of human beings is always functioning in the background. A diversity of views, especially in assessing certain challenges, is normal, desirable, and generally beneficial for a team, so long as difference does not generate hostility. Individuals must employ reason and be open to varying interpretations of the truth, even when what is true for one is not necessarily true for others: bioethics is a school of tolerance that must not deny any viewpoint genuinely advanced. Nobody owns truth; the conscience that this is true avoids constructing barriers against the acceptance of the new.

Innovation often leads to a new paradigm in thought or practice which is never brought about from nothing. There is some wisdom in recognizing the continuity presented by historical discontinuities, as in the elevation of religious transcendence through the plurality of religions, or the seriousness of researchers from very different domains of reality. History never repeats itself; for that reason, we trust that somehow the future will always be more interesting. Bioethicists recognize the common foundations of diverse challenges and are able to synthesize different approaches to meet the unique demands of each case. Every being is unique and human beings are no exception. Before any case, the question is always: what can experience bring to this event and what novel or exceptional factors can this event bring?

27.4 Economic and Social Costs

The proclamation of a new social-sanitary order from the *leitmotiv* declared that citizens "have a right to health" (a utopian exaggeration, but a typical one), and it is therefore incumbent on public institutions to provide for individuals when necessary and to finance such systems. History shows that this radical socialist project is almost unfeasible in practice. It was unsuccessful in the Soviet Union, and its benefits, maybe relative in Cuba, are costly and are financed by neglecting the provision of other social necessities. The satisfaction of bioethical concerns cannot proceed without consideration of its economic import, even if political ability or ignorance of budgetary constraints encourages its disregard. Who is concerned about the millions or billions of social security deficits? All social progress has an economic cost; the problem lies in appropriately selecting which funding sources are the most advisable and effective.

Thus, once we look at the history of bioethics, we perceive an oscillation between project and accomplishment, ideal and feasibility, the ultimate long-term vision and the concrete conditions for immediate improvement of the situation. If health demands an increase in investments and expenses, it is an urgent concern to determine how to identify and select financial resources and how to command economies in marginal sectors. In many countries, the useless repetition of lab tests and unnecessary consultations are common practice. A country whose external debt surpasses 30% or 50% of its GNP must accept restrictions on frivolous travel for modest savings. It is necessary to consider sectors other than public health, such as education and training, in which savings could be gained without damages. The maturity of a developed nation is evaluated by its rates of investment in scientific research, especially in biomedicine, but the fruits of this research mostly only benefit the elite populous.

Let us remember the solidarity of biomedicine with other public necessities, as shown by the proposals made to the government by the French ecologist, Nicolás Hulot: to make the environment the State's main priority; name a deputy prime minister in charge of sustainable development; create and apply a progressive carbon tax until carbonic gas emissions are four times less than at current; consult people about the direction of sustainable development, making clear they are to adhere to the chosen restrictions; promote people sensibly to ecology and public health (Hulot 2006).

To paraphrase Ségoléne Royal: The true challenge consists in reconciling the tensions between a better atmosphere and social urgency and sustainable development, which would allow for the suppression of privileges that impose high costs on society, such as artificially extending the survival of the babies of affluent families. The socialist ex-candidate to the presidency of the French republic had three high priorities: the environment, economic problems, and a concern for social problems in which public health would be increasingly more important (see Royal 2007).

Chile, the country having the best politico-social health system in the region, is associated with a deep-rooted attitude for the rejection of social security by capitalization, which demands a State contribution for benefit of the poorest, which has motivated a number of prejudices against Chile (the criminal acts of Pinochet are not to be considered here).

In order to protect the environment, Iceland has decided to fuel its public transportation system with hydrogen, a good replacement for oil when the reserves have been depleted. In a short time, the high costs of such innovations will be reduced and several additional benefits regarding public transportation and health will be acquired. The *Boeing-Spectrolab* society, supported by the North American Energy Department, developed photovoltaic models that can transform solar radiation at an incredible rate of 40.7% when the European records have not exceeded 37%. All such advances have a cost and most depend on research and investment options that are not feasible for all countries. The concentration of wealth and ability, both nationally and internationally, negatively affect the future prospects of some. This provides for the risk of achieving a future where the medical treatment of the rich and the poor differs significantly based on the quality of treatment affluency was able to secure for them.

Despite a few noble actions establishing international foundations or non-governmental organizations (NGOs) aimed at the public good, one must recognize that the advances of biomedicine have benefited primarily the wealthiest members of society. Promises of mutual benefit for all are stronger in discourse than actualized in practice. The relationship between the public and private sectors, in each country and the world generally, is not stable, and one risks falling into dogmatism when proposing what one considers the best solution, because solutions are always context dependent. Except for Monaco and a few extremely wealthy islands, the State will never be able to realize the promise of absorbing all costs required to maintain its citizens at an acceptable level of well-being.

Equality of treatment is merely a dream or an election promise. Few entrepreneurs or professionals from the public or private sectors earn more than a million euros, or three million dollars, in Latin America. The members of the wealthy elite (traditional or recent, of honest or fraudulent origin) sponsor works or foundations whose utility and generosity could be expanded to all nations. Reliance on the government for everything, whose members are the elite, does not help the dynamics of necessary social progress. Dom Fragoso, a former bishop of Crateús in the northeast part of Brazil, refused donations from a rich German diocese because, he said, this would turn the poor members of his community into beggars.

What magnitude of change will affect concentrations of wealth that privilege only a few companies, individuals, or families? After the end of oil reserves and the loss of energy and dynamism for North America, what would a world-wide Chinese domination look like? What would a fundamental Islamic imperialism, whose radicals show no signs of wanting peace, be like? In addition, what would happen if these two forces clashed in the near future? How would the Chinese or Islamic react to the current accomplishments of bioethics?

Bioethics, ecology, and economy are interconnected. They should be recognized as factors in the promotion of a universal, concrete, common good, in spite of the traditional blindness of potentates. Generally, a mysterious connection exists between the *closest* and the *most distant* factors: more than one invention has been the product of the sudden and accidental integration of data that were not traditionally considered in relation to each other.

In his chapter on historical introduction, Diego Gracia calls attention to the possibility of enriching the principles of justice and non-maleficence that seem relevant in this context. The *economic factor weighs ever more* on the sanitary challenge, not so much regarding the population multiplication (especially of the unfortunate migrants who flee their own countries), but mainly concerning increasing sanitary costs for curative and preventative measures.

The theme of justice is the object of a general ethics of the population which becomes unintelligible when powerful elites are caught in the performance of indiscretions and are publicly exonerated by ethics commissions or the courts. Once again, the recommendation must be reinforced, that to maintain a wise social security system and a just allocation of the health budgets to aid the rich and the poor, the privilege traditionally afforded to the rich must be eradicated. The essence of an effective social security system cannot be provided here, as the challenge must be faced country by country, state by state.

Regarding the argument of "non-maleficence," it is not a simple subject, because largely harmful actions caused by the rich and powerful appear to be more acceptable than small infractions by individuals of lower status who are unable to defend themselves. Asking for reparations is a difficult, long, and risky process for the poor. Aside from allowing successive appeals, legal cases can be affected by the defensive reactions of medical organizations. This problem also relates to the principle of patient autonomy. Discussions of autonomy require consideration of the importance of sociological factors, the condition of the patient, and the information patients receive about their condition, because they can all be limiting factors on one's real autonomy. Regarding the miserable sanitation conditions of the poor in the past, a number of studies have been completed; however, a bulk of them only reflect the conditions of Northern countries to the disadvantage of others (Lepargneur 2003).

Principlism entered Fidel's Cuba, primarily since the publication in 2002 of "Bioethics for Sustainability," a collection of essays edited by J. R. Acosta, with an emphasis in J. A. Martínez Gómez's chapter, "Projects for a Global Bioethics." This assimilation took place by adapting the principle of individual autonomy and emphasizing that the principle of beneficence constitutes the highest expression of justice. Cuba's sanitary system is its most successful accomplishment, even though potential damage may have been done to other socio-economic domains, but the system does deserve recognition for its altruistic application in countries facing hardship and lacking doctors (Chile in 1960, Algeria in 1963, Kashmir in 2005, Indonesia in 2006, Venezuela in 2007). Araujo proposed to substitute "accessibility, participation, and fairness" for the triad "beneficence, autonomy, and justice," but this is only a detail.

27.5 General Evaluation

At the end of so broad a historical survey, there is no point in emphasizing the relevance and quality of the project, concluded at the right time: that is, after exactly 30 years of innovative research experience in Spanish–Brazilian America, 30 years of conquests in lands not always prepared for joint research work; these discussions have aimed towards a common good that still demands new expansion efforts. Such efforts have already had some good results, not only for people's health, but also for the political–cultural development of those societies. Detailed monographs and bibliographies have been published in three of the primary languages.

With or without anti-Americanism, an attitude that prevails in contemporary times (for several reasons, the Latin character has always differed from the North American one), Latin Americans have had difficulties with the reception, understanding, and application of the four famous American "principles" of bioethics: autonomy, beneficence, non-maleficence, and justice. The problems arise because of the individualistic and analytical character of the principles that are foreign to Latin (and African and Asian) communitarianism. Every country has its own conceptions and preconceptions. To change a country's values is something more radical than the acceptance of a technological invention.

In this work on the history of bioethics in the Ibero-American region, it was expected that the collaborators would emphasize the originality of one's own country, region, and perhaps one's own contribution. A reflection on the South American foundations pays tribute to the Northern hemisphere, primarily North America, in a time of globalization in which knowledge spreads quickly due to the increasing number of specialized journals and congresses, and other instances of interchange, such as the Internet. Cultural and historical influences intervene inevitably but fortunately; every country, every collaborator, can be proud of the heritage they helped to create and all of them share.

In addition to Argentina – the continent's institutional pioneer in bioethics – Venezuela and Colombia deserve special mention, the latter because of its early efforts to integrate humanism and medical practice in the education of physicians. Despite the ideal of a universally accessible health care, cultural pluralism will always exist because of the central role of medicine in all cultures: all human beings, all people, must defend their own vitality and survival. These cultures have different ways of accepting and understanding recent advances in bioethics. The fast success of transplants in Latin America and mainly Brazil was not guaranteed at the beginning; it was certainly due to the ability of some surgeons, but no less to the taste for risk, more prominent here than on the European continent.

The influence of Catholic morality in Latin America should also be discussed, both because of its benefits (by means of the positive contribution of some university schools and some theologians) and its impediments. In addition, it seems – as shown by Alfonso Llano Escobar – that the order of the arrival of bioethics in Latin America was as follows: Argentina (that sponsored the Second World Congress of Bioethics in 1994), Colombia, Peru, Chile, Mexico, and Brazil (a country that stands out for sponsoring the First Latin-American Congress of Bioethics in 1988 and the Sixth World Congress of Bioethics in 2002 – Brasilia, DF). The PAHO also has a strong positive influence, along with Chile and its main university where PAHO has its office.

The collaboration of Latin America within the global context is important because developed countries along with the Earth itself are in a risky situation. Bioethics and ecological concerns, if only because of preventive public health measures, are ultimately joint efforts. A few years ago, René Dumont, an experienced agronomist said:

> The threats are becoming clear. They are serious and they put in danger the very existence of Earth inhabitants. The exhaustion of resources is illustrated by the rise in prices of oil and raw

materials. The soil, the air and the water are contaminated, sometimes in an irreversible way; an increasing number of vegetal and animal species vital for life are disappearing. There are four billion human beings [currently more than six billion], three quarters of which live in great poverty at a moment when rich countries almost monopolize available resources.[1]

More recently, he said, "Four billion human beings suffer from the lack of water, whereas others are afflicted by floods" (Dumont 2007).

Suggestions for improvement have been made and include those of the French ecologist, Nicolás Hulot, who supported: creating a progressive carbon tax until carbonic gas emissions are four times less; appointing a deputy prime minister in charge of sustainable development; consulting people about the direction of sustainable development, making clear they are to adhere to restrictions; promoting people's sensibility to ecology and public health; reforming agricultural sites; improving or universalizing education and professional training (Hulot 2006).

These circumstances make clear the interdependence between bioethics and politics in general, which also must consider the most urgent question of health policy and its alarming increase in cost: in all countries, researchers request more funds for maintaining their research and laboratories. The influence of drug manufacturers and their sound commitment to maximizing profits should also be mentioned.

The seemingly consensual relationship between bioethics and social–political evolutions is favorable, at least in some Latin American countries. Consider, for instance, the effect of the authoritarian management of the health care sector within bioethics and its gradual incorporation of democratic practices. (Although not all is good, because, as Francisco Batista Jr. warns, "social control is a project in construction"; besides, regarding HIV/AIDS, in Brazil "we have 18 [infected] girls for every ten boys.") Anyway, "A Latin-American perspective of solidarity must be created with concrete projects, as the environmental problem, which particularly affects the poor population" (De Lavor 2007). Will these concerns be part of a more encompassing Mercosur program someday?

With the documentation already obtained, we see that the main differences between countries have to do primarily with the socio-juridical, that is to say, the institutional place of bioethics, naturally taking into account the relative proportions of the different ailments and operations. No less apparent are the differences in the frequency of professional meetings and the existence of bioethical centers, as well as the pace of transformations in the acceptance of bioethics, the receptivity of new scientific perspectives, access to new knowledge and the flexibility of institutions to accommodate new practices. Comparative monographs will emerge to

[1] Les menaces se précisent. Elles sont graves et mettent en danger l'existence même des hommes sur la Terre. L'épuisement des ressources est illustré par la hausse du prix du pétrole et des matières premières. Les sols, l'air et l'eau sont souillés, parfois de manière irréversible; des espèces animales et végétales indispensables à la vie disparaissent en nombre croissant. Il y a déjà quatre milliards d'humains dont les trois quarts vivent dans le dénuement, alors que les pays riches se gorgent de la plupart des ressources mondiales. Source: http://www.planetecologie.org/ENCYCLOPEDIE/Pionniers/ReneDumont.htm. Translator's Note.

provide complete local and national information. The idea that bioethics goes hand in hand with social and cultural evolution reinforces the beliefs put forward by the founders of bioethics in Latin America. With the consistent establishment of additional national bioethics committees (advisory boards or commissions), it is inevitable for an Inter-American, Iberian–Brazilian Commission to arise to facilitate information exchange and the establishment of common rules, such as exists in the European Union, whose experience has revealed how difficult it is to reconcile different sanitary practices and ethical traditions.

In the United States, there is a wealth of literature regarding procedures for allocating scarce sanitary resources in particular contexts or circumstances. This shows that theoretical and principlist considerations on the subject are not lacking. In Latin America, it seems that the focus of the question is political: even though rules exist for the provision of obvious necessities, these are not always adhered to. Different segments of the population are unequally represented and the power of lobbying is as important in Latin America as it is in the United States. It is not uncommon that certain social classes are given preference over the most needy, who are frequently overlooked, and for federal governments to favor some States more than others, or even individual cases, according to the interests of powerful politicians or the needs of a political party. As one can see, the problem is essentially political and cultural (therefore, linked to education). Political habits are also not readily changed, oftentimes resisting the force of laws and regulations due to their interpretation according to the preferences of dishonest judges and politicians.

The context of the application of the *principle of non-maleficence* to patients and citizens is the same. Cases against doctors are generally judged by professional commissions whose rulings are self-interested; a claim not requiring much effort to prove. In several countries, assiduous covert practices of torture under authoritarian governments, even after their abolishment and their prosecution in court, lead ultimately to amnesties, acquittals, or the indefinite postponement of the final judgment until the death of the victim or the statute of limitations is exhausted. Gathering evidence, performing long sterile interrogations, covering costs, blackmail of several types, and the protection of and veracity of witnesses make it difficult for affected poor people to be properly assisted, whereas some lawyers receive, for insignificant injuries or so-called "moral damages," significant compensation. This subject is also related to the autonomy principle, which varies according to the importance of the sociological context in which the patients live or lived (Lepargneur 2003).

It is not impossible that the economic question Latin America is faced with will someday have the prominence it now has in India, even when most people there remain under the poverty line. In Brazil, in spite of waiting lists, organ transplants are already remarkably numerous, so much so that their costs, cheaper than in North-America, are designed to attract foreign patients. In India, in 2005, some 30 respected private hospitals welcomed about 150,000 "sanitary tourists" eager to benefit from prices 5–10 times less than those in the United States or Great Britain. In an estimate, 5 years from now "medical tourism" will provide India with two or three billion dollars, that is to say, equivalent to half of the country's income gained by computer "outsourcing."

27.6 Before Planetary Threats: By Means of Bioethics and Beyond

The return to a hypothetical horizon of a common morality would best be founded by bioethics because it is more immune to the influence of ideologies than other cultural sectors. With his well-informed and confident judgment, the journalist and ecological investigator Washington Novaes raised the issue of fast growth in biotechnological industries linked to combating possible bioterrorism, which was remembered by Kofi Annan shortly before he left the position of UN Secretary-General. Annan talked about the possible "catastrophic results" of recent advances in biotechnology falling into the wrong hands; he was referring primarily to genetic manipulation and viral research. According to Annan, in January 2007, such threats would grow exponentially and there would be no country, rich or poor, assumed to be protected. The distribution of preventative instruments or remedies has not been guaranteed. The risks indicated by researchers are not in check and the eagerness of the pharmaceutical companies to ensure the protection of the poor sectors of the population has not been assured, despite numerous meetings and conventions. The World Health Organization appears to be alone in its concern for avoiding a pandemic similar to chicken pox. The vulnerability of wealthy nations in the face of pandemic risks calls into question whether less prosperous countries in Latin America or Africa could expect much aid. Other dangers come from the future concerns of neo-nanotechnology (Novaes 2007).

The inevitable limitation of bioethics encourages our reflection on how to extend physical life, the undeniable basis for the standard of human life. However, what profound reason does one have to consider so important one's physical existence on this planet? In childhood, many human beings intuit the existence of a higher purpose, an abstract world of spiritual values that distinguishes human beings from other animals, enabling them to live happier, more demanding, and more visionary lives. This is transcendence. Some recognize religiosity as irreducible to the emotiveness of a utopian dream and some think it advisable to invest in a constituted religion. This is the argument of the *sense of life* which is foreign to the perspective of bioethics as a science/art that believes that all human beings return to the Earth from whence they have come. Whether they return entirely or not is the problem, or better, the mystery, that reason or science cannot solve and that we trust to our mystical or anti-mystical intuition, through faith or disbelief.

The difficulty of adhering to a religious faith resides in the fact that it always demands ritual ethical requirements that exceed a simple, but necessary, secular social ethics; an ethics of coexistence and harmony in a community. Such a perspective is able to give powerful human beings a sense to life, although it is far from explaining and justifying everything that surrounds us. A perception that can come to any one of us and may be rejected and not easily return seems to be like the wind: we do not know from whence it comes or where it goes. In it, we find the very question about the sense of life and, perhaps, the world. Everything seems to depend, from the beginning, on our awareness and interpretation of beauty and life, or suffering, disease, and the unavoidable fact of death. Nobody will deny that such questions are implicit in bioethics, in both its operations and its concern with health and sickness. In the bioethical domain, however, it is advisable to stay away from these issues so one does not introduce divergences that would harm the more urgent service. During the Middle Ages, theology was considered the "Queen of Disciplines," the oldest one, along with medicine, in the establishment of the first universities. On the one hand, theology judged the mysterious dualism of being and nothing in the context of metaphysics; on the other, it gave opinions about the no less mysterious dualism of life and death. Between both poles there is Time, the mysterious time of being and life. Could not we imagine bioethics as at the center of disciplines that radiated from it in modern times, like a fundamental star of the galaxy of being and knowledge? When attesting to the evolution of the irradiations of bioethics and their ramifications – especially of ecology, that worries our civilization and conditions for mankind's health and survival – let us imagine the effect of this outstanding place of bioethics beside elementary particle physics, itself related to evolutionary cosmology, that is to say, to the mystery of the entire cosmos and its evolution.

Bioethics expresses in a particularly obvious way the transitory and fragile character of our temporary life conditions in constant struggle with destructive forces and death. Everything that is progressively revealed illuminates that which has been ignored, serving not only to arouse our curiosity but to encourage our research and scientific efforts, as well as our religious aspiration to believe in some "there" that will always be hidden to the travelers of this time and planet that look to it only with their very eyes.

Would it not be foolish to think that bioethics, which unites a fundamental biological knowledge with life-saving actions to defeat death and decrepitude, ultimately actualizes Henri Bergson's ideal that consists in making acting men think and thinking men act? When they integrate rational and critical thought with action, are not true bioethicists, who entertain abstract discussions about life and make concrete decisions in committees, simultaneously thinking at the level of mankind as a whole (the aspiration to universality) while acting to preserve the life and the health of a concrete human person?

References

De Lavor A (2007) A saúde na política e a política na saúde. Radis 53 (Janeiro):30–33

Dumont R (2007) Hommage à René Dumont [Online] Available: http://www.planetecologie.org/ENCYCLOPEDIE/Pionniers/ReneDumont.htm. Accessed: 4-28-2009

Graziano X (2007) Pobreza e ecologia. O Estado de Sao Paulo, 16 de Janeiro

Hulot N (2006) Nouvel Observateur, December 30

Lepargneur H (2003) Principio da autonomia. In: Urban CA (ed) Bioética clínica. Revinter, Rio de Janeiro, pp 15–26

Novaes W (2007) As Ameaças que vêm do mundo invisível. O Estado de São Paulo, 5 de Janeiro

Royal S (2007) Putting Europe to the test. Social Europe 2(1):101–106

Rushdie S (2006) Salman rushdie stresses the meaning of words. Le Nouvel Observateur, December 21

Chapter 28
A Critical Reading of Latin American Bioethics

Germán Calderón Legarda

28.1 Searching for an Approach

The title of this text may appear pretentious, and this charge is not completely inaccurate. However, we should qualify it by saying that we do not intend to recount the entire history of bioethics in Latin America, but rather to emphasize some of its most significant aspects and to elucidate how its strengths and weaknesses have served to influence consequent developments. Any serious attempt at a critique must necessarily be dialogical in nature and therefore is indebted to those who engage us with questions from the start. In this sense, one must understand that by proposing a critical reading one is also paying tribute to those who established the practice of bioethical reflection in Latin America. We do not attempt to suggest how the development of bioethics should have occurred. Alternatively, we begin by recognizing the importance of the founders' work and proceed by suggesting an interpretation of the development of Latin American bioethics from which principles of form and content can be extracted to guide future development.

The history of Latin American bioethics has already begun to be written, and even rewritten, allowing for us to listen to the "other voices" that have constituted its prehistory (Lolas Stepke 2000, p. 49). It is impossible not to appreciate and respect the founders of bioethics, but one would pay them poor tribute if one allowed reverence to become consecration by asking only those questions whose answers have already been determined. If bioethics exists within our continent, it is because those who established it worked so hard to refine the exercise of their critical capacities. And it is by using these capacities that one is capable of interpreting their work.

G.C. Legarda
Ph.D. Pontificia Universidade Javeriana, Instituto de Bioética, Bogotá, CO
e-mail: german.calderon@javeriana.edu.co

L. Pessini et al. (eds.), *Ibero-American Bioethics: History and Perspectives*, Philosophy and Medicine 106, DOI 10.1007/978-1-4020-9350-0_28,

28.2 Recognizing the Work of the Pioneers of Medical Humanism

In the first phase of development, one observes a complex situation within which a justified restlessness motivates an initially discrete response not only to theoretical problems but also to the complex social and political conflicts arising throughout the region. Therefore, the tension between an uncritical acceptance of a North American bioethics, which centers around autonomy and patient's rights, and a Roman-Catholic perspective, which promotes a paternalistic approach to medical practice, is understandable during the foundational moments of this movement, as is perceived by Mainetti (2005).

The search for a "medical humanism," not necessarily from the Anglo-Saxon tradition, continued to motivate reflections on medicine as a social practice. Thus, it is to the credit of the founders of Latin American bioethics that the Mediterranean tradition of medical anthropology (Laín Entralgo) and the North American contributions to the medical humanities (H.T. Engelhardt, Jr. and Edmund Pellegrino) became part of the reflection. While this is not the place to describe an attempt to establish a particular way of thinking, it should be indicated that what would become Latin America bioethics (a concept that may have many meanings) began as a highly theoretical and philosophically oriented means of reflection, which sometimes engaged in legal–philosophical reflections (humanist doctors). The influences mentioned here serve to counter the thesis that the absence of a distinctively Latin American philosophical tradition served to impede the development of bioethics (Figueroa and Fuenzalida 1996). Regarding this thesis, three aspects can be emphasized:

1. While it may be true that those who established the medical humanities movement and bioethics proper were not professional philosophers, it should be noted that they were individuals with strong intellectual backgrounds in the classical humanist tradition.
2. Theoretical aspects were present from its beginnings, which have been reflected in the establishment of Latin American bioethics as a flexible, versatile, and liberal enterprise with all the strengths and weaknesses this implies.
3. The political and social realities of Latin America were not alienated from reflection, even though there were some advocates for the adoption of a distinctively North American model of doing bioethics.

A particular *ethos*, which was not conducive to a strict demarcation of problems or the establishment of a disciplinary specialization, allowed for the inclusion of social problems within the purview of Latin American bioethics, giving it a distinct openness not found in other bioethics. The following three characteristics of this newborn bioethics are acknowledged as controversial, and we are aware that some may consider them untenable generalizations. Nevertheless, these characteristics include:

1. A theoretical discipline close in character to the humanities
2. An inclusive character favoring the participation of a broad group of subjects to solve a diverse set of problems
3. A social movement accompanied by certain forms of activism and employing different discourses, including those of feminism (arguing for the rights of

women and minorities), ecological concerns, and professional defense (particularly relating to health professionals who were forced to defend their interests against what they called the "proletarization of medicine")

In addition to the intellectual interests of bioethics, its practices were also influenced by other factors. Nevertheless, this does not degrade the importance of its reflections nor the causes that were championed. As previously mentioned, the history of Latin American bioethics was written (or at least it has begun to be) by different authors at different times (e.g., James Drane, Pedro Laín Entralgo, Diego Gráacia, Alfonso Llano, José A. Mainetti, and Fernando Lolas).

28.3 A Respectful Retrospective Examination

A retrospective examination reveals the influence of the restoration of democracy on the revival of broader debates within medical ethics and health care, in addition to the introduction of new medical technologies made possible by a reflective framework similar to that of North American bioethics. However, it is a partial similarity, because the Latin American reality is marked by deep inequalities and a significant stratification regarding quality of life. This is seen in those cities where highly sophisticated intensive-care units exist in wealthy areas, while at the same time there exists a lack of even basic medical care for other populations, undoubtedly causing moral conflict. Due to the existence of social problems of this kind, it became clear to those engaged in bioethical reflection that the North American model was not wholly appropriate to Latin American concerns. However, one might want to note that the United States of America also has their own underdeveloped world within its borders, as was exposed by the consequent events of Hurricane Katrina in 2005. In addition, a number of US citizens are not protected by the health care system, demonstrating that there are issues of poverty and injustice in the developed world as well.

Returning to considerations of the Latin American reality, the inevitable tension between the liberal individual rights of the North American medical *ethos* and the "second generation" economic and social rights defined a significant concern for Latin America's political future. Given this, those who advocated for the inception of bioethics did not lack moral sensitivity because they acknowledged the inappropriateness of proposing a bioethics that only mirrored the North American and European perspectives. However, they could not ignore the benefits of adopting a new field capable of addressing the gap between the sciences and the humanities.

In fact, individuals such as José A. Mainetti (Argentina), Augusto Leon (Venezuela), Alfonso Llano, S.J. (Colombia), Fernando Sanchez Torres (Colombia), Armando Roa (Chile), and Manuel Velasco-Suárez (Mexico) have much to their credit in this way.[1] Their essential idea of integrating the sciences and social

[1] I apologize for the omission of many others in this list. My only defense is to point out that this essay does not claim to provide a comprehensive history of bioethics, an effort which has been better accomplished elsewhere (Lolas Stepke 1998).

humanities into medical theory and practice in their own political and geographical contexts is worthy of recognition.

As a newly established discipline, the purview of bioethics is not always easy to distinguish. This allows one to perceive how the interdisciplinary nature of bioethics allowed it to respond to the contextual needs of Latin American countries. At this point, with 20 years distance from its birth, one is able to retrospectively analyze the evolution of Latin American bioethics.

The nature of this exercise must be respectful, but it should be remembered that the founders of bioethics did not have the advantages of institutions dedicated to bioethics education and web sites, specialized databases, libraries, congresses, and seminars particular to bioethics. That is to say, they did not have the benefit of the tremendous efforts that have been put into its management. In light of this, one can see that their initial efforts took great courage and persistence.

A retrospective analysis will also allow us to reflect on the current state of bioethics and to make a prospective analysis of its crucial elements – including a proposal for what bioethics *ought* to do – which will allow for the coexistence of several conceptions capable of dialoguing among themselves to benefit from experience.

28.4 The Emergence of a Bioethical Reflection on Latin American Questions

Bioethics undoubtedly served to confront doctors and health professionals with the political and economic realities implicit in their professional practices. In Colombia, the professional association of nurses also played a vital role in bioethical developments. While it is certain that bioethics brought to the forefront concerns relating to patients rights, it was not entirely successful in cultivating a deeper reflection, beyond autonomy and beneficence, concerning the social problems of sanitary justice, access to basic health care, and the establishment of public health policies. Even today, these social issues have not sustained themselves in deep and lasting reflections, although bioethics does serve as a mediator for the dialogue between the economy, health as a public good, and theories of justice (Gargarella 1999). Perhaps this can be attributed to the excessive emphasis on principlism or particular interpretations of principlism that cloud one's perspective by preventing discussion of sanitary justice within the context of the realities of the developing world and the interrelation among nations. Here it must be recognize that justice cannot be seen as one principle among others; it must instead be recognized as *the* great problem to be solved within Latin American societies (Berlinguer 2002). Some authors have maintained that bioethics is necessarily more than just the conjunction of two or more fields of knowledge creating a third (Calderón 2004). Much more is required. In the specific case of sanitary justice, we need to establish a broader and deeper relationship between economics, health economics, political philosophy, and public health as a means for establishing more precise tools for analysis.

From the beginning, Latin American bioethics demonstrated an inclination to address global topics, which comes as no surprise and is indicative of future developments.

Although it sounds trivial, it is important to recognize that bioethics is a "life ethic" that requires an integrated perspective.

After all, bioethics must serve the citizens and contribute to a communitarian *ethos*. Nevertheless, one must acknowledge that mere appeal to moral ideals such as justice and fairness does not constitute by itself a rigorous analysis capable of deepening one's understanding of reality and precipitating change. Fernando Lolas was right in stating that the "simple uttering of good goals – bioethics has them – seems to be enough to attribute purity of means to those who declare an intention to cultivate them," which is not always the case. The notion of an intellectual discipline with its corresponding "wise men, experts, and politicians" needs to be well defined in an influential field like bioethics (Lolas Stepke 2005, p. 162). Furthermore, "intellectual strength is not a guarantee of moral kindness, nor is the latter a guarantee of rigorous thought" (Lolas Stepke 2005, p. 163).

28.5 The Appeal to Moral Ideals and the Risk of Bioethical "Pamphletism"

An appeal to general principles and the supplanting of a rigorous ethical–political analysis with the mere proclamation of moral ideals (e.g., condemning injustice and denouncing inequality) are not always effective. In this way, the pamphletism of certain developing countries, which serves to condemn without appropriate reflection, can be harmful because it misleads one into thinking that the denunciation of poverty, environmental damage, or injustice in international relationships is comparable to genuine intellectual contribution. The adoption of a "politically correct" language is not commensurate with advancement in one's analysis and reflection or with contributing to the empowerment of a social movement. Sometimes one is taken aback by the repetition of stock phrases at some bioethics conferences, which are, unfortunately, accompanied by a genuine astonishment when some are confronted with the attacks on human dignity taking place in some corners of the world or even within one's own country.

Nevertheless, this should not discourage us; global concerns have allowed bioethics to situate itself deeper within the context of a difficult reality, at times a risky one, which cannot be accommodated by a strictly North American liberal ethos. When addressing the Latin American reality of justice and sanitary resources, one realizes that a precise account of the situation serves as a gain, making the principlist understanding of justice as one principle among many principles misguided.

One's understanding of justice must go beyond its distributive nature to recognize its abilities as a reparative or restorative means, particularly in regions where citizens have been the victims of violence related to armed conflict. Leaving aside talk of principles and values, there are certain moral ideals present in the development of Latin American bioethics that constitute virtues, not defects. Concern is only appropriate when certain forms of demagogic proselytism attempt to supplant rigorous analysis by repeating mere slogans. But, so long as bioethics continues to employ an interdisciplinary analysis resultant of rigorous academic discourse, there is no reason it cannot be seen to engage in activism, to motivate social reform, or to contribute to the establishment of suitable legislation. In this vein, we must recognize the endemic evil that affects Latin American societies; that is, since the dawn of our republics, legal developments do not correspond to the reality in which we live. Recently, an esteemed Colombian geneticist commented that the governments legislating about human cloning in Colombia and other countries did not have a basic understanding of what the procedures consisted or the real possibilities of their applications. While this may appear anecdotal, it nevertheless reflects the reality of how questions are discussed, decided on, and legislated about. In addition, it is inadvisable to accept the unappealing stereotypes of Latin America's "magical realism" or "tropicalism," because these are harmful to our cultures. However, it is necessary to remember that many of the debates to which the label "bioethical" is applied often lack the inclusion of real scientific facts and ethical perspective, making them the subject of media sensationalism.

28.6 The Opening of Bioethics to the Great Themes Related to Life

The consideration of biotechnological themes, environmental impacts, and the implications of the medical practices of private and state health care systems allows bioethics to be considered a cultural and political movement. In this way, we must celebrate the passing of the stage that Mainetti calls "recreation," a stage that corresponds to the institutionalization of bioethics in Latin America (beginning in the 1990s), which reveals the similarities and particularities among individual countries.

On the other hand, Mainetti contends, "Bioethics has become the territory of new challenges for Latin America. An apparent uniformity masks rich heterogeneous activities. It should be realized that it is not only the European and Christian influences affecting the development of bioethics in Latin America, but also those of the indigenous intellectual traditions. While the latter does not have its own philosophy, as the Anglo-American tradition does, it does have its own narrative style and literature" (Mainetti 2005).

A way to make this reading feasible is to interpret it as a call from the author to focus on integrating different perspectives and to interpret bioethics with the respectful attitude of one who thinks and acts within a multicultural society. Aside from the increased articulation of environmental sciences and cultural anthropology in daily communication, some sectors have made an effort to understand the communal and medical practices of indigenous peoples, but one cannot say that these traditions have played an integral part in the development of bioethics. It is important to call attention to this fact, because it is necessary to recognize it as a pending task.

More interesting is the suggestion that our literature and narrative style can function as a source of knowledge. In a similar vein, Fernando Lolas has proposed the understanding of bioethics as a critical narrative. As such, bioethics is understood primarily as an anti-dogmatic discourse, essentially critical and characterized by a dialogic and pluralist attitude. From this perspective, the aim of a bioethics narrative is capable of conceiving of arguments such that they reveal the axiological architectures of those participating in a dialogue and thus establish connections between them.

A suggestive insight would be to regard bioethicists as experts capable of translating discourses. This is a beautiful conception that may be attainable for future bioethicists, although it is not the current reality. However, it is difficult to disagree with Lolas' weaker claim that bioethics is capable of mediating between dialogues. Bioethics makes engagement possible between different dialogues and disciplines, and it may even be said "between realities" (Calderón 2004). In this sense, the fear of Victoria Camps is at least understandable when she states that the term "bioethicist," understood as a hybrid between the scientist and the humanist, is inappropriate because bioethics must maintain a dialogue that "provides for an understanding between languages and worlds that have evolved independently from each other" (Camps 2001). One may sympathize with the concerns of Camps, but it is difficult to question bioethics' role in the practical integration of facts and values.

It is also stimulating to think of bioethics as a set of conceptual tools that allow one to engage in interdisciplinary dialogue among different realities. For this reason, bioethics cannot be the mere application of abstract principles to concrete situations. The term "applied ethics" can be confusing when understood as endorsing cultural relativism or contextualism, because extreme cultural relativism can be just as hollow as subscribing to a set of absolute principles purporting to have universal validity.

Bioethics must operate with concepts that admit to degrees and allow for different interpretations and emphases. We acknowledge that notions such as dignity and mutual respect exist in all societies and that filial relationships, for example, play important roles, but the structure and form they take vary interculturally. Although this is a simple example, we can acknowledge the varying meanings the concept of "family" has within different geographical contexts. Similarly, the degree of reverence for a society's elderly varies between those who value their wisdom and those who disregard them completely. What this illustrates is that societies have different conceptions of value, but they all employ a kind of evaluation.

This is not the place to define the "ought" of bioethics, but it is necessary to remember that one's fallible and insufficient knowledge of other cultural contexts requires us to employ a moderate relativism, because the common aspirations of mankind (universal values) are always inherently present. One must realize that it is very difficult to build anything upon a foundation of extreme relativism. In this way, bioethical reflection achieves its first mediation by rejecting the imposition of absolute principles but also by not becoming incapacitated by the plethora of cultures and ways of life (Macklin 1999, p. 109ff; Nussbaum 2001; Heller 1990).

The classical liberal ethos of North American principlism is somewhat exotic when considered within the Latin American context heavily influenced by Catholic and Mediterranean traditions. Aptly stated by Lolas, "one of the great problems caused by ‘importing’ intellectual disciplines consists in their being mostly incompatible with local traditions and cultures” (Lolas Stepke 2005, p. 69).

One must note that what is being advanced is not an argument for the truth of principlism or a situational ethics, but should instead be understood as an attempt to determine how a particular society at a particular time can be illuminated in terms of a particular theory. The purpose is to delimit various cultural contexts, to examine their argumentative strengths and weaknesses, to explain why something is successful only in certain cultural contexts, and to determine how intellectual traditions become compatible or incompatible with others. These are all honest exercises of reflection that must not be alien to bioethics and, in fact, may be the primary deliberative exercise constituting its main function.

However, one cannot help but notice that the use of the phrase “ethical dilemma” persists in the Latin American, as well as European, bioethics literature. By nature, dilemmas either lead to new problems, in which case they become diluted, or they place those who attempt to solve them in a predicament where no course of action is satisfactory. In this way, we should be more careful with the use of terms. Strictly speaking, bioethics examines problems that include both evaluative and empirical elements, as well as descriptive and prescriptive language. Those who consider bioethical problems to be dilemmas from the start run the risk of finding a dead end.

As an example, consider the decision of one of the highest-ranked officials of the Ministry of Health to choose the latter when presented with the “dilemma” of providing necessary medications to an adult HIV patient or administering vaccines to a group of children to prevent a prevalent disease. Some may interpret this scenario as a bioethical dilemma. However, if we analyze it more closely, we can see that no dilemma exists. There is simply a decontextualization of the problems pertaining to the distribution of resources. Similarly, the same official may have to face the dilemma of providing potable water or investing in the specialties of select students at state medical schools. The dramatic handling of these apparently insoluble dilemmas, combined with the embellishments of media coverage, prevents a deeper understanding of reality.

The problems of bioethics are complex, requiring an interdisciplinary approach and often times an urgent solution. On the one hand, bioethics engages in theoretical discussions about general principles, but primarily seeks to establish criteria for practical decision making. On the other hand, if we speak of dilemmas as the problems that persist once the initial situation has been examined, then the role of bioethics becomes useful if and only if it is capable of providing the conceptual tools necessary for analyzing and responding to highly difficult situations, situations in which evaluative judgments are intermixed with normative and experiential judgments (Mouliness 1991; Rescher 1999, p. 73ff).

28.7 The Search for the Epistemological Structure of Bioethics

In examining the epistemological structure of bioethics, one is encouraged by its apparent maturity, as evidenced by the existence of a collective reflection (Garrafa et al. 2005). However, one would be naïve to attempt to define a univocal epistemology of bioethics. The fact that bioethics is still an evolving discipline makes difficult a singular conception. Additionally, and most importantly, bioethics does not consist of a single subject of knowledge serving to exclude all others, nor does it address problems that are exclusive to its discipline. Therefore, to accurately reflect on its epistemological structure and its task as a discipline, one must approach it from the perspective of a work in progress. It should be treated as a progressive movement within which certain assumptions are apt to change and, when needed, new epistemic possibilities can be elaborated without negatively affecting the rigor or value of its analysis and without losing contact with other disciplines.

The question of an epistemological structure of bioethics is not the object of an agreement, nor is it the result of an exercise explicitly oriented towards this goal. Rather, it is established by the encounter of different discourses and the possibility of their interconnections. This allows for the expansion of cognitive horizons, but it does not require the full realization of an interdisciplinary practice. The close connection of bioethics with the life sciences, philosophy of medicine, philosophical anthropology, and its necessary reflections on biotechnology has allowed for the generation of an identifiable discourse, but the problem of inclusion (what pertains to bioethics) remains unsolved. One is incapable of determining once and for all the question of what does and does not fall under the purview of a new discipline. This occurs progressively over time as the discipline slowly becomes defined by a particular set of problems relevant to a given epoch, which problems shape the field of study and deepen the roots of its discourse. It is likely that, as a discipline, bioethics is more deeply indebted to its antecedents and other intellectual currents than it generally recognizes (Lolas Stepke 1998, p. 24).

It has been mentioned that bioethics cannot be conceived of as the simple sum of two or more disciplines. A more sophisticated relationship is required to be able to support a knowledge that is the product of interdisciplinary dialogue and is capable of closing the gap between theory and practice. Examples of this type of reflection include the work of Miguel Kottow, who faces the problem of moral epistemology and critiques the blind adoption of principlism in Latin America; Volnei Garrafa, who warns against forms of simple reductionism opposed to a new paradigm of complexity (Garrafa et al. 2005); and León Olivé, who addresses the descriptive and normative dimensions of ethics, bioethics, and epistemology and argues for a kind of "naturalized normativism" capable of recognizing the changing nature of norms. Fermin Roland Schramm acknowledges the existence of many legitimate bioethics, but searches for one that is uniquely Latin American because "the attempt to account for all moral problems when human praxis concerns vital processes as a whole leads one to forget that specific problems still exist, such as those moral problems that relate not to biomedicine, but to underdevelopment and extreme poverty, that is, problems related to the development of scientific and technoscientific practices, but not to the persistent problems resulting from already known conditions" (Schramm 2005, p. 172). This allows one to recognize that the reality of the southern Latin American countries does not require a lack of academic rigor or a parochialism that rejects all influence from the developed world based on the argument that it must consist in some form of imperialism, be it political, economic, or cultural.

28.8 A Final Remark

It is always worth the effort to reflect on and creatively engage in dialogue with other traditions and narratives because, as a result, one benefits from the products of real integration through the enrichment of one's perspective and a superior ability to understand other cultural contexts. One might say that, like interdisciplinary dialogue, engagement among cultures is just a difficult, but not an impossible task. Now that Latin American bioethics is more aware of its challenges, it fortunately has a good number of well-able thinkers eager to face them.

References

Berlinguer G (2002) Bioethics, power and injustice. Trans. Sobral A, Gonçalves MS. In: Garrafa V, Pessini L (eds) Bioética, poder e injustiça. Ed. Loyola & Centro Universitário São Camilo, São Paulo, pp 45–58

Figueroa PR, Fuenzalida H (1996) Bioethics in Ibero-America and the Caribbean. J Med Philos 21(6):611–627

Camps V (2001) Una vida de calidad: reflexiones sobre bioética. Arez y Mares, Barcelona

Gargarella R (1999) Las teorias de la justicia después de Rawls: un breve manual de filosofía política. Paidós, Barcelona

Garrafa V, Kottow M, Saada A (2005) Estatuto epistemológico de la bioética. Red Latinoamericana y Del Caribe de Bioética de la UNESCO, México, Instituto de investigaciones jurídicas

Heller A (1990) Mas allá de la justicia. Critica, Barcelona, pp 11–66

Calderón G (2004) La ambivalência de la bioética: cinco tesis para superar la vergüenza. In: Orientaciones Universitárias, n. 35, pp 107–122

Lolas Stepke F (1998) Bioética: el diálogo moral en las ciencias de la vida. Universitária, Santiago

Lolas Stepke F (2000) Bioética y antropologia médica. Mediterrâneo, Santiago

Lolas Stepke F (2005) Rehistoriar la bioética en Latinoamérica. La contribución de James Drane. Acta Bioética 11.2:162

Macklin R (1999) Against relativism: Cultural diversity and the search for ethical universals in medicine. Oxford University Press, New York

Mainetti JA (2005) Desarrollo de la bioética en América Latina. Revista Electronica de bioética I:1

Mouliness U (1991) Hechos e valores: falacias e metafalacias. Um ejercicio integracionista. Isegoria. Revista de filosofia moral y política, 33

Nussbaum MC (2001) Women and human development: The capabilities approach. Cambridge University Press, New York, pp 34–110

Rescher N (1999) Razón y valores en la era científico-tecnológica. Paidós, Barcelona

Schramm F (2005) Bioética sin universalidad? Justificación de una bioética latinoamericana y caribeña de protección. In: Garrafa V, Kottow M, Saada A (eds) Estatuto epistemológico de la bioética. Instituto de investigaciones jurídicas: Red Latinoamericana y Del Caribe de Bioética de la UNESCO, México, pp 165–185

Chapter 29
What Kind of Future Awaits Us? Some Challenging Questions for the Future of Bioethics in Ibero-America

Leo Pessini and Christian de Paul de Barchifontaine

29.1 Introduction

When one reflects on the historical perspective that has characterized the development of Latin America bioethics, one can distinguish a continuity, not without problems, among its three stages: (1) the 1970s, when North-American bioethics was transplanted and received; (2) the 1980s, a period of assimilation and evolution in accord with Latin American culture; and, (3) from the 1990s on, the re-creation phase involving the assertion of a uniquely Latin American perspective and practice that not only interprets bioethical contributions from other parts of the world, but enriches their meaning by engaging in a dialogical process. Fundamental to understanding this Latin American perspective is an examination of its epistemological foundations (cf. Garrafa et al. 2006) to bring to light those challenges that require more than just reflection. Among these challenges to be faced are concerns about ecology and the environment, research on human beings, public policies, legislation and law, and dialogue between secular and religious spheres.

The beginning of bioethics in the United States was primarily concerned with those ethical dilemmas created by the extraordinary technological developments of the life and health sciences, which included research on human beings, the humane use of technology, and end-of-life issues. This set of issues was eventually expanded to include those particular problems pertaining to values that arose within different health care professions, including nursing, public health, mental health, and others. In addition,

L. Pessini
Ph.D. Researcher and Professor of Bioethics at Centro Universitário São Camilo in the stricto sensu Master course in Bioethics, São Paulo, Brazil
e-mail: pessini@saocamilo-sp.br

C. de Paul de Barchifontaine
Researcher and Professor of Bioethics at Centro Universitário São Camilo in the stricto sensu Master course in Bioethics, São Paulo, Brazil
e-mail: cpb@saocamilo-sp.br

L. Pessini et al. (eds.), *Ibero-American Bioethics: History and Perspectives*, Philosophy and Medicine 106, DOI 10.1007/978-1-4020-9350-0_29,

larger social issues were introduced as broad bioethical themes, which included the allocation of medical resources, women's health, and ecology (Pessini 1999).

In Latin America and the United States, medical technology also motivated the development of clinical ethics. The initial questions prompting its development pertained to research involving human beings, the use and non-use of new medical equipment, and issues of informed consent. The existence of cutting-edge medical technologies and advanced medical care in some Latin American countries also raises issues of discrimination, injustice, and exclusion in health care. Additionally, issues related to access in health care in the region have proven more difficult to address than those related to the ethical use of medical technology. In light of this, Latin American bioethics has a strong social consciousness demonstrated by its commitment to the important cultural concepts of justice, equity, and solidarity, which enjoy a status similar to that of autonomy in the United States.

According to James Drane, Latin Americans are less inclined to understand the doctor–patient relationship within the context of consumerism and do not share the individualist perspective of North Americans. However, it would be a mistake to think that practices like informed consent and its benefits are unimportant to Latin Americans. The challenge is to learn from the experiences of the United States and Europe without naively imitating or integrating their practices, which are appropriate to a reality different from that of Latin America (Drane 1996). In this vein, some important points worthy of reflection are provided in the following sections.

29.2 Broadening the Ethical Perspective: From an Individualistic to a Communitarian Approach

A "macro" level approach to bioethics (concerned with society as a whole) must be proposed as an alternative to the "micro" level approach, which dominates the Anglo-American tradition and seeks only to resolve clinical issues. More specifically, a bioethics restricted to a technological "bios" and an individualistic "ethos," concerned primarily with issues like privacy and informed consent, must be carefully integrated with the humanist "bios" and communitarian "ethos" of Latin America, which takes solidarity, equity, and respect for the other as primary concerns.

The greatest challenge is to create a Latin American bioethics that will mitigate the exaggerated emphasis on the perspectives of others and allow for the redemption and valuation of the unique aspects of Latin culture as a means to providing a truly multicultural dialogue. It must also be recognized that Latin American bioethics is necessarily marked by poverty and social exclusion. To elaborate, a bioethics that only operates on the "micro" level and neglects to take into account this reality would be incapable of responding to the desires and needs for leading a dignified life. In terms of the global perspective, one cannot lose sight of the fact that Latin America is essentially excluded, and within this reality lives are affected (Pessini 2004).

For contemporary cultures, modern medicine has acquired a status similar to that of religion in the Middle Ages. The issues of concern within bioethics have become ever more central and have stimulated a growing interest within the general public.

At the peak of bioethical controversies, basic concepts are being redefined in all corners of the world, including those of life, death, family, disease, father, and mother. Increased communication between individuals with different outlooks can be immensely productive in terms of cultivating a deeper understanding of each culture and the means by which superior solutions can be decided upon to alleviate similar problems. Dialogue can bring together different regions and cultures to work towards integrating sociological, historical, and philosophical differences as a step in creating a set of bioethical standards that are coherent, respectful of difference, and capable of being shared by both secular and religious peoples.

According to Mainetti (1995), Latin America offers a unique bioethical perspective due to its humanistic traditions and its social status as a group of peripheral countries. However, for this Argentine bioethicist, European medical ethics, with its three main branches (medical anthropology, epistemology and axiology), may be better equipped to transform clinical and academic medicine into a new humanistic biomedical paradigm. This approach is favored because it would avoid the criticisms frequently directed at medical ethics, which claim that bioethics emerged to make medicine more humane, but it fails to recognize the true dehumanization of the system. For example, discourse about autonomy can mask the depersonalization of medical care and the related risks of iatrogeny, including exploitation of the body and the alienation of health. Additionally, in a technological era concerned with the development of biomedicine, bioethics should play a critical role in this process instead of remaining wholly optimistic and complacent about progress.

The Latin American reality is one of cholera, AIDS, and measles, which demands a communitarian ethic concerned with common welfare, justice, and equity before individual rights and personal virtues. The greatest need of impoverished countries is for equity in the allocation of resources and the distribution of health services. As a result, a "macro" ethics in public health can be proposed as an alternative to the Anglo-American tradition of "micro" or clinical ethics.

While reflecting on Latin American bioethics, it is informative to consider the perspective of Diego Gracia (1995), who states:

> Latin Americans feel deeply uncomfortable with rights and principles. They are [accustomed] to judging things and actions good or bad instead of right or wrong. They prefer benevolence to justice, friendship to mutual respect, excellence to rights.... Latinos seek virtue and excellence. I do not believe they reject or think little of principles ... As the Latin cultures traditionally were oriented by the ethics of virtues, the principlist approach may be very helpful in avoiding some traditional defects of our moral life, such as paternalism, the lack of respect for laws and tolerance. In the search for virtue and excellence, Latin American countries by tradition have been intolerant. Tolerance has not been included as a virtue in the ancient catalogue of Latino virtues. The true virtue was intolerance, and tolerance was considered a vice.... Anglo-Saxons discovered tolerance as a virtue in the [seventeenth] Century. Perhaps this is the most significant difference with other cultures. The most important moral issue is not the language we use to express our moral feelings, but the respect for moral diversity, the choice between pluralism and fanaticism. Fanaticism states that values are total and absolute and objective and should be imposed forcefully upon others, whilst tolerance defends moral autonomy and freedom for all human beings and the search for a moral agreement through consensus (Gracia 1995).

The recent growth of the initiative for a global bioethics has prompted the consideration of ethical issues that concern many Latin American and Caribbean scholars.

Daniel Wikler, former President of the International Association of Bioethics (IAB), in his closing address at the Third World Congress on Bioethics (San Francisco, USA, 1996) entitled "Bioethics and Social Responsibility," stated, when we look at the birth and development of bioethics, we clearly detect four phases: The first phase includes professional codes of conduct and an understanding of bioethics as a practical medical ethics (Wikler 1997). In the second phase, the doctor–patient relationship is incorporated, and paternalism and the rights of patients begin to be debated, including issues of autonomy, freedom, and truth. During the third phase, questions arise about health care systems, including their structure and organization in addition to their funding and management, which prompt the study of the economics and politics of health by bioethicists (cf. Callahan 1980). Last, in the fourth phase, which Latin America entered during the 1990s, bioethics begins to deal primarily with population health and the social sciences, humanities, human rights, equity, allocation of resources, and other important issues, all of which become topics of debate.

29.3 Challenges in Developing a Horizon of Meaning for Bioethics

One's reflections will be incomplete if the challenging necessity of developing a broader horizon of meaning, or a mystique, for bioethics is neglected. It may appear strange to suggest a need for a mystique within a discipline marked by pragmatism and the maximization of efficiency, but bioethics needs such a horizon of meaning to be able to develop its reflections and proposals. Additionally, one cannot establish a bioethics divorced from a world of human relationships. This, by itself, is an indication of the need for some type of mystique, or of a set of fundamental meanings, upon which an idealism can be cultivated and options and organizing practices can be established (Pessini 2005).

It is difficult to define this broader horizon of meaning in a few words. It must necessarily include a firm belief in the transcendence of life, which rejects the notions of disease, suffering, and death as absolutes that cannot be tolerated. It must include an acknowledgement of others as partners capable of living in solidarity, and an understanding and acceptance of life as a gift. This horizon would also serve as a witness to ensure that egoistic individual interests do not prevail by silencing the voices of the excluded and vulnerable, masking their needs. In addition, this horizon would monitor technological discoveries in health care and the life sciences by challenging the techno-scientific imperative, "I can do," by forcing it to reconcile with the ethical imperative, "therefore, ought I do?" More than this, it would serve as a means to motivate individuals and groups, from the most diverse social, political, cultural, and economic backgrounds, to unite in the enterprise of guaranteeing a dignified life for all by establishing an economic, technological, and scientific paradigm guided by the demands of human solidarity (Anjos 1994, 1996).

29.4 Beyond Principlism

The principlist model of theoretical analysis, which was initiated by the Belmont Report and implemented by Beauchamp and Childress, is one among many ethical languages. It is neither exclusive nor the only one. The expression of ethics is possible in a number of different theoretical languages, paradigms, or models, including, for example, those of virtue, the casuistic, the contractual, the liberal autonomist, the model of care, the anthropological humanistic, and the model of liberation. This type of pluralism demands a dialogue respectful of differences and the recognition of tolerance as a primary characteristic. All of these models are intrinsically interrelated, but each one is also intrinsically incomplete and limited. A model may deal well with a definitive aspect of moral life, but cannot deal effectively with all others. One cannot consider models as exclusive, because they are incapable of completely capturing the moral dimensions of human experience and should rather be understood as complementary. This should come as no surprise, because the vast wealth of human experience always escapes the reach of any theological or philosophical system. Adopting this modest perspective will free one of the virus of "isms" and the partial truths upon which one attempts to construct a full reality.

29.5 Justice and Equity in Health Care

The bioethical problems of utmost importance in Latin America and the Caribbean are those of justice, equity, and the allocation of medical resources. Large sections of the population do not have access to medical technologies, and there is even less of a desire to emancipate the sick. A great deal of paternalism is also still being disguised as charity. In light of this, it is imperative that justice, equity, and solidarity are given priority over the principle of autonomy, which is so deeply important to the Anglo-American perspective (Barchifontaine, Pessini 1996).

The bioethics of the developed world (the United States and Europe) ignores, for the most part, the basic issues that affect millions of excluded individuals in Latin America and focus, instead, on those issues that are, at best, of marginal concern for this population. For example, in the developed world death with dignity is a significant topic of bioethical discussion. In the Latin American context, one is impelled to demand that human dignity should first seek to provide a life with dignity and not simply a state of degrading survival, before being concerned with a dignified death. The reality of the undeveloped world is one with an unjust and premature death that cuts short and destroys thousands of lives, including those still in their childhood. However, in the developed world, one dies after having lived and enjoyed a life of elegance, even in old age. The question remains, would a painful survival warrant a dignified death?

The former president of IAB, Campbell (1998), in considering the future of bioethics found that a key issue to be addressed will be justice in health and health care. As a result, a greater research effort seeking to address this issue and to develop a bioethical theory is a necessary step. Bioethics cannot become a "chaplain in the real kingdom of science," thereby losing its critical role regarding techno-scientific progress.

29.6 Bioethics and Religion

A characteristic of the Latin American and Caribbean regions is the deep Christian Catholic heritage, which has been strongly impacted by fundamentalist sects in the media. The process of secularization has begun among the educated bourgeoisie, but it has not yet reached people in general. Therefore, the morals of these regions remain primarily religious and confessional and wholly unaware of the characteristic pluralism of developed countries throughout the world. From this, a challenge arises as to how a dialogue is to take place between a secular, civil, pluralist, autonomist, rational bioethics and the religious perspective deeply rooted in these lands.

Edmund D. Pellegrino, a notable pioneer of American bioethics, raises three questions for bioethics to face in the future. The first is how to decide among diverse opinions what bioethics is and what its field should be. The second is how to relate the various models of ethics and bioethics among themselves. And the third is what the precise role of religion and theological bioethics is in the public debates of abortion, managed care, etc. Up until now, religion has remained in the penumbra of philosophical debates. However, authors like Thomasma and Pellegrino (1997) predict the gradual emergence of religious values in public debates as the awareness of cultural diversity increases. They emphasize the need for a methodology capable of accommodating the increasing polarization of perspectives brought about by authentic convictions and, also, the need to live and work together even when philosophical and religious convictions are in irreconcilable conflict.

29.7 A Final Note

It is necessary to cultivate a wisdom capable of prophetically challenging the ethical imperialism of those who regard their truth as the only one, in addition to the ethical fundamentalism of those who refuse to enter into an open and genuine dialogue with others in a pluralistic and secular context.

The intuition of V. R. Potter (1971), in coining the concept of bioethics as a "bridge to the future," needs to be reinterpreted in this new millennium as a bridge towards multi- and transcultural dialogue. It should be a new dialogue among different people and cultures that will enable one to recover the humanistic tradition, a respect for life and the transcendence of life in its maximum magnitude (cosmic and ecological), as well as being able to enjoy it both as a gift and a conquest with dignity and solidarity.

References

Anjos MF (1994) Bioethics in a liberationist key. In: Dubose ER, Hamel RP, O'Connell LJ (eds) A matter of principles: ferment in US bioethics. Pennsylvania Trinity Press International, Valley Forge, pp 130–147

Anjos MF (1996) Medical ethics in the developing world: A liberation theology perspective. J Med Philos 21(6):629–637

Barchifontaine CP, Pessini L (1996) Bioética a partir de América Latina. In: La vida vale: bioética : nuevos caminos. Centro de Estudos Y Publicaciones, Lima, Peru, pp 33–42

Callahan D (1980) What obligations so we have to future generations? In: Patridge E (ed) Responsibilities to future generations. Prometheus, Buffalo pp 73–85

Campbell AV (1998) A bioética no século XXI. Saúde Heliópolis (April/May):9–11

Drane JF (1996) Bioethical perspectives from Ibero-America. J Med Philos 21(6):557–569

Garrafa V, Kotow M, Saada A (eds) (2006) Bases conceituais da bioética: enfoque latino-americano. Editora Gaia, São Paulo

Gracia D (1995) Hard times, hard choices: Founding bioethics today. Bioethics 9(3, 4) (July):192–206

Mainetti JA (1995) History of medical ethics: The Americas – d. Latin America. In: Reich WT (ed) Encyclopedia of bioethics, rev. ed., vol 5. Macmillan, New York, pp 1639–1644

Pessini L (1999) Bioethics: a horizon of hope for a new time. O Mundo da Saúde 23(5):259–262

Pessini L (2002a) Bioethics, power and injustice: Some personal thoughts from a Latin American perspective. IAB NEWS 13 (February):9–14. Available: http://www.bioethics-international.org/news/iabnews-feb2002.pdf

Pessini L (2002b) Building a new culture of ethics in research involving humans in Brazil. Notizie di Politéia XVIII.67:101–112

Pessini L (2004) O desenvolvimento da bioética na América Latina. Algumas considerações. In: Pessini L, Barchifontaine CP (eds) Fundamentos da bioética, 2nd edn. Paulus, São Paulo, pp 9–29

Pessini L (2005) Bioética e seu futuro: alguns desafios a partir de uma perspectiva Latino-americana. In: Neves M, Lima M (eds) Bioética ou bioéticas na evolução das sociedades. Edição Luso-brasileira, Gráfica de Coimbra – Centro Universitário São Camilo, São Paulo, pp 357–360

Potter VR (1971) Bioethics bridge to the future. Prentice-Hall, Englewood Cliffs, New Jersey, USA

Thomasma DC, Pellegrino ED (1997) The future of bioethics. Cambridge Quart Health Ethics 6:373–375

Wikler D (1997) Bioethics and social responsibility. Bioethics 11(3/4):185–186

Part V
Postscript

Chapter 30
The Many Beginnings of Bioethics: A Comparison of American and Ibero-American Bioethics and the Possibility of a Global Bioethics

Jennifer A. Bulcock

Ibero-American Bioethics: History and Perspectives allows one to contrast the establishment and development of a distinctly Ibero-American bioethics with that of the American tradition. Essays such as, "The Environment and Bioethics: A Brazilian Perspective," immediately stand out to the American reader because, as is mentioned in a number of the essays in this volume, American bioethics has defined itself as a distinctively medical, or biomedical, ethics in contrast with the Ibero-American or Latin American approach, which espouses more of a "life ethic." From the Ibero-American perspective, bioethics not only includes medical ethics, but also focuses on ecology and human values. Thumbing through any American anthology of bioethics one will find topics relating to reproductive issues, genetic enhancements, end-of-life issues, resource allocation, research ethics, organ donation, and more, but one will be hard pressed to find an essay on environmental ethics, for instance. In addition to issues of social justice, such as poverty or world hunger, environmental ethics would be found in an "applied ethics" anthology or as an independent topic of study. This seemingly insignificant observation, serves to indicate a discontinuity in the term "bioethics" as it is used by the two traditions in addition to an alternative understanding and structure of what bioethics is and what it consists of.[1]

The differences observed become especially important when trying to conceive of a global bioethics because the different conceptions determine different and sometimes exclusive sets of relevant bioethical issues, making the definition of a global bioethics implausible. Considering the issues of bioethical importance for a developed versus a developing country, the content of the two sets of concerns may be entirely exclusive of each other. The primary concerns of a developing country may include the provision of basic medical care, sanitation standards, and economic

J.A. Bulcock
Rice University, Houston, TX, USA
jb7@rice.edu

[1] This narrower, biomedical understanding of bioethics continues to be the case in much of the American bioethics literature, but there appears to be a growing recognition that issues involving ecology and the environment are within the purview of bioethics. For example, Howard Brody acknowledges environmental concerns as one of the future issues of American bioethics in his book, *The Future of Bioethics* (2009).

L. Pessini et al. (eds.), *Ibero-American Bioethics: History and Perspectives*, Philosophy and Medicine 106, DOI 10.1007/978-1-4020-9350-0_30,

justice, while a developed country may focus primarily on issues of clinical equipoise, genetic enhancement, euthanasia, and the moral status of advance directives. One can see how the primary concerns of one country in comparison to those of another can be not only dissimilar to, but also irrelevant for one another. In this way, the varying concerns and independent conceptions of bioethics that exist among the different countries and regions of the world reveal legitimate challenges to the ideal of a global bioethics. They serve to undercut the possibility of understanding all bioethics on the model of American bioethics. While family resemblances may exist among all bioethics, it is important to recognize that distinctively different conceptions are determined and motivated by the varying political, economic, social, and religious influences of the local society.

Returning to the comparison of the American and Ibero-American perspectives, it should be noted that it is unproductive to ascribe a limited and particular definition of bioethics to all of the countries included under the classification of "Ibero-American." As it has been noted by a number of the authors in this volume, there are as many similarities as there are differences among the distinctive bioethics that have been developed by the individual Ibero-American countries, which require independent consideration and treatment. With this being noted, there are some similarities which surface in the essays of this volume. These can be considered general characteristics of Ibero-American bioethics, but should not be considered indicative of definitive characteristics of every Ibero-American country. One should also recognize that the influence of American bioethics has varied widely in its impact depending on the economic, social, and political context of a country when American bioethics was initially received and the various developmental stages that have constituted its evolution.

There are four general features of the development of Ibero-American bioethics that can be readily contrasted with those of the American tradition. Included among these features are: (1) a communitarian versus individualistic (autonomy-centered) ethics; (2) a particular and ad hoc establishment guided by physicians and theologians versus an academic and institutional establishment motivated by philosophers and academics; (3) bioethics as a social/political movement versus bioethics as an institutionalized academic discipline with practical applications; and (4) the determination of the content of bioethics by the social, economic, cultural, political, and religious history and development of a region or country.

1. *Communitarian versus individualistic (autonomy-centered) ethics* The establishment of a distinctively individualistic approach can, in great part, be attributed to the primacy afforded to the concept of autonomy in American bioethics. In an effort to establish foundational principles to guide the character of bioethical policies, the National Commission for the Protection of Human Subjects of Biomedical and Behavioral Research (NCPHS) espoused a "trinity" of ethical principles including, autonomy, beneficence, and justice. According to the Belmont Report, these "basic ethical principles" were to be understood as "those general judgments that serve as a basic justification for the many particular ethical prescriptions and evaluations of human actions" (National Commission for the

Protection of Human Subjects of Biomedical and Behavioral Research 1979). The adoption of these principles was the result of extracting from H. Tristram Engelhardt's essay, "Basic Ethical Principles in the Conduct of Biomedical and Behavioral Research Involving Human Subjects," the principles of autonomy ("respect for persons as free moral agents") and beneficence ("concern to support the best interests of human subjects in research"), in addition to the use of Tom Beauchamp's account of distributive justice in his essay, "Distributive Justice and Morally Relevant Differences" (Jonsen 1998, p. 103),[2] a point that Engelhardt does not celebrate (Engelhardt 2000, p. 66).[3]

This trinity of principles set forth by the Commission was quickly ingrained in bioethical policies and theory as a result of their publication in the Belmont Report (1979). It became even more entrenched with the publication of Beauchamp and Childress' *Principles of Biomedical Ethics*, which espoused a theory centered on the four principles of autonomy, nonmaleficence, beneficence, and justice. Contrary to the intention of Beauchamp and Childress, autonomy has repeatedly been designated as the primary bioethical value to which all others should be subordinate. Given the importance it has been granted, the concept of autonomy is employed in all areas of bioethics, including research ethics, the right to die, abortion, consent, and patient rights. This absolute priority was never intended in the basic definition put forth by Engelhardt, making the current definition and meaning of autonomy foreign to that of its initial articulation. However, its privileged status in bioethical evaluations and its emphasis on the freedom of one's will have made it the defining characteristic for determining the nature of American bioethics as individualistic. The appeal to autonomy has also been undertaken as a default strategy in the face of moral pluralism (Engelhardt 1996).

Alternatively, Ibero-American bioethics adopts a communitarian approach where the rights of the individual are neither the only nor the primary concern. The principle of solidarity is endorsed and an inclusive ethic meant to foster unity has been an important focus. For example, the participation of family, community, religious, or cultural members in the decision-making processes within the context of medical ethics is encouraged. This is evidenced in some countries by the direct participation of family members, among others, in decisions about a patient's care during the hospital ethics committee's consultation process. The family is recognized as possessing an integrity and authority. While it is true that most committees around the world would allow for this type of participation by family members, the point to be emphasized is that this type of involvement is the standard, not the exception in the Ibero-American context where participation is sincerely encouraged and expected.

---

[2] Albert R. Jonsen's book, *The Birth of Bioethics* (1998), presents a historical account of the emergence of bioethics in America. For a somewhat different account, see M.L. Tina Steven's book, *Bioethics in America: Origins and Cultural Politics* (2000).

[3] In addition to Beauchamp and Engelhardt, essays from Kurt Baier, Alasdair MacIntyre, James Childress, and LeRoy Walters (all ethicists) were also considered (Jonsen 1998, p. 102).

Although the example chosen here is one from medical ethics, it should be stressed that Ibero-American bioethics is also concerned with issues well beyond this genre of topics. One might have also chosen an example involving the genetic enhancement of plants or other farming techniques that may affect an entire community or biosphere. The focus on the impact for the community in this context demonstrates the communitarian ethic. One might also note the topics of poverty, pollution, and sanitation mentioned in the articles of this volume, as additional support for the Ibero-American claim that an ethic should focus on the community and its collective protection, consideration, and maintenance.

Given the privilege and primacy awarded to autonomy in American bioethics, it is important to note the distinctive communitarian approach that is widely adopted in Ibero-American bioethics as a differentiating characteristic.

2. *The particular ad hoc establishment of bioethics guided by physicians and theologians versus the academic and institutional establishment motivated by philosophers and academics* Bioethics was initially conceived of in the United States as an academic and institutional endeavor aimed at addressing the rapid technological advancements of medicine and the related concerns of patients and medical professionals. The Kennedy Institute of Ethics was founded at Georgetown University in 1971 with the support of a grant from the Joseph P. Kennedy, Jr. Foundation. Many of the founding members of the institute were professors from Georgetown University making the establishment of the institute and its vision for bioethics an organized, institutionalized, academic approach. Additionally, in 1978, the Kennedy Institute published the four-volume *Encyclopedia of Bioethics* (Reich 1978) that helped to establish the academic character of the field of bioethics, which, at the time, remained generally undefined. A year later, in 1979, Beauchamp and Childress advanced a distinctively philosophical theory of biomedical ethics, in the first edition of *Principles of Biomedical Ethics*, which heavily influenced the development of American bioethics and still continues to do so. The establishment of the Kennedy Institute and the publication of Beauchamp's and Childress' monograph within the span of a decade lead to an effective and well-structured introduction of bioethics in America. Consideration of these events, in total, serves to demonstrate the academic and institutional character of the foundations of American bioethics, which was motivated and accomplished primarily by philosophers and academics.

   Alternatively, the development of bioethics in the Ibero-American region was, for the most part, rather ad hoc and depended heavily upon the initiative of physicians and scholars who were exposed to its tenets at foreign universities or conferences and consequently took a personal and professional interest in it. As mentioned in a number of the essays in this volume, it was often the case that only a few individuals pursued the development of bioethics in their community through self-education and association with scholars and physicians from other countries. These pioneers also made persistent efforts at establishing and developing interest in bioethics at the educational, governmental, and health care levels of their country.

In addition to the interest and passion of particular physicians and scholars, many Ibero-American religious institutions maintained significant influence in the educational and public policy arenas of many Ibero-American countries during the introduction of bioethics, and often times served to sculpt the contours of its content. For example, many theologians and religious institutions used their influence to shape the reception of bioethics by preventing the reconsideration of certain controversial issues (e.g., abortion, euthanasia, etc.) and tailoring its objective. It should also be noted that while religious educational institutions participated to some extent in the shaping of bioethics, its integration into the university community and other educational institutions was generally slow.

While the involvement of religious institutions and theologians in the Ibero-American context was explicit, this is not to suggest that the development of American bioethics was entirely without the influence of theology. For example, theologians such as Paul Ramsey and Richard McCormick played formative roles in the initial development of bioethics. Ramsey's book, *The Patient as Person* (1970), preceded the formal establishment of bioethics, and addressed relevant issues, such as the definition of death, organ transplantation, and research on human beings, from the perspective of a distinctively Christian ethics. According to Stanley Hauerwas, Ramsey thought that "medicine became the practice that exemplified the moral commitments of Christian civilization, and the goal of the ethicist was to identify the values that were constitutive of medicine" (Hauerwas 1995, p. 11). In this way, Christian ethicists were able to find a voice in the developing field of bioethics. Although the perspectives of theologians were initially incorporated in the founding of bioethics, it did not take long for explicitly theological and religious concerns to be marginalized. Even so, some with theological backgrounds, such as Warren Reich and James Childress, played secular roles in the development of bioethics. Taking this into consideration, it is easy to see that the influence of theology was present in the development of American bioethics, but its role and influence were minimal in comparison to the Ibero-American situation.

These circumstances frame an important contrast between the academic and philosophic establishment of American bioethics, and the more religiously motivated bioethics driven by the role of particular personalities that was developed in Ibero-American countries. The bioethics of America and Ibero-America became distinctively different from one another, due to the different players and institutions involved and the channels by which each was established.

3. *Bioethics as a social/political movement versus bioethics as an institutionalized academic discipline with practical applications* Given the different developmental paths bioethics took in America and the Ibero-American region, it has come to operate in different capacities within each society. In America, its formal introduction via the Kennedy Institute and the philosophical theory of Beauchamp and Childress gave it a philosophical and doctrinal function. This, in turn, has lead to an understanding of the role of bioethics as a set of governing beliefs meant to guide the aims and practices of medicine. In the words of Engelhardt:

> Public bioethical reflection produced the secular equivalent of a content-full moral theology, which delivered secular guidelines for a secular pastoral ethics (a bioethics that could guide secular "ethicists" in giving advice regarding particular cases), along with a kind of secular canon law (e.g., secularly morally justified regulations for research involving human subjects) (Engelhardt 2000, p. 27).

In this way, bioethics has become institutionalized through hospital ethics committees and institutional review boards (IRBs), allowing for one to bring vexing ethical questions before a committee with an expectation that a solution to one's case will be provided. If the committee is unable to provide such an answer, because the governing rules have yet to determine the relevant doctrine to resolve the issue, philosophers are expected to produce relevant analyses and arguments with the hope that after some debate an initial consensus will be reached capable of defining appropriate guidelines for practical use.

A significant historical example of the philosophical nature and doctrinal function of American bioethics is provided by the set of overarching rules developed by the National Commission for the Protection of Human Subjects (NCPHS),[4] whose aim was to establish ethical guidelines for such pressing issues as research on prisoners, children, and fetuses and the founding of IRBs. The NCPHS relied heavily on the scholarship of philosophers when establishing ethical guidelines for defining the appropriate conduct of investigators conducting research involving human subjects. In all of this, there was a heavy reliance on philosophically structured reflection, even when undertaken by non-philosophers, which characterized the emergence of American bioethics as an academic discipline with practical applications.

In contrast, the introduction of bioethics in Ibero-America was not born of a formal educational or institutional endeavor and instead has taken on the character of a social/political movement. One can see this characteristic in Ibero-American bioethics in the way it identifies problems and understands the role of bioethics in solving them. To begin, it should be mentioned that Ibero-American bioethics takes more readily to Van Renssalaer Potter's original conception of bioethics as a humanistic field concerned primarily with the preservation of environmental and biological systems (Potter 1988). The focus of Potter's concern was to sustain life in general. Understanding bioethics in this way, the Ibero-American perspective is more appropriately conceived of as a mechanism for change and a tool through which one can guarantee and protect certain rights and the means for flourishing. Ibero-American bioethics understands problems of unsanitary conditions and insufficient medical treatment as social issues requiring solutions achieved through the reorganization of institutional priorities and the creation of rights for individuals. In this way, bioethics is seen as a vehicle for change meant to move towards ensuring life and the conditions necessary for thriving.

Comparatively, one can see that American bioethics is unable to account for the type of social function that is called for within the Ibero-American context.

---

[4]The NCPHS was created by an act of the United States Congress in 1974 to shape bioethical policy in the United States.

However, this is not to deny the influence of particular ideological or political perspectives on American bioethics. For example, the undeniable influence of the social–democratic commitments of political philosopher, John Rawls, is evident in the development of bioethics, as well as those of other early bioethicists. What one should acknowledge is that American and Ibero-American bioethics serve different purposes within their cultures and therefore cannot help but have dramatically different ways of impacting and motivating change.

4. *The determination of the content of bioethics by the social, economic, cultural, political, and religious history and development of a region or country* This circumstance is not only a defining factor separating American and Ibero-American bioethics, but, as already noted, it shapes the creation and development of bioethics by any community, country, or region. Even among the many countries that comprise the Ibero-American region, the development of bioethics within an individual country is affected by the influence of particular historical and contemporary influences, including those of a social, economic, cultural, political, or religious nature. Bioethics is a discipline meant to respond to the needs and ethical concerns of a particular society and its interactions with the world around it. It therefore reflects the intricate relationship between the contextual conditions of a society and the questions and issues it raises. What must be emphasized is the particular way in which a socio-cultural context frames bioethics and how one comes to understand one's place within it, as it shapes one's goals, desires, and behaviors, and, consequently, the content, structure, and function of bioethics as a means to serving and preserving the collective.

While it is clear that there are a number of differences between Ibero-American and American bioethics, one should not be misled in thinking that there are no similarities. As is evidenced by the essays in this volume, a number of Ibero-American countries have adopted a practice of informed consent and have established research and hospital ethics committees under the influence of American bioethics. This has directed their consideration of the relevant issues for integrating advanced technologies into their medical practices (including various forms of genetic engineering) and has reshaped the doctor–patient relationship. These few examples represent only a small portion of the issues addressed by Ibero-American bioethics that correspond with concerns in contemporary American bioethics. While these issues are approached in ways tailored to the Ibero-American culture, they remain points of similarity between the two cultures, and, at times, their formulation and treatment may even echo American principles.

The final point to be made is that Ibero-American bioethics takes on a uniquely complex character when one considers the demographics, history, and culture of the region, which serve to distinguish it from American bioethics. While the dissimilarities are numerous, one can still observe the influences of American bioethics on that of Ibero-America and can use this comparison as a means for understanding how bioethics functions to exemplify the relevant and pertinent issues of a community. In this way, the contributions of this volume are invaluable in recording the distinctive history of Ibero-American bioethics in addition to preserving the individual bioethical histories of many countries within the region. Beyond this goal, this volume allows the recognition of the nature and development of bioethics in different societies and the challenges these differences present for the establishment of a global bioethics.

References

Beauchamp TL, Childress JF (1979) Principles of biomedical ethics. Oxford University Press, New York

Brody H (2009) The future of bioethics. Oxford University Press, New York

Engelhardt HT Jr (1996) The foundations of bioethics, 2nd edn. Oxford University Press, New York

Engelhardt HT Jr (2000) The foundations of Christian bioethics. Scrivener Press, Salem, MA

Hauerwas S (1995) How Christian ethics became medical ethics: The case of Paul Ramsey. Christian Bioethics 1(1):11–28

Jonsen AR (1998) The birth of bioethics. Oxford University Press, New York

National Commission for the Protection of Human Subjects of Biomedical and Behavioral Research (1979) The Belmont report: Ethical principles and guidelines for the protection of human subjects of research. US Government Printing Office, Washington, DC

Potter VR (1988) Global bioethics: Building on the Leopold legacy. Michigan State University Press, Lansing

Ramsey P (1970) The patient as person: Explorations in medical ethics. Yale University Press, New Haven, CT

Reich WT (ed) (1978) Encyclopedia of bioethics, vols 4. Free Press, New York

Stevens MLT (2000) Bioethics in America: Origins and cultural politics. Johns Hopkins University Press, Baltimore, MD

Index

Q

R

Lightning Source UK Ltd.
Milton Keynes UK
05 March 2010

150936UK00004B/62/P

9 781402 093494